Nutritional Psychology

Nutritional Psychology: Understanding the Relationship Between Food and Mental Health provides a broad look at the intersection between food and mental health and offers a comprehensive approach to effectively prioritize nutrition as a powerful component to maintaining overall wellbeing. Each of the 16 chapters deeply informs about a broad range of nutritional factors including those that promote stable blood sugar levels, optimize brain functioning, and contribute to the microbiome and hormone levels so important to the brain–gut connection. There are useful insights into the dynamics of food selection, eating disorders, obesity, body image, and nutrition quality that can stabilize or destabilize mental and emotional disorders. Additionally, environmental influences that shape eating behaviors are fully explored.

Nutritional Psychology: Understanding the Relationship Between Food and Mental Health combines psychology, nutrition, and medicine to form a framework for optimizing the relationship between diet and mental wellbeing. This textbook is designed for undergraduate and graduate psychology and nutrition college courses for students pursuing careers as psychologists, dietitians, nurses, social workers, and a variety of health professionals who want to incorporate nutrition and eating behavior into their discussions with patients.

Dr. Cook and Dr. Champion are both clinicians who work directly with clients with psychological and physical health issues and utilize a blend of nutritional and psychological interventions in their work, providing useful clinical applications for nutritional psychology.

Nutritional Psychology

Understanding the Relationship Between Food and Mental Health

Andrea Cook, PhD and Jennifer Champion, DCN

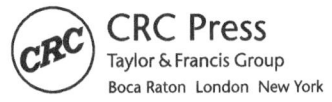

CRC Press
Taylor & Francis Group
Boca Raton London New York

CRC Press is an imprint of the
Taylor & Francis Group, an **informa** business

Designed cover image: Shutterstock

First edition published 2025
by CRC Press
2385 NW Executive Center Drive, Suite 320, Boca Raton FL 33431

and by CRC Press
4 Park Square, Milton Park, Abingdon, Oxon, OX14 4RN

CRC Press is an imprint of Taylor & Francis Group, LLC

ISBN: 978-1-032-64760-9 (hbk)
ISBN: 978-1-032-64014-3 (pbk)
ISBN: 978-1-032-64764-7 (ebk)

DOI: 10.1201/9781032647647

Typeset in Times
by KnowledgeWorks Global Ltd.

Contents

SECTION I   Foundations of Psychology

SECTION II   Foundations of Nutrition

SECTION III   The Emergence of Nutritional Psychology

SECTION IV   Nutrition and Mental Health Challenges

SECTION V   Eating Behaviors

SECTION VI   Where Do We Go from Here?

About the Authors

Andrea Cook, MA, PhD, FMCHC, is a Licensed Clinical Psychologist with a telemental health private practice where she provides individual therapy to adult clients. Dr. Cook incorporates nutrition as an important part of all her therapy work and often recognizes clear improvements in clients when they include dietary changes as part of their treatment. She has a doctorate in Clinical Psychology and a master's degree in Counseling Psychology. She is a Functional Medicine Certified Health Coach (FMCHC), a Diabetes Educator, and has completed training in Advanced Nutritional and Integrative Medicine for Mental Health Professionals. She is a faculty member at the University of California at Santa Cruz (UCSC) where she teaches Nutritional Psychology, Health Psychology, Clinical Psychology, and Psychopathology undergraduate courses. The Nutritional Psychology course is taught as a large lecture class for 180 students and is a course that she proposed, developed, and has taught both as a remote synchronous course using Zoom as well as a live in-person class. It was the development of this course that clarified the need for a textbook on this topic.

Jennifer Champion, DCN, CNS, CN, LDN, is a board-certified Nutritionist, Health Coach, Educator, Speaker and the Owner of NeoGenesis Nutrition, a Functional & Integrative Nutrition program that emphasizes individuality and whole-person health. The focus of her nutrition program is education on the connection between food choices and health status, and empowering individuals to make better choices and know that they are worthy of having the best life possible. Dr. Champion's specialties include digestive diseases and disorders, autism, autoimmune, inflammatory conditions, hormone balance, PCOS, adrenal health, thyroid health, diabetes, genetic testing and coaching, mitochondrial function, ADHD, anxiety, trauma work through HeartMath, and hypnotherapy.

Acknowledgments

Andrea Cook

I first want to thank the many people who have offered kind words of support and enthusiasm for my work over the years. I feel so grateful to be surrounded by such a generous community.

To Erika Torres and Bela Medellin, I am so grateful for your ability to roll up your sleeves and support me in getting the book written. Your work really helped move the project forward.

To my children Gabriella Cook, Tim Cook, Janet Cook, Josie Lake, and Megan Happe-Cook, thank you for continuing to provide love and affection to lift my spirits and give me strength to get the book finished.

To my parents Bob and Phyllis Neumann, thank you for teaching me to believe in myself enough to chase my dreams. It means so much that you have always been there encouraging me that this is an important book for me to write.

To my Publishing Consultant Nancy Hancock, you have been my essential ally these many months, diligently working by my side to both examine every detail as well as to keep the big picture in mind. I cannot thank you enough for your kind and knowledgeable guidance on how to take this spinning mass of ideas and get them into print in an organized and thoughtful way that makes them accessible to others.

To my dear sister Cindy Davis, you taught me how to be a better writer and kept reminding me that I had something important to say. Thank you for believing in me and for your endless enthusiasm to talk with me about nutrition and health.

To my co-author Jennifer Champion, what an amazing partner you are! When I would start to panic, you would stay calm. When I was tired, a conversation with you always helped renew my enthusiasm. I would get stuck in the weeds, and you would see a way to move forward. It has been such a joy and an honor working with you on this project.

To my amazing husband Bill Cook, after writing so many words to create this book, I can hardly find the words to express my appreciation for your support. It has meant so much to me that your belief in this project has been unwavering and passionate since the beginning when I first came up with the idea. You believed and sacrificed more than anybody else to make sure this book was completed. You kept me fed and gave me massages to keep me strong, held me in your arms and comforted me when I was exhausted and overwhelmed, handled things so that I was free to write, remained interested but not pushy about how the writing was progressing, and never chastised me about the endlessly moving deadlines. This book would not have happened without your support and hard work!

Finally, to my therapy clients and students at the University of California Santa Cruz (UCSC), thank you for continuing to inspire and push me to be a better therapist and teacher. Your curiosity, drive to learn and grow, challenging questions, insightful comments, enthusiasm, and desire to make the world a better place clarified for me that writing a nutritional psychology textbook was a worthy quest.

Jennifer Champion

I would like to express my deepest gratitude to Andrea Cook, PhD, for her incredible understanding and flexibility throughout this journey. Your unwavering support has been invaluable in making this endeavor possible.

To Tamra, your continuous love, encouragement, and support have been my foundation. Thank you for being by my side through every step, cheering me on when I needed it most.

To Jaeden, your presence in my life has been a gift beyond measure. Thank you for helping me heal mentally and for offering me your unconditional love. You've shown me the importance of resilience, trust, and inner peace.

Lastly, to my clients, thank you for showing up as your most authentic selves in our sessions. Your courage and vulnerability have not only allowed me to guide you, but have also given me the privilege of learning and growing with you through empathy and understanding.

I am truly grateful for each of you and the role you have played in this journey.

Section I

Foundations of Psychology

1 Psychology Basics

The field of psychology is very broad and examines many aspects of human functioning. People often think psychology only considers how you feel (i.e., your emotions), how you think (i.e., your cognitions), and how you act (i.e., your behaviors). Your daily experience with aspects of each of these are all ideas we expect to discuss when talking about psychology. While you may sometimes feel intensely sad, anxious, or frightened, there is a great deal of nuance about how and why we experience these emotions and cognitions and then act on them with behaviors. Why do some people suffer when others do not? What environmental and genetic factors affect how we experience the world? What actions can we take to help ourselves and others feel better? The new field of Nutritional Psychology explores the influence of nutrition and lifestyle on emotions, cognitions, and behaviors, and thereby provides avenues of treatment and self-care that can help alleviate difficult psychological challenges for many people.

This chapter provides an overview of how we currently approach mental illness in the United States You will learn about how and why we diagnose mental disorders and some of the benefits and challenges of that process. The focus of this textbook is on new approaches to treating mental disorders, so we have included a discussion about the education pathways to becoming a mental health clinician.

DEFINING THE FIELD OF PSYCHOLOGY

According to the American Psychological Association, psychology is "the study of the mind and behavior" (APA, 2023). It is a diverse scientific discipline that includes both research about why and how people do what they do, as well as the applied side of psychology which focuses on how we use what we know about humans to improve things like individual functioning, group dynamics, and societal patterns. Major branches of psychological research include experimental, biological, cognitive, lifespan developmental, personality, and social psychology. Applied psychology branches, including clinical, industrial/organizational, educational, health, neuropsychology, forensic, sports, and cross-cultural, focus on applying psychological theory to understand and treat mental, emotional, physical, and social dysfunction and to enhance behavior and functionality in various settings of human activity (e.g., home, school, workplace, battlefield, courtroom, sports arena, and medical office).

A FOCUS ON CLINICAL PSYCHOLOGY

Clinical Psychology will be the primary psychological focus in this textbook, so let's start with a definition. The American Psychological Association (APA) defines the clinical psychology specialty as focused on providing "comprehensive mental and behavioral healthcare for individuals, couples, families, and groups; consultation to agencies and communities; training, education and supervision; and research-based practice" to address a wide range of mental and behavioral health problems (APA, 2022a). I would offer a second definition Andrew Pomerantz uses in his textbook *Clinical Psychology: Science, Practice, and Diversity*, "Clinical psychology involves rigorous study and applied practice directed toward understanding and improving the psychological facets of the human experience, including but not limited to issues or problems of behavior, emotions, or intellect" (Pomerantz, 2019, p. 5).

In simple terms, this major branch of psychology focuses on human functioning across the lifespan and includes diagnosing, preventing, and treating mental illness, which is where we focus in this textbook. We use the terms mental illness, mental disorders, psychiatric illness, and psychiatric disorders interchangeably in this textbook since they all describe the same focus of

DOI: 10.1201/9781032647647-2

challenges to human functioning. Other terms, such as mental health challenge, psychiatric issue, and mentally unwell, are general terms that are more loosely defined and not necessarily tied to a psychiatric or mental health diagnosis where the symptoms match the established diagnostic criteria. You will also note that we use the term *client* rather than *patient* to describe a person receiving treatment services from a mental health clinician or nutritionist. The term patient is more often used in a medical setting whereas client is more often used in a mental health setting. In a setting that is both medical and mental health, such as a psychiatric hospital, the term patient is more likely to be used.

EXPANDING CLINICAL PSYCHOLOGY

This textbook delves into how and why we diagnose and treat mental illness in the U.S. population. It explores common risk factors for mental illness, current treatment approaches in the mental health field, and a new treatment paradigm that focuses on the important impact of food and nutrition on mental health. You will have a chance to consider research demonstrating the strong links between food and emotions, cognitions and behavior, and the exciting ways we can improve mental health by making changes to our food.

DIAGNOSING MENTAL ILLNESS

Let us begin by examining how we define mental illness. Unlike most medical illnesses, mental illness does not have a lab test to confirm or deny a diagnosis. You do not go in and have your blood drawn, and a week later find out that you have bipolar disorder. Or walk away from a doctor's visit saying, "Yep, I caught a bad case of crazy this week!" Instead, mental illness is diagnosed based on gathering information about a person's behaviors, thoughts, and emotions. A thorough diagnosis begins with a trained mental health clinician coming up with a plan for how to assess their client. This can include several features including: carefully listening to a person describe their symptoms; asking the person to complete a survey with questions about different mental health symptoms; hearing from other people who describe that person's symptoms such as a family member, friend, teacher, coach, medical provider, or former therapist; and observing the client's behavior and attitudes in the therapy sessions or other environment such as a classroom or clinical setting. Yet, even after gathering all that information, identifying which symptoms and behaviors are sufficiently problematic and thereby can be defined as a mental illness requires consideration of multiple factors.

THE FOUR DS

In their textbook *Psychopathology: Science and Practice* (12th edition), the authors explain that psychopathology is hard to define and that no single definition has won total acceptance. However, most of the definitions have features in common often called the "Four Ds" which are deviance, distress, dysfunction, and danger (see Figure 1.1). These concepts help us to clarify the basic tenets by which we judge others as psychologically unwell (Comer & Comer, 2024).

Deviance is generally determined by cultural norms. Each society decides what is and what is not considered "normal." When a person's behavior, thoughts, and emotions are markedly different from what that society deems as normal for proper functioning, then that person is labeled as deviant. For example, many of us talk to ourselves. Come on, you can admit it. There are often long conversations when we are alone in the car where we have the chance to argue our perspective without any interruptions. At what point would that behavior be considered deviant? Is it only if we get caught talking to ourselves by accident? Or is it only deviant if we do it openly in public while others are watching? There is some subjectivity in the decision about where the line is between deviant, acceptable, and optimal behavior.

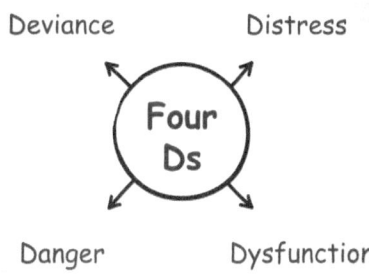

FIGURE 1.1   The Four Ds of psychopathology. Adapted from dizain (Shutterstock).

Distress is a very common symptom of mental illness. Many people experience symptoms of mental illness that they find very distressing. Anxiety symptoms of worrying, loss of sleep, and feeling tense and sick to your stomach are very unpleasant and people are often desperate to relieve those symptoms. When someone is terribly unhappy due to their psychiatric symptoms, most cultures consider that person unwell, in poor health, or mentally ill. Yet not all people are distressed by their symptoms. In some cultures, a hallucination where one sees ghosts may be considered a pleasurable spiritual experience rather than a disturbance that should be mitigated. In this case, we can acknowledge that culture plays a big part in determining mental illness if there is limited or no distress experienced by the person demonstrating the symptoms.

Dysfunction focuses the ability to carry out activities of daily living. Societies expect adults to manage their basic needs such as providing food, shelter, and clothing for oneself and one's children, while appropriately interacting with other people and not destroying other's property. Behavior outside of these expectations is considered dysfunctional and often falls within the definition of mental illness. Some would argue that amplified distress which leads to progressively more dysfunction is a more important feature of diagnosing mental illness than deviance since many people function outside of social norms, but if they are wealthy or famous then they are not crazy, they are just eccentric (Bergner & Bunford, 2017).

Danger considers whether a person is at risk for harming themselves or harming others due to their psychiatric symptoms. While this is a feature of diagnosing mental illness, it is actually pretty rare for it to be a substantial part of a person's mental health challenges. Risk of harm to self is the most common form of danger, and is the primary reason for psychiatric hospitalization (Dunseith, 2020). Most often harm to self refers to suicidal thoughts, planning and actions (see more in the section on Suicide and Mental Health in Chapter 2), which goes against common cultural taboos about taking your own life. Danger in the form of harm to others includes threats or actions that harm people or their property. This can include command hallucinations where a person hears a voice that tells them to hurt someone, or a criminal with an antisocial personality disorder who repeatedly participates in violent and unlawful behaviors.

CHALLENGES WITH DIAGNOSING

Clearly with such broad definitions of what constitutes a mental illness, there is a great deal of room for differences of opinion, especially when we consider the complex and varied nature of human functioning. For example, where and when you see a person often changes your perception of their outlook and behavior. We are all a little uptight and tense in a doctor's office compared to how we act and feel when surrounded by loved ones sharing a good meal or playing our favorite game.

Clinicians need to account for those situational differences when considering a diagnosis by assessing a person on different days ideally in different ways, such as asking them to complete a survey, doing an in-depth interview, asking for feedback from family or teachers, neuroimaging, and sessions where the person has some time to talk about their life and what troubles them (Merrell, 2008). This is especially true with children, who have less ability to sit with an adult and talk about their concerns, so limiting the clinician interaction to an office visit risks an incomplete understanding of the child's behavior and challenges in different settings (Tackett et al., 2013).

DIAGNOSTIC AND STATISTICAL MANUAL OF MENTAL DISORDERS

Even with a careful assessment, that still leaves a lot of interpretation by the individual clinician to decide whether this person is mentally ill, whether or not they need treatment, and which is the best treatment approach. To minimize this bias and standardize the way we diagnose and treat clients, the field of psychology in the U.S. utilizes a manual based on decades of clinical research and clinician experience titled the *Diagnostic and Statistical Manual of Mental Disorders (DSM)*. The DSM organizes common mental health symptoms into a long list of possible diagnoses that practitioners use to more accurately diagnose mental disorders.

The DSM is the most widely used mental health classification system in the U.S. and is the basis of almost every official mental illness diagnosis given in our healthcare system. It is relied on heavily for insurance coverage and to create a common language among professionals. If a person is diagnosed as having schizophrenia, major depressive disorder, or generalized anxiety disorder, each is directly tied to a specific DSM code, which is accompanied by the symptoms presented in each disorder. Most other countries primarily use the *International Classification of Diseases (ICD)*, which was developed by the World Health Organization and is a more comprehensive listing of both medical and mental health disorders.

The American Psychiatric Association published the first DSM in 1952. The content from the original version has changed significantly over time, with formal updates and revisions to the DSM published every 6–13 years based on updated research, the need for more specific classifications, and feedback from professionals in the field. The latest full edition, the DSM-5 (which changed the numbering system from Roman with DSM-IV to Arabic with DSM-5), was published in 2013. In 2022, the APA published the DSM-5-TR, an interim text revision of the fifth edition, meaning the diagnostic concepts were not changed but there were clarifications and changes made to some of the language. For example, "natal male/natal female" was used to replace "individual assigned male at birth" or "individual assigned female at birth," and "cross-sex treatment regimen" was replaced with "gender-affirming treatment regimen" (American Psychiatric Association, 2023; First et al., 2022).

It is important to remember that the DSM describes symptoms, and the statistical occurrence of reported cases associated with mental health symptoms. It is essentially a catalog of the many challenges and maladies that can occur in human mental health. However, it does not explain *why* people experience these symptoms. There are many different reasons and contributing factors that trigger a person to experience mental health symptoms. One person who struggles with depression may have a very different background or life experience when compared to someone else who struggles with very similar symptoms.

BENEFITS OF THE DSM

One benefit to having a shared diagnostic manual is that it creates continuity through shared language when describing common ways that people feel, think, and behave. This creates opportunities to compare our experience with the experience of others. It can help answer the questions: What does it mean to be depressed or anxious? Am I the only one who feels this way or do other people struggle with the same feelings? At what point should I consider myself crazy? What is acceptable and at what point does it become unacceptable?

Media portrays extreme forms of mental illness like trying to take your own life or kill someone else because you hear voices (hallucinations) and have bizarre thoughts (delusions) that make you believe these actions are rational and appropriate. That is one side of mental illness, but certainly not the whole picture. Mental health falls on a broad spectrum with lots of diversity in how and why we do what we do. The DSM helps us look at the nuances behind labels like "depressed" and "crazy" to come to a deeper understanding how mental health symptoms are experienced and to create descriptions that represent typical and atypical behaviors and thought patterns.

The common language provided by the DSM enables researchers to study and observe various groups of people exhibiting similar symptoms. We can examine which symptoms often go together (e.g., agitation and avoidance are both common symptoms of anxiety) so that we can better understand how and why those symptoms began, why they sometimes reliably cluster, and what feeds or maintains their existence. Clinicians use that information to design and standardize treatments that demonstrate effectiveness for specific mental disorders. Standardizing how we diagnose clients helps ensure that clients receive appropriate, effective treatment across a wide variety of mental health practitioners and settings. It also allows for coding and billing within our current healthcare system so that clients can receive health insurance coverage for the mental health services they receive (Fritscher, 2023).

For many people, the value of diagnosing lies in their newfound ability to understand themselves through the lens of a diagnosis. Applying clear and descriptive language to vague or confusing sensations, thoughts, and behaviors can help a person conceptualize and clarify those experiences. Made aware through diagnosis, people can gather information about their mental health disorder in books, journals, online, and by seeking out support groups and social media pages to connect with like-minded people who have lived a similar experience. While mental health disorders often carry a social stigma, being part of a group or tribe that all share that trait can decrease the impact of the stigma they perceive, fear, or experience. A diagnosis can also increase optimism that a person has a recognized disorder with some predictable patterns as well as some clearly research-based treatment options.

PROBLEMS WITH THE DSM

The DSM also has some problems. Reliability is one of those problems. In this context, reliability means that if different clinicians assess the same patient using the same system (i.e., DSM-5), they will come up with the same diagnosis. Unfortunately, that is not always the case, which raises the question of how realistic the diagnoses are when used in the real world. While efforts were made to increase the reliability of the DSM-5 compared to previous versions (Moran, 2012), some of the research that examined the reliability of DSM-5 diagnoses found relatively low consistency among clinicians (Cooper, 2014), while others found it to be satisfactory (Rice et al., 2022). Cooper argues that the DSM-5 task force used an unacceptably low Cohen's kappa statistic of 0.4–0.6 as an acceptable level of agreement of diagnosis between clinicians (known as interrater reliability), where a value of 0 represents chance agreement and a value of 1 represents perfect agreement. This means that if two clinicians gave a diagnosis to the same person, there was a 40–60 percent chance they would give the same diagnosis. This was low compared to the use of a Cohen's kappa of 0.7 to represent an acceptable level of agreement during the development of the DSM-III. In contrast, the article by Rice et al. found the DSM-5 to have high interrater reliability for autism spectrum disorder (ASD) diagnoses with Cohen's kappa scores ranging from very good (0.60–0.79) to excellent (≥0.80).

Many clinicians feel the DSM attempts to oversimplify human behavior (Allsopp et al., 2019; Fritscher, 2023) and has limited clinical value due to the overlap of clinical symptoms. Clients often meet diagnostic criteria for two or more diagnoses (known as comorbidity), such as a depressive disorder and a substance abuse disorder. A more complex patient with comorbid disorders requires a broader approach to treatment beyond the diagnoses that addresses multiple issues at the same time (Bakker, 2019; Raskin et al., 2022).

Despite questions regarding the clinical usefulness of diagnosing clients, since the health insurance system requires a DSM diagnosis, clinicians must provide a diagnosis to receive payment for mental health services, even if it does not guide their therapy process. Many clinicians who do not accept insurance do not establish a formal diagnosis, since it is often less relevant for complex clients and is not necessary to design an effective treatment plan. They are also resistant because they know there is stigma associated with receiving a psychiatric diagnosis that can be troublesome for some clients (see section on Stigma later in this chapter).

Another concern with the DSM is over-diagnosing. Recent changes made in the DSM-5 have made it likely that more people will receive certain diagnoses than in the past. For example, a person can be diagnosed with mild neurocognitive disorder based on symptoms that many consider to be normal age-related forgetfulness. Similarly, a diagnosis of prolonged grief disorder (recently added in the 2022 DSM-5-TR) includes a person struggling with the death of a loved for more than a year (American Psychiatric Association, 2022). In this case, the question becomes, "What is the appropriate reaction to death? What is healthy bereavement?"

Bereavement is a normal reaction to the death of a loved one often expressed by feelings of sadness, low energy, changes in sleeping and eating, and not feeling pleasure from one's usual activities. Imagine that your grandfather died, and your grandmother responded to the loss of her best friend and life partner for over 50 years with the bereavement symptoms described above and continued to experience those symptoms one year after his death. Is she mentally ill for responding to his death in this way or is she reacting in an understandable healthy way to a difficult life transition? This addition of the diagnosis of prolonged grief disorder makes it more likely that your grandmother will be diagnosed with a mental illness and encouraged to begin mental health treatment such as antidepressant medication. In this way, we are at risk for pathologizing appropriate behavior and calling it a mental illness.

Numerous clinicians, researchers, and professional groups have spoken out against the DSM-5. The depth of concern about the accuracy and usefulness of the DSM-5 was highlighted in the decision by the National Institute of Mental Health (NIMH), one of the largest international funding sources for mental health research. In 2013, right before the launch of the DSM-5, NIMH announced that they were moving away from funding clinical research based on DSM-5 diagnoses (Winerman, 2013). Instead, NIMH is promoting the neuroscience-focused tool called the Research Domain Criteria (RDoC) which they developed as a classification guide for researchers, a move that has been criticized for redirecting funds away from essential psychiatric clinical trials that evaluate current treatment interventions to focus on potential future uses of neuroscience in clinical treatment (Markowitz & Milrod, 2022).

The RDoC incorporates more behavioral and neuroscience evidence than the DSM-5. The goal of the RDoC is to promote an interdisciplinary approach to mental illness that better integrates psychology and biology, especially genetics and neuroscience, by focusing on observable behavior and neurobiological measures such as scalp electroencephalography (EEG) and functional magnetic resonance imaging (fMRI) (Kozak & Cuthbert, 2016; Patrick et al., 2019). For example, when studying addiction to alcohol, a researcher might examine "reward seeking behavior" (i.e., drinking alcohol to feel relaxed) and then use neuroimaging to see how that shows up in the brain and in what ways it activates dopamine receptors in the brain's pleasure center. Treatment might then focus on changing behavior variables (e.g., only drink alcohol with other people) to see if changes in behaviors favorably impact brain processing of information that reduce unpleasant sensations like cravings, known to often drive excessive alcohol consumption.

Criticism about the DSM-5 has also focused on the suspected bias of the authors due to their financial ties to the pharmaceutical industry. A person with financial ties receives income from a pharmaceutical company in one of many forms that can include a salaried position or research funding. When the DSM-4 was published in 1994, 57 percent of the task force members who wrote the manual had financial ties to the pharmaceutical industry. That number increased to 69 percent of the DSM-5 task force, meaning that over two-thirds of the authors of the DSM-5 disclosed a potential financial conflict of interest that had "the potential for bias" to support the use of medication as the primary treatment option. This was especially true for DSM panels that were responsible for writing about the diagnoses "for which pharmacological treatment is the first-line intervention" such as mood disorders and psychotic disorders, where a larger portion of the DSM task force members had financial ties to "pharmaceutical companies that manufacture the medications used to treat these disorders" (Cosgrove & Krimsky, 2012). These concerns persisted after publication of the DSM-5-TR in 2022, where 60 percent of the DSM panel members had financial ties to the pharmaceutical industry. It is important to keep in mind that potential financial conflicts of interest are not evidence of wrongdoing, but they do create concerns about bias in the research process and can undermine public trust (Cosgrove, 2024).

STIGMA AND MENTAL ILLNESS

The terms mental illness and psychiatric disorder are loaded with negative concepts of human weakness and disgust that can separate and spark ridicule and mistrust rather than encourage compassion and effective help and support. People with mental illness often feel blamed and shamed for their symptoms feel marginalized and worry that they are seen as unreliable by their groups and communities. Projection, labeling, and resulting discrimination show up in many social settings that support healthy functioning such as the job market, housing, and healthcare. Often employers are reluctant to hire and promote people with declared mental illness, even though many are fully capable of doing a good job, especially as employers increasingly improve support through flexible paid time off, family leave, and increased mental health coverage and support. Without support, psychiatric illness can lead to homelessness because landlords will not rent to them or work with them when adjustments need to be made, such as more flexible payment schedules, or access to premises for repairs or even more respectful notice when there is a deviation in expectations. To make matters worse, discrimination in the healthcare systems frequently offers psychiatric patients a lower standard of care that interferes with their ability to stabilize their treatment and to better manage their symptoms (American Psychiatric Association, 2020).

Mental health stigma remains a globally persistent issue that interferes with our ability to understand mental health disorders, access treatment, and empathize with people suffering from severe symptoms, especially symptoms that include peculiar behaviors associated with highly stigmatized diagnoses like schizophrenia and substance abuse disorder. We have known about the stigma and stereotypes toward mental illness for centuries, with research confirming the harmful effects on individual sufferers and the greater community (Rossler, 2016). Yet knowing that stigma is a problem does not remove the stereotype of people with mental illness being dangerous, irresponsible, and incompetent due to their weak character and dependent nature (Fox et al., 2018).

CULTURE AND STIGMA

Stigma has changed over the years. A 2021 study of U.S. adults analyzed participant perceptions and attitudes about mental health disorders across two time periods: 1996–2006 and 2006–2018. Responses during the first period reflected an increase in "scientific attributions" such as genetics to explain the cause of mental illness. Then, perhaps largely due to this shift in thinking of mental illness using more of a disease model focused on a genetic cause, there was a decrease in stigma around certain diagnoses, in particular around major depression (Pescosolido et al., 2021), which also tied into the rapid rise of prescribing antidepressant medication by primary care providers in the medical system, including people's family doctors and pediatricians.

Culture also has an impact on attitudes and stigma about mental illness. In a study of Asian American participants, younger participants reported that, while they recognized the value of mental health services, they felt pressure to avoid using those services due to cultural expectations (Do et al., 2020). Other empirical studies focused on differences between Eastern and Western cultural attitudes toward mental health. For example, a study performed in Vietnam noted Eastern cultural perceptions of hallucinations (seeing or hearing things) and delusions (strange beliefs) associated with schizophrenia as forms of "behavioral deviance and illness" caused by spiritual or supernatural influences, which carries less stigma and blame, and allows patients to pursue spiritual treatment as well as medical support for physical discomfort such as headaches associated with these symptoms. This differs markedly from the Western belief that schizophrenia symptoms are associated with an illness that needs to be cured (Gaines, 2014). The author notes that attributing symptoms to a supernatural influence removes the attitude that the person is sick or weak, which may be influenced by the Eastern collectivist culture to protect family members and their virtue and creates pressure to avoid admitting that there is a problem.

NEGATIVE IMPACT OF STIGMA

Stigma is associated with reluctance or refusal to enter mental health treatment. More than half of all people with mental illness do not receive treatment for fear of being treated disrespectfully, being thought less of, and/or losing their job and their livelihood. As a result, stigma decreases the likelihood that someone will seek out and find appropriate treatment and then adhere to the treatment recommendations, thereby increasing their psychiatric symptoms (American Psychiatric Association, 2020; Fox et al., 2018).

As a society our general stigma around mental illness reflects our projection of perceived weakness, flaw, or personal failings resulting in fewer resources dedicated to providing treatment relative to other areas of healthcare, which is more commonly accepted as necessary and as correcting something that needs to be addressed to return to optimal functioning. The perceived difference makes accessing necessary mental health services often difficult and daunting. After diagnosis, people with mental illness, due to their symptoms, are less likely to adhere to the treatment protocol recommended for them, which can worsen symptoms and contribute to feeling bad about themselves (e.g., guilty for not doing what they are told and getting better) and internalizing (starting to believe) the stigma that people are directing toward them (e.g., that they are a lazy, disgusting, flawed person) (Lim et al., 2019; Pescosolido et al., 2021; Tanaka et al., 2003).

Stigma impacts not only individuals with mental health conditions but also the community at large. Prejudice and discrimination due to misunderstanding and fears about mental illness cause reluctance in community members to engage with or support people with mental illness. Community rejection causes alienation of people struggling with a psychiatric illness and further isolates them from seeking out support and treatment. Delays in treatment at the onset of the disorder, when someone first starts to really struggle with their symptoms, make it more likely that the symptoms will become severe before they finally receive any treatment services (Tanaka et al., 2003). Now the community feels the impact. When the severity of mental illness in untreated community members rises, more and more members end up joining the swelling ranks of people who are unemployed, homeless, or in prison due to their mental health issues (see further discussion about housing and psychiatric care in Chapter 9).

Recently, stigma has shifted to trivializing and glamorizing certain mental health conditions in the media, diminishing the seriousness of these conditions. Attention-deficit/hyperactivity disorder (ADHD) and obsessive-compulsive disorder (OCD), for example, are associated with providing beneficial personality traits. The belief by people who do not really understand the extent of the difficulties or suffering caused by these disorders perceive them as an advantage, where someone with ADHD has a lot of energy and someone with OCD is highly organized (Pavelko & Myrick, 2019). This distortion of understanding appears to be largely coming from social media sites marketed as educational that distribute misinformation and contribute to confusion about psychiatric diagnoses and inaccurate attempts to self-diagnose (Clark, 2023).

The need for better dissemination of accurate information about psychiatric illness continues to be a challenge. "Media coverage of mental illnesses has been consistently and overwhelmingly negative and imprecise" (Rossler, 2016, p. 1251). However, it is worth the struggle to keep putting good information into circulation. Research shows us that when mental health professionals provide accurate information to people not directly associated with the mental health field, there is increased understanding about the symptoms and challenges of different disorders, better support for seeking psychiatric treatment, and decreased overall stigma (Tanaka et al., 2003). Thus, general information about mental health may act as a protective barrier to stigmatization and stereotypical beliefs about mental health, its treatment, and those who suffer from its conditions.

Of Note . . . "TAKE A BREATH"

Why do people tell you to take a breath in a stressful moment? Likely it is because slowing down and taking a few deep breaths during a crisis can help us to think more clearly and to act more rationally than when we are in a highly aroused and emotional state. That one-minute pause to regroup can sometimes make all the difference to creating happier outcomes.

Deep breathing is a tool commonly taught in psychotherapy, coaching, and any form of stress management training. This is a powerful tool to have in your self-care toolkit! You can handle so many difficult situations more effectively when you can calm yourself and focus on solving the task at hand rather than becoming immobilized by emotions of fear and overwhelm. When you are sitting down to take that final exam, taking some deep breaths can be a life saver because it helps your brain to function better and to remember all those great facts you reviewed when you studied.

Practicing deep breathing on a regular basis when you are not in crisis helps train the body how to slow down and slip into that calm state more quickly upon request so that you can get quiet and open yourself to new information. It is deeply embedded in many religious and spiritual practices, as well as sports psychology, psychotherapy, and stress management training, and will be discussed in more detail in Chapter 16. Like building a muscle, the more we practice deep breathing, the better we are at leaning into it during difficult times. Consider adding a few minutes of deep breathing to your daily habits starting today.

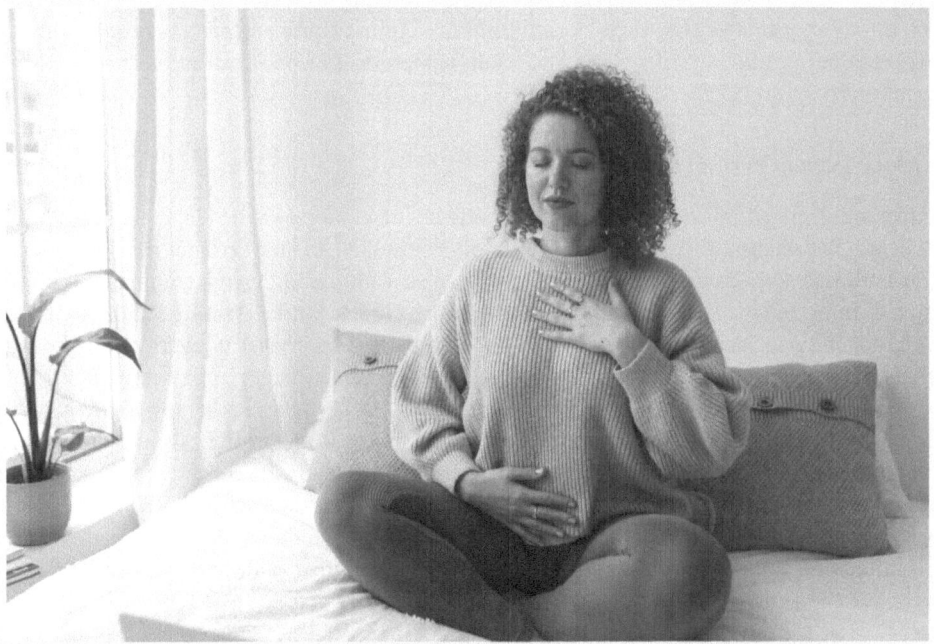

FIGURE 1.2   Take a breath. Credit: shurkin_son (Shutterstock).

SCOPE OF PRACTICE AND EDUCATION PATHWAYS

As mentioned at the beginning of this chapter, we will be focusing on clinical psychology in this textbook. The term clinical psychology describes the general field of mental health treatment as well as a specific educational pathway to become a Clinical Psychologist. In either case, the overarching question is, "How do we help people to improve their mental health?" Toward that end, there are many different educational pathways to become a mental health clinician.

Mental health clinicians are required to complete a Master's or Doctoral level graduate school program and to complete supervised clinical hours to become licensed to treat clients (Careers in Psychology, 2023). These programs include coursework, comprehensive exams, writing a thesis or dissertation, and working with clients in a supervised setting.

MASTER'S DEGREE PROGRAMS

A master's level license involves two to three years of coursework and up to 4000 hours of post-degree supervised clinical work (American Psychological Association, 2021). Some programs require completion of a master's thesis, which is an in-depth research paper. After a student has completed the course work and supervised clinical hours, they are eligible to sit for the licensing exam required by the state in which they want to provide therapy.

Master's level licenses vary by state and include Marriage and Family Therapist (MFT), Licensed Clinical Social Worker (LCSW), Licensed Professional Counselor (LPC), Licensed Mental Health Counselor (LMHC), Licensed Clinical Professional Counselor (LCPC), Licensed Clinical Mental Health Counselor (LCMHC), and Licensed Professional Clinical Counselor (LPCC), and Licensed Pastoral Counselor (LPC) (Caldwell, 2022; Jones, 2022). All these programs prepare a practitioner to provide psychotherapy to clients. They differ in their emphasis on the type of therapy (e.g., individual, couples, family, group), clinical setting (e.g., community clinic, locked psychiatric unit, medical hospital, prison, school), client population (e.g., children, family, older adult) and clinical issue (e.g., substance abuse, relationships, cognitive function, access to resources such as housing). For example, an MFT provides short-term psychotherapy to individuals, couples, families, and groups in an outpatient setting such as a community clinic or private practice office, with a focus on topics including emotional disorders and relationship issues (American Association for Marriage and Family Therapy, 2023).

DOCTORAL DEGREE PROGRAMS

Four doctoral degrees allow you to become a mental health clinician in the United States: PhD, PsyD, EdD, and MD (Broudy, 2019). The PhD (Doctor of Philosophy) and PsyD (Doctor of Psychology) can both be pathways to becoming a Licensed Psychologist, with the PhD having a greater emphasis on research training and the PsyD having a greater focus on clinical work. Training requirements vary by state and generally include four to five years of coursework and supervised clinical training to graduate (Michalski & Fowler, 2016). Intellectual, personality and neuropsychological assessments are primarily performed by psychologists, who also provide a wide range of psychotherapy services in various settings. The EdD (Doctor of Education) has an education focus and is often the path to becoming a School Psychologist. The MD (Medical Doctor) goes through medical school and then specializes in psychiatry during residency to become a psychiatrist. Most students enter a doctoral program with a bachelor's degree and complete their doctoral program and clinical hours in five to seven years (APA, 2022b), after which they must pass both state and federal licensing exams to be licensed to see clients.

INTERNSHIPS AND FELLOWSHIPS

Completion of an *internship* is a requirement for both master's and doctoral-level clinicians. An apprenticeship of sorts, the internship starts after the course work and pre-internship (practicum) clinical work is complete. Similar to a medical residency, this is the transition from student to professional. At the doctoral level, the internship is generally a year of full-time supervised clinical experience in an applied setting that is a requirement for graduation.

The *fellowship* takes place after the student has completed their doctoral degree. It typically lasts one or two years and a licensed practitioner still provides supervision but with more independence (such as being a group leader without a more experienced co-leader) and opportunities to train and supervise interns. The fellowship is generally where a clinician receives more specialized training in topics such as health, forensics, child, or neuropsychology. The additional clinical hours achieved during the fellowship complete the 2000–4000 hours required to be eligible to sit for the licensing exams.

For example, one California program to become a Licensed Clinical Psychologist with a PhD is a five-year program that trains students to both perform research and provide psychotherapy. The first three years focus on coursework, which includes the completion of a research project. At the same time, students work part-time in a clinical setting to complete 1200 hours of supervision and training for their practicum placement. The fourth year is generally when students focus on writing their dissertation, a 100-to-200-page report that details original research performed by the student. Finally, the fifth year is a 1500-hour clinical internship. After graduation, the student must complete an additional 1500 hours of supervised clinical work in the form of a one- or two-year fellowship to complete the 3000 hours required to sit for the national licensing exam. After the student passes the national licensing exam, they must pass the smaller state licensing exam. At the end of this long journey, the student is now a Licensed Clinical Psychologist and can work with a variety of clients in a broad range of settings and supervise interns who are training to become psychologists.

Prescribing Psychotropic Medication

Prescribing psychotropic (mental health) medication is predominantly the realm of psychiatrists, although this is expanding. Due to a shortage of psychiatrists, there has been a movement to allow properly trained psychologists to have *prescriptive authority* that allows them to prescribe medication in approved regions of the country, symbolized as *RxP*. In 1998, the California School of Professional Psychology (CSPP) (now Alliant International University) established the nation's first Postdoctoral Master of Science in Clinical Psychopharmacology program, an online two-year program for licensed psychologists. Upon graduation, these psychologists can prescribe psychotropic medication in states or regions who have passed regulatory legislation that allows RxP. Currently these include: six states (New Mexico, Louisiana, Illinois, Iowa, Idaho, Colorado), U.S. territory of Guam, military healthcare systems (i.e., the Department of Defense), Indian Health Services (IHS), and the Commissioned Corps of the United States Public Health Service (USPHS cares for patients in underserved communities). The purpose of the prescriptive authority movement is to provide psychotropic medication to patients with mental health issues while also providing psychotherapy to maximize the effectiveness of the medication by assisting with lifestyle changes that include tapering or discontinuing other medications (e.g., opioids and sleep medications) for patients who are over-medicated (DeAngelis, 2023).

Continuing Education

Licensed clinicians are required to attend continuing education training programs in order to stay licensed. Each state licensing board establishes the minimum number of ongoing training hours their clinicians are required to complete. For example, a Licensed Psychologist in New York must complete 36 hours of approved training every three years. In Arizona, a Licensed Marriage and Family Therapist (LMFT) must complete 30 hours of continuing education every two years (American Association for Marriage and Family Therapy, 2023).

WHAT DO MENTAL HEALTH CLINICIANS DO?

Psychotherapy (also known as talk therapy) is the most common professional activity performed by mental health clinicians. Other activities include assessment, prescribing medication, teaching, supervising interns, research, and writing. With psychotherapy, whether meeting with individuals, couples, families, or groups, the focus is on helping clients to feel better through a variety of methods based on the needs of the client and the theoretical orientation of the practitioner. One of the key ingredients of this work is creating a safe environment where the client can express their thoughts and feelings and explore current and past challenges to better understand them. There are numerous theoretical models for psychotherapy including: cognitive, behavioral, psychodynamic, and humanistic therapies.

FOOD FOR THOUGHT: THE FIELD OF PSYCHOLOGY NEGLECTS NUTRITION

Emerging research about the interaction between food and the human body has been demonstrating a strong correlation between dietary nutrition and overall health, especially concerning nutrition's impact on individual mental wellbeing. However, originating less than two decades ago, the field of nutritional psychology remains in its infancy (CNP, 2024). Thus, until only recently, psychological research has offered minimal consideration of nutrition-related factors and their impact on mood and behavior.

Psychological research and education have largely neglected recognizing that nutritional intake is a major contributor to mental wellbeing, which has left the field and the public with a lack of accurate and adequate information. Outside of eating disorder and substance abuse treatment training, mental health clinicians receive no training about nutrition. The same is true for medical doctors, which includes psychiatrists. Western medicine often takes a neutral stance about the interrelationship and resulting consequences between nutrition and physical health, with the common lukewarm recommendation to "eat better and exercise" given at many medical visits, with little to no follow-up or referrals to a nutrition specialist or support group. Healthcare training leaves many medical and mental health professionals unaware and unequipped to effectively act upon the potential healthcare treatment options associated with nutritional improvements, especially preventive care before diseases fully develop (Campbell-McBride, 2018).

A survey of medical students reported they want nutrition education and feel they have insufficient knowledge and skills to provide appropriate nutrition education to effectively support dietary behavior change in their patients (Crowley et al., 2019). The U.S. National Academy of Sciences recommends a minimum of 25 hours of nutrition education for medical providers; however, the majority of medical schools offer little to no training or education in nutrition, leaving medical students, residents, and physicians feeling that the nutrition education they received is inadequate to feel confident in providing nutrition education to their patients (Caldow et al., 2022; Danek et al., 2017).

Additionally, medical insurance coverage for both medical and mental health treatment continues to exclude nutritional support as part of mental health treatment protocols because the Western model of healthcare fails to recognize poor nutritional habits as a primary driver of illness (Downer et al., 2020). This model ignores the expansive data demonstrating links between nutrient deficiencies caused by the consumption of inflammatory nutrient-poor foods and the manifestation of psychiatric symptoms including symptoms associated with depression and anxiety. Mental health disorders are on the rise, yet mental health treatment has not changed significantly to understand and meet this growing need. The focus has remained attached to using pharmaceuticals and talk therapy, with a lack of consideration for the contributory effect of poor nutrition on developing and maintaining psychiatric symptoms.

This lack of awareness and neglect occurs both within and outside of the healthcare system. Social media continues to exist as a platform with the ability to quickly spread mass information, which has led to an uptick in the spread of misinformation related to nutrition and health. Individuals with little to no credentials or training easily disseminate inaccurate information to their viewers. Social media has popularized "health" trends and fad diets in mainstream culture. When surveyed, over half of participants acknowledged that social media somewhat encouraged healthier choices, despite some mistrust due to the conflicting information that was presented, which caused them to doubt their choices (International Food Information Council, 2023).

But things are beginning to change. We are seeing more and more recognition of the primary importance of good nutrition for both physical and mental health. The mental health field continues to explore nutrition treatment options as primary or adjunctive support for psychiatric treatment protocols. Professional psychology organizations such as the APA and the American Psychiatric Association have published numerous articles, books, and continuing education courses that support nutrition training for mental health clinicians. The current trend indicates that increased nutrition training will continue to be incorporated into our healthcare practices, much to the benefit and appreciation of all future mental health clients.

REFERENCES

Allsopp, K., Read, J., Corcoran, R., & Kinderman, P. (2019). *Heterogeneity in psychiatric diagnostic classification*. https://doi.org/10.1016/j.psychres.2019.07.005

American Association for Marriage and Family Therapy. (2023). *Marriage and family therapist license requirements*. https://www.aamft.org/Advocacy/State_Resources/Arizona.aspx

American Psychiatric Association. (2020). *Stigma, prejudice and discrimination against people with mental illness*. https://www.psychiatry.org/patients-families/stigma-and-discrimination

American Psychiatric Association. (2022). *Prolonged grief disorder*. https://www.psychiatry.org/patients-families/prolonged-grief-disorder

American Psychiatric Association. (2023). *DSM history*. https://www.psychiatry.org/psychiatrists/practice/dsm/about-dsm/history-of-the-dsm

American Psychological Association (APA). (2022a). *Clinical psychology*. https://www.apa.org/ed/graduate/specialize/clinical

American Psychological Association (APA). (2022b). *State licensure and certification information for psychologists*. https://www.apaservices.org/practice/ce/state/state-info

American Psychological Association (APA). (2023). *Psychology*. American Psychological Association. https://dictionary.apa.org/psychology

American Psychological Association. (n.d.). *State licensure and certification information for psychologists*. https://www.apaservices.org/practice/ce/state/state-info

Bakker, G. M. (2019). A new conception and subsequent taxonomy of clinical psychological problems. *BMC Psychology, 7*(1), 46. https://doi.org/10.1186/s40359-019-0318-8

Bergner, R., & Bunford, N. (2017). Mental disorder is a disability concept, not a behavioral one. *Philosophy, Psychiatry, & Psychology, 24*, 25–40, https://doi.org/10.1353/ppp.2017.0004

Broudy, M. S. (2019). *What do all those letters mean? Guide to therapist's credentials*. https://www.e-counseling.com/self/guide-to-therapist-credentials/

Caldow, G., Palermo, C., & Wilson, A. N. (2022). 'What do doctors think they need to know about nutrition?'— A qualitative study of doctors with formal nutrition training. *BMC Nutrition, 8*(1), 85. https://doi.org/10.1186/s40795-022-00577-w

Caldwell, B. (2022). Decoding Counselor Alphabet Soup: LPC, LPCC, MLHC, and more. *Psychotherapy notes*. https://www.psychotherapynotes.com/decoding-counselor-alphabet-soup-lpc-lpcc-lmhc/#:~:text=Licensed%20Clinical%20Professional%20Counselor%20(LCPC,largest%20of%20which%20is%20California

Campbell-McBride, N. (2018). *Gut and psychology syndrome: Natural treatment for autism, dyspraxia, ADD, dyslexia, ADHD, depression, schizophrenia*. Chelsea Green Publishing.

Careers in Psychology. (2023). *Psychology licensure requirements by state*. https://careersinpsychology.org/psychologist-license-procedures-by-state/

Clark, A. (2023). *Social media and mental illness identity formation: The role of community culture and misinformation*. The George Washington University.

CNP. (2024). *The history of nutritional psychology: A new field of study to support a new model of mental healthcare.* The Center for Nutritional Psychology. https://www.nutritional-psychology.org/the-history-of-nutritional-psychology-a-new-field-of-study-to-support-a-new-model-of-mental-healthcare/

Comer, R. J., & Comer, J. S. (2024). *Psychopathology: Science and practice* (12th ed.). Worth Publishers.

Cooper, R. (2014). *How reliable is the DSM-5?* Mad in America: Science, Psychiatry and Social Justice. https://www.madinamerica.com/2014/09/how-reliable-is-the-dsm-5/

Cosgrove, L. (2024). Financial conflicts of interest in the DSM—A persistent problem. *BMJ, 384*, q36. https://doi.org/10.1136/bmj.q36

Cosgrove, L., & Krimsky, S. (2012). A comparison of DSM-IV and DSM-5 panel members' financial associations with industry: A pernicious problem persists. *PLoS Medicine, 9*(3), e1001190.

Crowley, J., Ball, L., & Hiddink, G. J. (2019). Nutrition in medical education: A systematic review. *The Lancet Planetary Health, 3*(9), e379–e389. https://doi.org/10.1016/S2542-5196(19)30171-8

Danek, R. L., Berlin, K. L., Waite, G. N., & Geib, R. W. (2017). Perceptions of nutrition education in the current medical school curriculum. *Family Medicine, 49*(10), 803–806.

DeAngelis, T. (2023). Prescriptive authority gains new momentum. *Monitor on Psychology, 54*(4). https://www.apa.org/monitor/2023/06/prescriptive-authority-psychologists

Do, M., McCleary, J., Nguyen, D., & Winfrey, K. (2020). Mental illness public stigma and generational differences among Vietnamese Americans. *Community Mental Health Journal, 56*, 839–853.

Downer, S., Berkowitz, S. A., Harlan, T. S., Olstad, D. L., & Mozaffarian, D. (2020). Food is medicine: Actions to integrate food and nutrition into healthcare. *BMJ, 369*, m2482, https://doi.org/10.1136/bmj.m2482

Dunseith, L. (2020). Study finds involuntary psychiatric detentions on the rise. *UCLA Newsroom.* https://newsroom.ucla.edu/releases/involuntary-psychiatric-detentions-on-the-rise

First, M. B., Yousif, L. H., Clarke, D. E., Wang, P. S., Gogtay, N., & Appelbaum, P. S. (2022). DSM-5-TR: Overview of what's new and what's changed. *World Psychiatry, 21*(2), 218–219. https://doi.org/10.1002/wps.20989

Fox, A. B., Earnshaw, V. A., Taverna, E. C., & Vogt, D. (2018). Conceptualizing and measuring mental illness stigma: The mental illness stigma framework and critical review of measures. *Stigma and Health, 3*(4), 348.

Fritscher, L. (2023). *Advantages and disadvantages of the diagnostic statistical manual.* Very Well Mind. https://www.verywellmind.com/dsm-friend-or-foe-2671930

Gaines, R. (2014). *Culture & Schizophrenia: How the manifestation of schizophrenia symptoms in Huế reflects Vietnamese culture.* Independent Study Project (ISP) Collection. 1826. https://digitalcollections.sit.edu/isp_collection/1826

International Food Information Council. (2023). *2023 Food & health survey.* https://foodinsight.org/2023-food-and-health-survey/

Jones, H. (2022). *Pastoral counseling: Everything you need to know.* Very Well Health. Retrieved September 7, 2024 from https://www.verywellhealth.com/pastoral-counseling-5270580

Kozak, M. J., & Cuthbert, B. N. (2016). The NIMH research domain criteria initiative: Background, issues, and pragmatics. *Psychophysiology, 53*(3), 286–297. https://doi.org/10.1111/psyp.12518

Lim, L., Goh, J., & Chan, Y.-H. (2019). Internalized stigma, disclosure and self-esteem among psychiatric patients in a general hospital outpatient clinic. *Australasian Psychiatry, 27*(6), 584–588.

Markowitz, J. C., & Milrod, B. L. (2022). Lost in translation: The value of psychiatric clinical trials. *The Journal of Clinical Psychiatry, 83*(6), 43385.

Merrell, K. W. (2008). *Behavioral, social, and emotional assessment of children and adolescents* (3rd ed.). Erlbaum.

Michalski, D., & Fowler, G. (2016, January 2016). *Doctoral degrees in psychology: How are they different, or not so different?* Retrieved December 18, 2024, from https://www.apa.org/ed/precollege/psn/2016/01/doctoral-degrees

Moran, M. (2012). *DSM-5 emphasizes diagnostic reliability.* American Psychiatric Association. https://psychnews.psychiatryonline.org/doi/full/10.1176/pn.47.5.psychnews_47_5_1-a

Patrick, C. J., Iacono, W. G., & Venables, N. C. (2019). Incorporating neurophysiological measures into clinical assessments: Fundamental challenges and a strategy for addressing them. *Psychological Assessment, 31*(12), 1512–1529. https://doi.org/10.1037/pas0000713

Pavelko, R. L., & Myrick, J. G. (2019). Measuring trivialization of mental illness: Developing a scale of perceptions that mental illness symptoms are beneficial. *Health Communication, 35*(5), 576–584.

Pescosolido, B. A., Halpern-Manners, A., Luo, L., & Perry, B. (2021). Trends in public stigma of mental illness in the US, 1996-2018. *JAMA Network Open, 4*(12), e2140202–e2140202.

Pomerantz, A. M. (2019). *Clinical psychology: Science, practice, and diversity.* Sage Publications.

Raskin, J. D., Maynard, D., & Gayle, M. C. (2022). Psychologist attitudes toward DSM-5 and its alternatives. *Professional Psychology: Research and Practice*, *53*(6), 553.

Rice, C. E., Carpenter, L. A., Morrier, M. J., Lord, C., DiRienzo, M., Boan, A., Skowyra, C., Fusco, A., Baio, J., Esler, A., Zahorodny, W., Hobson, N., Mars, A., Thurm, A., Bishop, S., & Wiggins, L. D. (2022). Defining in detail and evaluating reliability of DSM-5 criteria for autism spectrum disorder (ASD) among children. *Journal of Autism and Developmental Disorders*, *52*(12), 5308–5320. https://doi.org/10.1007/s10803-021-05377-y

Rossler, W. (2016). The stigma of mental disorders. *EMBO Reports*, *17*(9), 1250–1253.

Tackett, J. L., Herzhoff, K., Reardon, K. W., Smack, A. J., & Kushner, S. C. (2013). The relevance of informant discrepancies for the assessment of adolescent personality pathology. *Clinical Psychology: Science and Practice*, *20*(4), 378–392.

Tanaka, G., Ogawa, T., Inadomi, H., Kikuchi, Y., & Ohta, Y. (2003). Effects of an educational program on public attitudes towards mental illness. *Psychiatry and Clinical Neurosciences*, *57*(6), 595–602.

Winerman, L. (2013). NIMH funding to shift away from DSM categories. *Monitor on Psychology, 44*(7). https://www.apa.org/monitor/2013/07-08/nimh

2 Overview of Common Mental Health Disorders

Research estimates that as many as one in five adults currently struggle with mental illness, which can include many different disorders and range in severity from mild to moderate to severe (NIMH, 2023a). This chapter gives a brief overview of some of the more frequently diagnosed mental health disorders. The diagnostic criteria offered throughout the chapter are based on the DSM-5-TR since that is the primary mental health diagnostic manual used in the U.S. Therefore, these diagnoses are intricately woven into our healthcare system as well as our basis for thinking about and understanding mental illness. The diagnostic criteria describe the symptoms of each disorder but do not discuss the etiology (origin, root cause) of these disorders.

The DSM describes various risk factors for mental health disorders including genetics (e.g., runs in families), temperament (e.g., childhood traits like anxiety), and environment (e.g., adverse childhood experiences). Nutritional psychology brings in a new approach that expands these risk factors to include the impact of nutritional deficiencies and gut dysfunctions as important factors as contributors to the root cause of these disorders.

It is helpful to have accepted terminology in the mental health field to categorize and discuss mental health issues in the population. Additionally, in this chapter, we discuss common mental health disorders to create a shared understanding so that when we discuss dynamics that positively or negatively impact mental health, we will have a frame of reference as to what is being helped or hurt. For example, if a research study says that eating more fruits and vegetables decreases symptoms of depression, you will have a shared understanding of what "symptoms of depression" refer to within context.

PREVALENCE OF MENTAL HEALTH DISORDERS

Current research estimates that 23 percent of U.S. adults have a mental illness, with the highest rates of that total (34 percent) found in young adults ages 18–25 (NIMH, 2023a; SAMHSA, 2024). Lower rates of mental disorders (about 17 percent) were found in children ages 5–17 (Zablotsky & Terlizzi, 2020). In the data collected on adults, two broad categories describe the level of impairment caused by a person's mental health symptoms: any mental illness (AMI) and serious mental illness (SMI). AMI includes all mental illnesses listed in the DSM. SMI is a subset of AMI and describes people with more severe mental health symptoms. Adults ages 18–25 accounted for the highest percentage of people struggling in both categories, AMI and SMI (see Figure 2.1).

Those with AMI and SMI are more vulnerable to major stressors, of which a pandemic certainly qualifies. A 2021 survey that asked about the impact of COVID-19 found that people with mental illness were more likely to report the pandemic negatively impacting their lives "quite a bit or a lot" compared to those with no mental illness who were more likely to respond they had been impacted "not at all" or "a little or some" (SAMHSA, 2022b). Those with SMI were especially hard hit and nearly half (48.9 percent) responded that COVID-19 had a significant negative impact on their lives compared to only 8.1 percent of people with no mental illness.

PREVALENCE BY DEMOGRAPHIC GROUP

Mental illness impacts some demographic groups more than others. For example, a person who identifies as American Indian or Mixed Ethnicity is more like to report a mental illness than

DOI: 10.1201/9781032647647-3

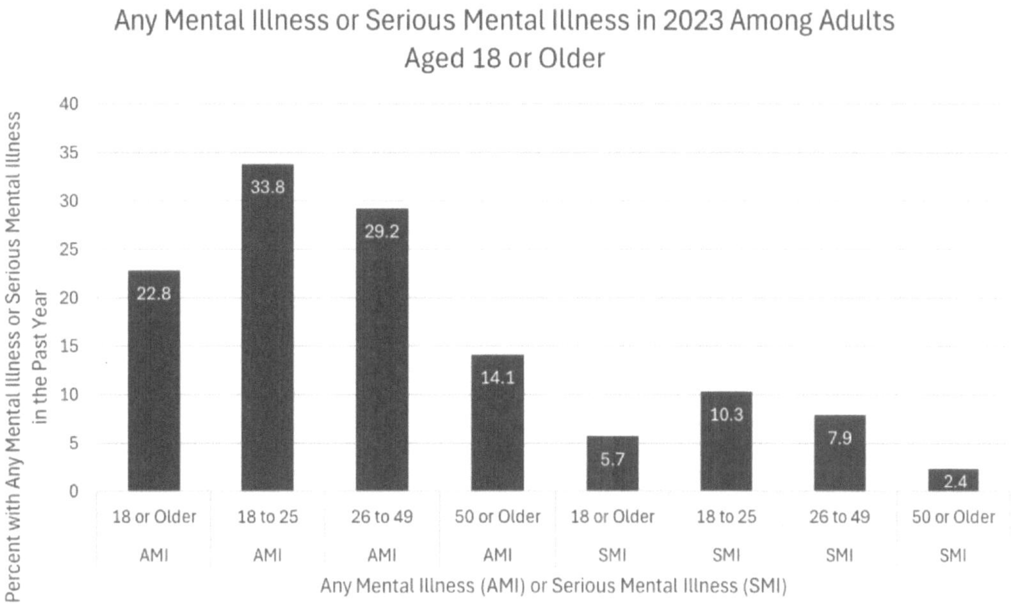

Any Mental Illness or Serious Mental Illness in 2023 Among Adults Aged 18 or Older

FIGURE 2.1   Any mental illness and serious mental illness among U.S. adults (SAMHSA, 2024). (Courtesy of the Substance Abuse and Mental Health Services Administration.)

someone who identifies as Asian, and a member of the LGBTQ community is much more likely to report a mental illness than a person who identifies as heterosexual (NAMI, 2023) (see Table 2.1).

There are objections in the mental health community that there is a lack of multicultural research in many of the diagnoses in the DSM. A multicultural perspective considers the impact of belonging to a cultural group that can include race, ethnicity, disability, sexual identity, age, and gender. Historically, clinical research has primarily used young white participants as the basis of developing mental health diagnoses, which did not recognize bias and the importance of different cultural experiences in how we respond to challenging situations. This potentially skewed perspective of normal human functioning shows up in many diagnoses. Of particular concern are diagnoses for personality disorders since they are founded on markedly deviating from the cultural expectations of who we should be and how we should act and are based on Western cultural values (Mulder, 2012). For example, the diagnosis of borderline personality disorder includes intense mood fluctuations, angry

TABLE 2.1

Annual Prevalence of Mental Illness among U.S. Adults by Demographic Group

Non-Hispanic Asian	16.4%
Non-Hispanic Native Hawaiian or Other Pacific Islander	18.1%
Non-Hispanic Black or African American	21.4%
Hispanic or Latino	20.7%
Non-Hispanic White	23.9%
Non-Hispanic American Indian or Alaska Native	26.6%
Non-Hispanic mixed/multiracial	34.9%
Lesbian, Gay, or Bisexual	50.2%

Source: SAMHSA (2022a, 2023). Courtesy of the Substance Abuse and Mental Health Services Administration.

outbursts, self-harm, fear of abandonment, and relationship challenges. Many theorists believe that gender and other cultural influences impact the development of these behaviors as coping strategies for feeling overwhelmed and disempowered. Frequently people diagnosed with borderline personality disorder have experienced adverse childhood experiences involving social inequalities like sexism, racism, and homophobia that can be causative to feeling powerless and marginalized, which makes their behaviors a more reasonable reaction to an unfair social situation rather than a psychological abnormality (Choudhary & Gupta, 2020).

PREVALENCE AMONG COLLEGE STUDENTS

Ongoing research shows college students are struggling with their mental health. According to the Healthy Minds Study, which collects data from 373 campuses nationwide, more than 60 percent of college students met diagnostic criteria for at least one mental health disorder in the 2020–2021 school year (Abrams, 2022). College counseling centers have been reporting large increases in demand over the last decade, with a high prevalence of eating disorders, compulsive disorders (including body dysmorphic disorder and obsessive-compulsive disorder), depression, posttraumatic stress disorder, and sleep disorders (Kang et al., 2021).

A long-term study of 190,000 college students in 180 college and university counseling centers identified mental health trends over the past decade (Center for Collegiate Mental Health, 2025). From 2013 to 2022, there were increased reports of concerns about anxiety and trauma, and decreased reports of concerns about relationship problems, with a rise and then fall of depression concerns before and after 2017 (see Figure 2.2). The trauma concerns were focused on childhood emotional abuse and a history of sexual violence more than current traumatic situations. Some of the increase in early trauma may be due to more openness and interest in this topic. Fortunately, students who stayed in school and did not drop out while they received counseling services generally experienced improvement across all areas of reported distress.

Untreated mental health disorders can have a devastating impact on individuals and their families. According to the World Health Organization (WHO), depression is the leading cause of disability worldwide, causing people to frequently call in sick to work and to miss out on time with friends and family due to their depressive symptoms (Friedrich, 2017). Anxiety is the sixth leading cause of disability and, like depression, affects more women than men.

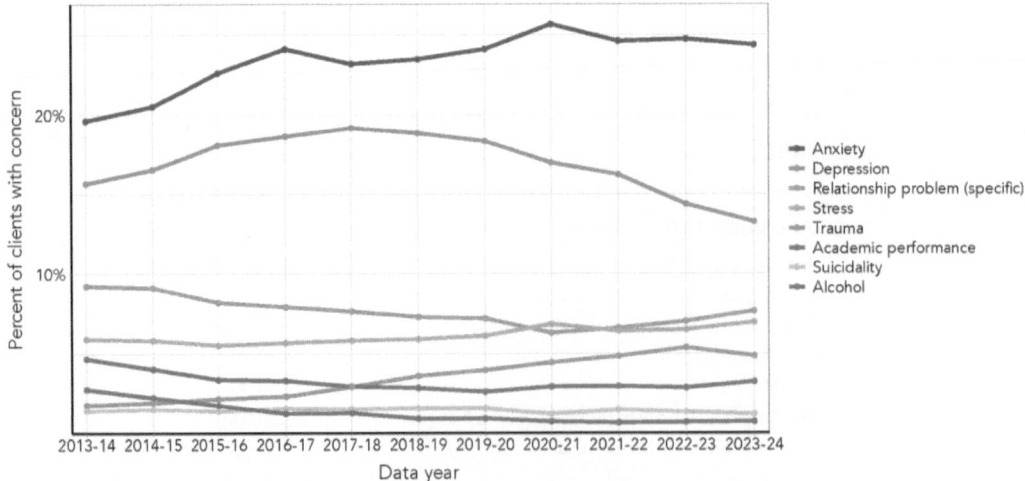

FIGURE 2.2 Top concern for college students in college counseling centers 2013–2024. (Courtesy of the Center for Collegiate Mental Health; Center for Collegiate Mental Health, 2025.)

Anxiety and depression are the most frequently diagnosed mental health disorders in the U.S. Annual estimates of the portion of U.S. adults diagnosed with some of the most prevalent psychiatric disorders are as follows (NAMI, 2023):

- Anxiety disorders: 19.1%
- Major depressive episode: 8.3%
- Posttraumatic stress disorder: 3.6%
- Bipolar disorder(: 2.8%
- Borderline personality disorder: 1.4%
- Obsessive compulsive disorder: 1.2%
- Schizophrenia: <1%

MOOD DISORDERS

Mood disorders primarily affect one's emotional state, and include intense feelings of fear, sadness, and anger. While there is a great deal of overlap of these strong emotions across different mood disorders, they are differentiated based on the predominant and most problematic emotions. It is important to remember that a person can receive more than one diagnosis at the same time, and that they may go through periods where one disorder is more distinct than the other. Anxiety and depression often go together and much of the mental health research includes these two mood disorders.

We now discuss three categories of mood disorders: anxiety disorders, depressive disorders, and bipolar disorders.

ANXIETY DISORDERS

Three of the most frequently diagnosed anxiety disorders are generalized anxiety disorder, social anxiety disorder, and obsessive-compulsive disorder. They all have fear as the primary characteristic, but the symptoms are expressed in different ways, which guide the treatment process.

The primary diagnostic criteria for *generalized anxiety disorder (GAD)* are at least six months of excessive uncontrollable worry about numerous matters which shows up as restlessness, fatigue, difficulty concentrating, irritability, muscle tension, and sleep issues. These symptoms cause significant distress and/or dysfunction in daily living(American Psychiatric Association, 2022). Around 4 percent of the U.S. population meet diagnostic criteria for GAD, the majority of whom are non-Hispanic white women (NIMH, 2023a).

While GAD is expressed as general fear about most things, *social anxiety disorder* is focused on fear related to interactions with other people. Clients report a pattern of tremendous fear of being criticized in social situations and therefore end up avoiding social situations due to their intense fears. The person's fears are out of proportion to the actual situation and usually include perceiving oneself as performing worse than is perceived by others. This can include speaking to people socially, eating in front of others, and performing poorly at work. Many people hide their fears by withdrawing when interacting with people in social situations which others sometimes interpret as lack of interest, snobbery, or hostility (Comer & Comer, 2024).

Of Note . . . SOCIAL MEDIA CAN EXACERBATE SOCIAL ANXIETY

Increasing data shows that social media can increase social anxiety and feelings of insecurity. There is intense pressure to post images that make you look good with the constant pull that those images will increase your popularity. We all want to be liked and admired. Yet social media also brings fears that someone else will post unflattering information or images about you, or that you will be ridiculed, criticized, or excluded from a social group. Research shows that many people feel worse about themselves after spending time on social media, often comparing themselves to others and finding themselves less capable and less interesting, which leads to feelings of envy toward others and dissatisfaction with ourselves (Abi-Jaoude et al., 2020).

Frequent and debilitating obsessions and compulsions are the primary focus of *obsessive-compulsive disorder (OCD)*. *Obsessions* are "recurrent and persistent thoughts, urges, or images that are experienced as intrusive and unwanted" and compulsions are "repetitive behaviors or mental acts that an individual feels driven to perform in response to an obsession or according to rules that must be applied rigidly" (American Psychiatric Association, 2013a, p. 235). *Compulsions* are an attempt to manage distressing obsessions by performing ritualized activities that help calm the fears associated with those obsessions.

Obsessions focus on a fear of germs (the most common), ordering and counting, and forbidden thoughts (e.g., an intense fear that you have become infected with a deadly disease and will either die or infect someone you love). Compulsions include hand washing, cleaning, checking, and counting. You can see how a natural reaction to feeling fear that you have been infected by germs is the desire to wash your hands. Due to the intensity and unremitting pressure of the fear and obsession about germs, someone with OCD can end up washing their hands for hours each day trying to calm themselves down to the point of making the skin on their hands red and raw from so much washing. To meet diagnostic criteria, the obsessions and compulsions must be time-consuming and cause significant distress or dysfunction in fulfilling their social and occupational responsibilities. Often clients have insight about their disorder and recognize that their obsessions are probably not true and that their compulsions are unnecessary and even a waste of time, yet they feel compelled to continue the behaviors during times of stress as their only means of managing the distress caused by their irrational obsessions.

DEPRESSIVE DISORDERS

We all have periods of feeling down, sad, unmotivated, and fatigued. Yet there is a difference between the colloquial use of the term depressed (e.g., "I got a B on the final exam. I am so depressed.") and the clinical use of the term. Clinical depression is longer lasting beyond an immediately stressful situation. Symptoms often include sadness, fatigue, poor concentration, and difficulty enjoying life (anhedonia). Clinical depression is also more severe in that it negatively impacts multiple areas of functioning: emotional, motivational, behavioral, cognitive, and physical. A person who is clinically depressed will often feel sad and hopeless, with little to no energy or inspiration to get even small things accomplished like bathing and interacting with family members. They often withdraw to a bedroom to be alone, unable to stay focused or to complete any meaningful tasks.

Major depressive disorder (MDD) is the most well-known diagnosis of depressive disorders. It is characterized by *depressive episodes*, which are distinct periods of at least two weeks (and often much longer) where there are clear changes in how a person feels, thinks, and functions (American Psychiatric Association, 2013a). A depressive episode primarily involves a person going from feeling pretty normal and functional to then having a depressed mood (sad, empty, hopeless) every day with a decreased interest in most activities. It can also include changes in appetite or weight (gaining or losing weight), sleeping too much or too little, agitation, fatigue, feeling worthless or guilty, poor concentration, and a repeated focus on death or suicide. Often insomnia (the inability to sleep as much as desired) and fatigue are the primary complaints that drive people to seek medical help. This is differentiated from grief or bereavement which focuses on feelings of emptiness and loss associated with the death of a loved one, and generally does not include the feelings of worthless-ness and self-loathing that are associated with depressive episodes. If the depressive episode does not lift over time and the symptoms are continuously present for at least two years, then the diagno-sis changes to *persistent depressive disorder (dysthymia).*

Premenstrual dysphoric disorder (PMDD) is a new diagnosis in the DSM-5. The diagnostic criteria require significant symptoms in the week before the onset of menses for the majority of menstrual cycles. Symptoms include mood swings, irritability, depressed mood, anxiety, anhedonia, poor concentration, lethargy, changes in appetite (overeating, food cravings) and sleep, overwhelm, and physical symptoms such as breast tenderness and bloating. The symptoms cause significant dis-tress and interfere with work, school, or relationships with others. This is a controversial diagnosis, with critics arguing that it pathologizes normal premenstrual discomfort as a psychiatric illness, and proponents arguing that it finally recognizes the distress felt by many women associated with their hormonal cycles and thereby expands support and treatment options (Hartlage et al., 2013).

BIPOLAR DISORDERS

Bipolar disorder (BD) was formerly known as manic-depressive disorder to describe someone with moods that swing from very high (manic) to very low (depressive). The word bipolar means two opposite poles, one high and one low. This is in contrast to depressive disorders (sometimes called unipolar depression) that only trend toward low mood with no periods of high mood. The key fea-ture of BD is the experience of at least one manic episode.

A *manic episode* is a period of at least one week of high mood with lots of energy that results in nonstop work or activity, a decreased need for sleep, racing thoughts, and talking fast. The epi-sode can come on over several days. When the mood is just starting to become elevated, known as hypomania, the feeling is very pleasurable. The person feels inspired, creative, and confident. Then as it progresses over multiple days with little to no sleep, the person feels more and more agitated and irritable, annoyed that other people cannot keep up or are trying to slow them down, and often drawn to involvement in high-risk behavior such as spending a lot of money and sexual infidel-ity. Unchecked, the manic episodes can lead to long-term impairment in social or occupational functioning.

BD is further differentiated into bipolar I and bipolar II. The two types of BDs primarily differ in the level of mania. A diagnosis of bipolar I requires the occurrence of at least one full manic episode. This is often followed by a depressive episode where the person collapses, exhausted, and feeling guilty and ashamed. Bipolar II is different from bipolar I in that it does not include a full manic episode and is more focused on depressive events. A person with bipolar II has had at least one hypomanic episode (a milder form of mania) and at least one depressive episode meet the diag-nostic criteria for this disorder.

TRAUMA-RELATED DISORDERS

Trauma-related disorders are diagnosed for people with symptoms that result from experiencing a life trauma, which is defined as a catastrophic or aversive event (American Psychiatric Association, 2013a). The threat can be to oneself or witnessing a violent or accidental event as it occurred to oth-ers. Complex or developmental trauma is exposure to multiple traumatic incidents over time such as childhood abuse versus a one-time event such as a hurricane.

BIG T AND LITTLE T

Trauma is sometimes categorized as *Big T* and *Little T* in the clinical world to describe different types of trauma experiences. A Big T trauma generally includes being exposed to war, a natural disaster, a serious car accident, physical or sexual abuse, and terrorism. Whereas Little T is used to describe an accumulation of less pronounced events that are not individually life-threatening. Little T events are more of a threat to our ego than our body and are experienced as overwhelming and disruptive. These include interpersonal conflict, infidelity, divorce, abruptly moving to a new home, legal trouble, and financial difficulties. These events are often overlooked by the individual and healthcare providers and dismissed as life challenges. However, over time, if a person does not have adequate support and coping skills, the grind of multiple or ongoing life challenges can add up and have a significant negative impact on a person's wellbeing (Barbash, 2017).

Our natural response to stress and traumatic situations is to activate our fight-or-flight response. (The fight-or-flight response will be discussed in more detail in Chapter 9.) When we are in fight-or-flight, our body is revved up and ready for action, which is a normal healthy response to smaller challenges or Little T events. The system is designed to handle an immediate threat that resolves relatively quickly. A person who suffers from a Big T event or multiple or ongoing Little T events can get stuck in this over-drive state, which is exhausting and leads to the body starting to break down due to the pressure. Many of the symptoms associated with PTSD are due to this over-activation of our emergency systems which leads to symptoms of over-arousal such as: hypervigilance (overly concerned with potential threats), reactivity (exaggerated startle response), poor sleep, poor concentration, and irritability. If the pressure continues beyond what can be handled in this high activation state, the body's systems become overwhelmed, and different coping mechanisms are initiated, such as withdrawal and dissociation.

DISSOCIATION

When a person becomes overwhelmed by a traumatic situation, an automatic coping mechanism that the brain sometimes uses is to detach from the situation mentally and emotionally. This can range from feeling slightly detached to a fully dissociative episode. *Dissociation* can include a distorted experience of the world. Typically, people feel like they are standing outside of themselves, watching their thoughts, feelings, and behaviors, like in a dream, or they feel okay or numb inside their own skin, but the world feels surreal, distant, and distorted.

When feeling detached a person might feel spaced out and unfocused, disconnected from others, with a loss of interest in previously enjoyed activities (anhedonia). A dissociative reaction includes gaps in memory where a person cannot later remember stressful moments or parts of traumatic events. Dissociation can become an ongoing coping function, where a person "checks out" when they become distressed, like during an argument where they become angry and irrational and then the next day cannot remember what they said or did during the argument. A dissociative episode also includes flashbacks, where a person is awake and completely loses awareness of their present surroundings, believing they are back in the middle of the traumatic event that they experienced (Wiginton, 2023).

Children respond to trauma in a variety of ways that are different from adults. Children often regress to behaviors that are expected for younger children but are not developmentally appropriate for older children. This can include bedwetting, thumb sucking, and tantrums. For example, trauma related irritability in children can look like angry outbursts, physical aggression, and extreme temper tantrums that are more intense than is developmentally appropriate or expected for their age. We are not surprised when a three-year-old throws themselves on the floor kicking and screaming. While we may not be happy about the behavior, it is developmentally normal for a child of this age to throw a tantrum. However, if a ten-year-old child displays the same behavior, we would be much more concerned since that is much less common.

POSTTRAUMATIC STRESS DISORDER

Posttraumatic stress disorder (PTSD) is the most commonly diagnosed trauma-related disorder. PTSD symptoms are the result of exposure to actual or threatened death, serious injury, or sexual violence. While it is normal to have a strong reaction to an upsetting event, not every reaction to a

TABLE 2.2

PTSD Symptom Categories

Exposure	Exposed to actual or threatened death or injury to self or others
Intrusive	Distressing memories, reminders of the event, nightmares, and flashbacks
Avoidance	Avoiding people, places, and thoughts associated with the event
Cognitions and mood	Inability to remember aspects of the event, frequent negative beliefs and emotions, anhedonia, detached from others, unable to feel happy
Arousal	Irritable, over-reactive, self-destructive behavior, poor concentration, difficulty sleeping

Source: Created by Andrea Cook.

traumatic event leads to PTSD. To meet the diagnostic criteria for PTSD, the client must experience significant distress or impairment due to symptoms that last more than one month after the event. Symptoms for PTSD cover five areas: exposure, intrusive, avoidance, cognitions and mood, and arousal (Table 2.2; American Psychiatric Association, 2022).

CASE STUDY: SURVIVING A FLOOD

Adrienne was 32 years old when the 100-year flood event struck their town. After an already wet winter, that freakish evening in February took things to a new level. The rain poured non-stop for hours while the wind ripped through the area, taking down trees and peeling open roof tops. In the middle of the night, the creek embankment behind Adrienne's house broke and her living room was filling with water. Adrienne decided to grab the kids and evacuate. Into the darkness they went. The power was out, and the water was rapidly rising. Fearing for their lives, she loaded the kids and their dog into their canoe, as she set off wading into the waste-deep water, and pulling the canoe, she followed the small beam of light from her flashlight out to the street and then up to higher ground.

It took over a year to repair their house from the flood damage and to replace their many destroyed belongings. Adrienne put on a brave face and tried to be calm and patient with her kids while organizing all the steps necessary to put their lives back together. During the day, she avoided talking about the flood with anybody, even though memories of that night were constantly replaying in her head. They had survived but so many things could have gone differently ending in even more disaster. Eventually, she avoided being around people as much as possible because she felt overwhelmed and unable to socialize. Her ability to talk about things that didn't matter to her diminished. She was tense and jumpy, and felt guilty for frequently losing her temper and shouting at her kids. While the days were hard, the nights were worse. Exhausted and desperate for rest, she often laid awake running through to-do lists, kept awake by waves of worry and guilt. When she did sleep, she was pummeled by nightmares about the flood and would awaken shaking and frightened. Adrienne felt like there was no end in sight, and life would never return to normal.

COMORBIDITY

Often there is overlap between mental health disorders where a person has symptoms that meet diagnostic criteria for more than one diagnosis, known as *comorbidity*. This does not imply that one causes the other, only that they exist at the same time in the same person. For example, someone who is both depressed and socially anxious might meet criteria for both and be diagnosed with comorbid MDD and social anxiety disorder.

Individuals with PTSD have a high comorbidity with other disorders, especially anxiety disorders, depressive disorders, BDs, and substance use disorders. For example, in addition to having PTSD symptoms of nightmares, avoiding reminders of the event, memory gaps about the event, and an increased startle response, a person may also have anxiety symptoms like restlessness, difficulty concentrating, irritability, and muscle tension. At the same time, they may also have depressive symptoms like sadness, fatigue, sleep issues, and anhedonia. Comorbid substance use issues are associated with PTSD, as people often turn to alcohol and other substances in an attempt to "self-medicate" and soothe their difficult and uncomfortable emotions and thoughts (American Psychiatric Association, 2013a).

Children with PTSD are at risk of acting out with anger and aggression because of their trauma experience which increases the likelihood of receiving a diagnosis of oppositional defiant disorder where they become extremely argumentative and angry, and regularly break rules. They might also go the other direction and withdraw and become insecure, which can develop into comorbid separation anxiety disorder where they feel extreme anxiety or panic when they are separated from their primary care givers.

Of Note ... DEFINING PSYCHOSIS

The term *psychosis* refers to a state where a person has some loss of contact with reality. This is referred to as a psychotic episode, during which there are changes in thoughts and perceptions, and often difficulty understanding what is real and what is not real (NIMH, n.d.-b). Psychotic symptoms include *delusions* and *hallucinations*, as well as incoherent speech and odd or inappropriate behavior. Delusions are false beliefs that are oftentimes paranoid or persecutory, focusing on the idea that people are talking about you and trying to harm you. Hallucinations are seeing or hearing things that other people do not see or hear, like hearing a voice that perhaps ties to a paranoid delusion and says things like, "Do you see how that person is looking at you? They hate you and want to kill you!" Psychotic episodes are often frightening and disruptive as the person struggles to make sense of what their mind is telling them while feeling confused and unable to explain or communicate their experience with others.

Psychosis can be a symptom of a diagnosis, such as with a diagnosis of MDD with psychotic features, where the primary symptoms are depressive and then the person's thinking at times becomes distorted to the point of being a delusion, such as "Everybody hates me and wishes I was dead." Or the psychosis can manifest into a full-blown psychotic disorder like schizophrenia, where the psychotic symptoms are the primary features of the overall presentation. In diagnosing psychosis, a clinician must rule out other possible causes for these symptoms, such as sleep deprivation, general medical conditions, side effects of certain prescription medications or combinations of medications, and the misuse of alcohol or other drugs.

The National Institute of Mental Health (NIMH) describes the following behavioral warnings signs of psychosis:

- Sudden drop in grades or job performance
- New trouble thinking clearly or concentrating
- Suspiciousness, paranoid ideas, or uneasiness with others
- Withdrawing socially, spending a lot more time alone than usual
- Unusual, overly intense new ideas, strange feelings, or no feelings at all

- Decline in self-care or personal hygiene
- Difficulty telling reality from fantasy
- Confused speech or trouble communicating

A person in a psychotic episode also may experience depression, anxiety, sleep problems, social withdrawal, lack of motivation, and difficulty functioning overall (NIMH, n.d.-b).

ADDICTIVE DISORDERS

How much is too much? Whether it is a substance, a behavior, or a food, what is the point at which when are engaging in too much or too often and it has become a problem? The term *addiction* can be defined as chronic use of a substance, behavior, or activity that has harmful physical, psychological, or social effects including uncomfortable or dangerous withdrawal symptoms and feeling out of control to stop using the substance or behavior. This describes changes in a person related to their continued use of a substance or behavior even though it is having a clearly harmful impact on their life.

The DSM-5 includes a new category of addiction that is not substance related called behavioral addiction. Gambling disorder is currently the only behavioral addiction disorder; however, internet gaming disorder is included for further study. This expansion describes shared characteristics in how people respond to addictive substances (e.g., alcohol) and addictive behaviors (e.g., gambling) in that they are consumed or participated in to excess due to intense activation of the brain reward system (feelings of pleasure, i.e., a "high") so that there is lowered self-control to the point where normal activities are neglected (American Psychiatric Association, 2013a). Addiction also includes *tolerance* where a person needs to consume increasing amounts of a substance or behavior over time to achieve the same pleasure/reward effect, and *dependence* where a person continues to consume a substance or perform a behavior even with conscious knowledge, some of which may include rationalization and/or recognition that the substance or behavior is in some way harmful to them.

A neuroscience approach to addiction recognizes that ongoing exposure to an addictive substance or behavior creates neuroadaptive changes in the brain that then contribute to maintaining the addictive behavior (Koob, 2012). Addiction can be seen as a chronically relapsing cycle that includes: cravings and a preoccupation with engaging in the addiction, loss of control in limiting intake, followed by a withdrawal or negative emotional state (e.g., dysphoria, anxiety, irritability). Elevated long-term substance use disrupts activity in multiple brain regions and circuits in ways that interfere with our ability to delay gratification. Each time an addictive substance is used the brain reward pathways are intensely activated in ways that change our ability to experience pleasure from less stimulating activities, which increases the risk of repeating the addictive cycle. For example, changes to the frontal region of the brain during cocaine use contribute to withdrawal symptoms that impact our ability to focus, remember, and think clearly, all of which impair our natural inhibitory control, which increases impulsivity and decreases our ability to delay gratification.

The DSM includes diagnoses for overuse of substances which include both legal and illegal substances. Substance-related disorders include abuse of alcohol, opioids (e.g., oxycontin and heroin), amphetamines, tobacco, and cannabis. Caffeine use disorder is listed in the DSM-5 under Conditions for Further Study, so it is not yet a diagnosis, however, the evidence is growing that caffeine can become a significant problem for some people where it contributes to a failure to fulfill obligations at work, home, or school, and increases irritability and related interpersonal problems (American Psychiatric Association, 2013b).

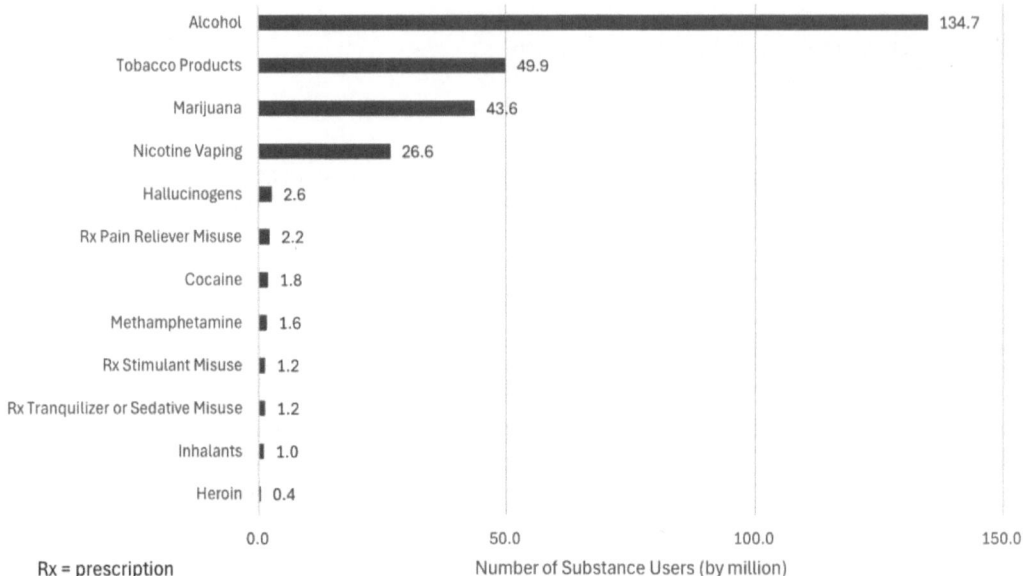

FIGURE 2.3 Substance use among people 12 or older. (Adapted from the results from the 2023 National Survey on Drug Use and Health; SAMHSA, 2024.)

PREVALENCE OF SUBSTANCE-RELATED DISORDERS

Substance-related addictions are abundant in the U.S., with alcohol and nicotine being the most frequently used substances (see Figure 2.3). Substance use disorders (SUDs) in the DSM include cannabis (marijuana), hallucinogens, inhalants, opioids, sedatives, stimulants, and tobacco. While caffeine is also a highly used substance and is included in the DSM as a potential SUD, it is generally not included in studies about substance abuse. The commonality among these disorders is that the substances are taken in excess and have direct activation of the brain reward system, which is involved in the reinforcement of behaviors that cause a person to neglect normal activities (American Psychiatric Association, 2022).

Similar to PTSD, people diagnosed with an SUD often have a comorbid diagnosis with another mental illness. In a 2021 national survey, of the 82.5 million adults who reported having either an SUD or any mental illness (AMI), almost a quarter of the participants (19.4 million) reported having both an SUD and an AMI (SAMHSA, 2022b). A history of physical or emotional trauma increases your risk of developing an SUD. "People with PTSD may use substances in an attempt to reduce their anxiety and to avoid dealing with trauma and its consequences" (NIDA, n.d., p. 8). Also, the use of one substance increases your risk of polysubstance use, where a person has comorbid SUDs for different substances. For example, among people with a cocaine use disorder nearly 60 percent also have an alcohol use disorder, approximately 48 percent are dependent on nicotine, and over 21 percent have a marijuana use disorder.

FOOD ADDICTION

There are growing arguments that some foods, in addition to caffeine, should be included in discussions about addiction. When we define addiction based on predictable reactions in the brain reward center, such as similarities between the effect of alcohol consumption and gambling, there is room to consider that some people go through comparable addictive cycles with certain foods, namely sugar, baked goods, and ultra-processed foods (Lustig, 2021). Push back against this line of thinking argues that food is different from other substances and behaviors because it is necessary for survival. The counterargument is that sugar and ultra-processed foods are different than whole foods because of the high level of processing. The processing chemically alters them from what is found in nature and impacts how they are utilized in the body, much the same way heroin is produced by processing the Asian poppy plant, which in its natural whole plant form is not addictive. From that perspective, ultra-processed foods can have a negative long-term effect on some people and their consumption is not necessary for survival. This topic is discussed further in Chapter 13.

OTHER MENTAL HEALTH DISORDERS

PERSONALITY DISORDERS

Personality disorders (PDs) are a group of diagnoses focused on rigid patterns of maladaptive thinking and behavior that repeats over time and in multiple relationships. Some of the most well-recognized PDs are borderline personality disorder (BPD) (big mood swings, fear of abandonment), narcissistic PD (strong desire for admiration and energy exchange), obsessive-compulsive personality disorder (OCPD) (rigidly focused on order, control, and perfection), and antisocial personality disorder (ASPD) (disregard for the rights of others). People with a PD often focus intensely on their own experience which impairs their capacity for empathy toward others and limits their ability to maintain any kind of intimacy (NIMH, 2023b).

People with a PD have a personality style that tends to be more extreme and dysfunctional than most other people, with a tendency to blame others for their unhappiness, known as *externalizing*. Externalizing behavior is really a problem because they are so focused on what others are doing wrong that it distracts them from taking any accountability and leaves them unaware of their own inappropriate behavior, thereby creating situations where people are constantly angry at them. They are not sure why everybody is always angry at them, which leads to distress and either withdrawing and shutting down or becoming defensive and angry themselves. They often form habitual thinking and react in ways that other people find offensive, all while being unable to change their ways. The hallmark of PDs is relationship issues, with impairments in social, occupational, and other areas of functioning where they have interactions with people (American Psychiatric Association, 2013a).

Research indicates that about 15 percent of U.S. adults have at least one PD, and many meet the criteria for more than one PD (American Psychiatric Association, 2013a). Patients with PDs are often seen in the healthcare system due to their chronic feelings of distress and dissatisfaction and their high comorbidity with other mental health disorders. They can be difficult patients, often quarreling with their doctor or therapist. PDs are not diagnosed in children, since they are still in the process of developing their personality.

NEUROCOGNITIVE DISORDERS

Neurocognitive disorders (NCDs) focus on cognitive deficits due to a number of different causes (known as etiologies) including Alzheimer's disease, traumatic brain injury, substance/medication-induced, and Parkinson's disease. NCDs, sometimes referred to as dementia, are unique among DSM diagnoses in that these are syndromes with some understanding of the underlying pathology like a disease or brain injury. With NCDs, the core features are deficits in cognitive functioning that are acquired as an adult rather than part of a childhood disorder and include disturbances such as difficulty focusing, making decisions, learning, and memory loss that impair independent functioning (American Psychiatric Association, 2022).

DISORDERS COMMON FOR CHILDREN AND ADOLESCENTS

Neurodevelopmental disorders such as attention-deficit/hyperactivity disorder (ADHD) and autism spectrum disorder (ASD) are the most frequent diagnoses in children and adolescents. Symptoms begin during childhood, often co-occur with intellectual disability or learning disorders, and may impact lifelong functioning. These disorders often result in impairment in personal, social, academic, and occupational functioning. Symptoms can include hyperactivity, impulsivity, inappropriate social behavior, and rigid maintenance of routines.

Children and adolescents tend to fall into two different ways of expressing discomfort and overwhelm. Some tend to *externalize* so that they get more active, bigger, louder, and more aggressive when they are distressed (which overlaps with how the word externalize is used with PDs). Others tend to *internalize* where they withdraw, get quiet, and turn toward self-harm behaviors when they are feeling overwhelmed. Along gender lines, those who identify as male tend more toward externalizing behavior including impulsivity, aggressiveness, hyperactivity, low frustration tolerance, and inattention (Cicchetti & Handley, 2019). Those who identify as female tend more toward internalizing behavior including depression, low self-esteem, helplessness, anxiety, and being overly self-critical and self-controlling (Liu et al., 2011). Those with externalizing tendencies are more at risk for disorders focused on impulsivity and aggression while those with internalizing tendencies are more at risk for disorders focused on social isolation and self-harm behaviors. This helps explain why the juvenile hall population are predominantly male, with estimates of the breakdown at 85 percent male and 15 percent female (Hockenberry, 2022).

DISRUPTIVE DISORDERS

Disruptive disorders focus on problems with self-control of emotions and behaviors. Poorly controlled anger and repeated behavior that violates the rights of others (e.g., destruction of property and bullying) are the foundation of these disorders. The two primary diagnoses in this category are *oppositional defiant disorder (ODD)* and *conduct disorder (CD)*. ODD includes angry irritable mood, argumentative, defiant behavior that is negatively impacting their social relationships and educational functioning. People with ODD often have comorbid ADHD and are at increased risk of anxiety, depressive, and substance use disorders. ODD symptoms tend to be less severe and dysfunctional than CD symptoms.

CD is a pattern of behavior where the basic rights of others or societal rules are violated. Diagnostic criteria include aggressive behaviors including bullying, physical fights, using a weapon, being cruel to people or animals, deliberately destroying property, theft, and serious violation of rules such as running away from home and being truant from school. This is the most prevalent diagnosis for youth in the juvenile justice system and is often seen as a precursor to an adult diagnosis of antisocial PD. It is important to keep in mind that these youth often have lives filled with chaos including dysfunctional families, abuse, and neglect. Sometimes the child runs away from home and steals to escape an abusive parent which can start them down a path with the justice system that is difficult to redirect.

FOOD FOR THOUGHT: SUICIDE AND MENTAL HEALTH

Suicide is defined by the National Institute of Mental Health (NIMH) as "death caused by self-directed injurious behavior with intent to die as a result of the behavior" (NIMH, 2023c). NIMH goes on to describe a *suicide attempt* as a non-fatal, self-directed, potentially injurious behavior with intent to die as a result of the behavior" that may or may not result in injury. In addition, the term to describe when a person is thinking about, considering, or planning suicide is *suicidal ideation*.

According to the Centers for Disease Control and Prevention (CDC), suicide is one of the leading causes of death in the U.S. In 2021, suicide was among the top nine leading causes of death for people ages 10–64, and the second leading cause of death for people ages 10–14 and 20–34. Between 2000 and 2021, suicide rates increased 36 percent. Over 48,000 people died by suicide in 2021, which is approximately one death every 11 minutes. Rates of suicide are disproportionately high in some racial/ethnic groups, with the highest rates in non-Hispanic American Indian and Alaska Native people and non-Hispanic White people. Males are approximately four times more likely to die by suicide than females. Males make up 50 percent of the population but nearly 80 percent of suicides. By age, suicide is highest for people 75 and older, followed by adults aged 25–34. Firearms are the most frequently used method in suicides and makeup over half of all suicide deaths (CDC, 2023a).

Suicidal thoughts and behaviors are quite ubiquitous. Many people think about, plan, and attempt suicide without dying. According to the CDC, in 2021, 12.3 million adults seriously thought about suicide, 3.5 million adults made a plan, and 1.7 million adults attempted suicide (CDC, 2023a). Young people in the LGBTQ+ community are at particularly high risk of attempting suicide. Estimates show that lesbian, gay, and bisexual youth are almost four times more likely to attempt suicide than their heterosexual peers (CDC, 2023b), and transgender adults are nearly nine times more likely to attempt suicide at some point in their lifetime compared to the general population (James et al., 2016). A prior suicide attempt is an important indicator that increases the likelihood of another suicide attempt and death by suicide (CDC, 2022).

Almost half of people who die by suicide have a diagnosed mental health condition (CDC, 2018). Suicidal thoughts and behaviors are more frequently associated with certain psychiatric disorders. Most notably, people diagnosed with depression, substance use, and psychosis are at the highest risk, especially those taking antidepressant medication. Other mental illness associated with a higher risk of attempting suicide are anxiety, personality, eating, and trauma-related disorders (Bachmann, 2018; Hengartner & Plöderl, 2019; Klein & Attia, 2017; Moutier, 2023; Yen et al., 2021).

For many people, suicide is preventable. Improving access to mental healthcare and suicide support services is a key first step toward suicide prevention. As part of this essential support, other important factors are increasing access to substance abuse programs, stabilizing housing, increasing symptoms and signs awareness in families, schools, communities, and healthcare settings, teaching coping and problem-solving skills, and promoting healthy social connections (Bachmann, 2018; CDC, 2022; Kiran et al., 2024). Also important is blocking access to high-risk means of suicide, such as medications, firearms, and bridges. For example, the Golden Gate Bridge in San Francisco has constructed a suicide deterrent system (known as the safety net) that has decreased the number of suicides from people jumping off the bridge (Rosenheim, 2023).

Please remember that if you or someone you know is having frequent thoughts about suicide, help is available, and it is possible to feel better with the appropriate care. Feeling suicidal is a treatable condition for most people. It is important to ask for help. The National Suicide Prevention Lifeline is available in the U.S. at 1-800-273-8255 or you can dial the 988 Suicide & Crisis Lifeline for free and confidential crisis support 24/7/365.

REFERENCES

Abi-Jaoude, E., Naylor, K. T., & Pignatiello, A. (2020). Smartphones, social media use and youth mental health. *Canadian Medical Association Journal*, *192*(6), E136–E141.

Abrams, Z. (2022). Student mental health is in crisis. Campuses are rethinking their approach. *Monitor on Psychology*, *53*(7). https://www.apa.org/monitor/2022/10/mental-health-campus-care

American Psychiatric Association. (2013a). *Diagnostic and statistical manual of mental disorders: DSM-5* (5th ed.). American Psychiatric Association. http://dsm.psychiatryonline.org/doi/book/10.1176/appi.books.9780890425596

American Psychiatric Association. (2013b). *DSM-5 fact sheets*. https://www.psychiatry.org/psychiatrists/practice/dsm/educational-resources/dsm-5-fact-sheets

American Psychiatric Association (2022). *Diagnostic and statistical manual of mental disorders: DSM-5-TR* (5th ed., text rev. ed.). American Psychiatric Association Publishing.

Bachmann, S. (2018). Epidemiology of suicide and the psychiatric perspective. *International Journal of Environmental Research and Public Health, 15*(7), 1425.

Barbash, E. (2017). Different types of trauma: Small 't' versus large 'T'. *Psychology Today.* https://www.psychologytoday.com/us/blog/trauma-and-hope/201703/different-types-trauma-small-t-versus-large-t

CDC. (2018). *Vital signs: Suicide rising across the US.* Centers for Disease Control and Prevention.. https://www.cdc.gov/vitalsigns/suicide/

CDC. (2022). *Suicide prevention: Risk and protective factors for suicide.* Centers for Disease Control and Prevention. https://www.cdc.gov/suicide/risk-factors/index.html

CDC. (2023a). *Suicide data and statistics.* Centers for Disease Control and Prevention. https://www.cdc.gov/suicide/facts/data.html

CDC. (2023b). *Youth risk behavior survey data summary and trends report: 2011-2021.* Centers for Disease Control and Prevention. https://www.cdc.gov/healthyyouth/data/yrbs/pdf/YRBS_Data-Summary-Trends_Report2023_508.pdf

Center for Collegiate Mental Health. (2025). *2024 Annual report.* https://ccmh.psu.edu/annual-reports

Choudhary, S., & Gupta, R. (2020). Culture and borderline personality disorder in India, *Frontiers in Psychology, 11,* 714. https://doi.org/10.3389/fpsyg.2020.00714

Cicchetti, D., & Handley, E. D. (2019). Child maltreatment and the development of substance use and disorder. *Neurobiology of Stress, 10,* 100144.

Comer, R. J., & Comer, J. S. (2024). *Psychopathology: Science and practice* (12th ed.). Worth Publishers.

Friedrich, M. J. (2017). Depression is the leading cause of disability around the world. *The Journal of the American Medical Association, 317*(15), 1517.

Hartlage, S. A., Breaux, C. A., & Yonkers, K. A. (2013). Addressing concerns about the inclusion of premenstrual dysphoric disorder in DSM-5. *The Journal of Clinical Psychiatry, 74*(1), 415.

Hengartner, M. P., & Plöderl, M. (2019). Newer-generation antidepressants and suicide risk in randomized controlled trials: A re-analysis of the FDA database. *Psychotherapy and Psychosomatics, 88*(4), 247–248. https://doi.org/10.1159/000501215

Hockenberry, S. (2022). *Juveniles in residential placement, 2019.* U.S. Department of Justice. https://ojjdp.ojp.gov/publications/juveniles-in-residential-placement-2019.pdf

James, S. E., Herman, J. L., Rankin, S., Keisling, M., Mottet, L., & Anafi, M. (2016). *The report of the 2015 U.S. transgender survey.* National Center for Transgender Equality. https://transequality.org/sites/default/files/docs/usts/USTS-Full-Report-Dec17.pdf

Kang, H. K., Rhodes, C., Rivers, E., Thornton, C. P., & Rodney, T. (2021). Prevalence of mental health disorders among undergraduate university students in the United States: A review. *Journal of Psychosocial Nursing and Mental Health Services, 59*(2), 17–24.

Kiran, T., Angelakis, I., Panagioti, M., Irshad, S., Sattar, R., Hidayatullah, S., Tyler, N., Tofique, S., Bukhsh, A., Eylem-van Bergeijk, O., Özen-Dursun, B., Husain, N., Chaudhry, N., & Hodkinson, A. (2024). Controlled interventions to improve suicide prevention in educational settings: A systematic review and network meta-analysis. *Clinical Psychology: Science and Practice, 31*(1), 85–93. https://doi.org/10.1037/cps0000179

Klein, D., & Attia, E. (2017). Anorexia nervosa in adults: Clinical features, course of illness, assessment, and diagnosis. *UpToDate.* https://www.uptodate.com/contents/anorexia-nervosa-in-adults-clinical-features-course-of-illness-assessment-and-diagnosis

Koob, G. F. (2012). Neuroanatomy of addiction. In K. D. Brownell & M. S. Gold (Eds.), *Food and addiction: A comprehensive handbook.* Oxford University Press.

Liu, J., Chen, X., & Lewis, G. (2011). Childhood internalizing behaviour: Analysis and implications. *Journal of Psychiatric and Mental Health Nursing, 18*(10), 884–894. https://doi.org/10.1111/j.1365-2850.2011.01743.x

Lustig, R. H. (2021). *Metabolical: The lure and the lies of processed food, nutrition, and modern medicine.* HarperWave.

Merriam-Webster Dictionary. (2023). *Addiction.* https://www.merriam-webster.com/dictionary/addiction

Moutier, C. (2023). *Suicidal behavior.* Merck Manuals. https://www.merckmanuals.com/professional/psychiatric-disorders/suicidal-behavior-and-self-injury/suicidal-behavior#v82347620

Mulder, R. T. (2012). Cultural aspects of personality disorder. In T. A. Widiger (Ed.), *The Oxford handbook of personality disorders* (pp. 260–274). Oxford University Press. https://doi.org/10.1093/oxfordhb/9780199735013.013.0013

NAMI. (2023). *Mental health by the numbers.* National Alliance on Mental Illness. https://nami.org/mhstats#card6

NIDA. (n.d.). *Why do substance use problems often occur along with other mental disorders?* National Institute on Drug Abuse. Retrieved December 19, 2024 from https://nida.nih.gov/research-topics/co-occurring-disorders-health-conditions#problems-occur

NIMH. (n.d.-a). *Mental health information: Statistics.* https://www.nimh.nih.gov/health/statistics

NIMH. (n.d.-b). *Understanding psychosis (NIH publication no. 20-MH-8110).* National Institute of Mental Health. https://www.nimh.nih.gov/health/publications/understanding-psychosis

NIMH. (2023a). *Mental illness.* National Institute of Mental Health. https://www.nimh.nih.gov/health/statistics/mental-illness

NIMH (2023b). *Personality disorders.* National Institute of Mental Health.

NIMH. (2023c). *Suicide.* National Institute of Mental Health. https://www.nimh.nih.gov/health/statistics/suicide

Rosenheim, J. (2023). *Decrease in golden gate bridge suicide jumps likely a result of prevention barrier.* CBS News Bay Area. https://www.cbsnews.com/sanfrancisco/news/decrease-in-golden-gate-bridge-suicide-jumps-likely-a-result-of-prevention-barrier/

SAMHSA. (2022a). *2020 National survey on drug use and health: Lesbian, gay, or bisexual (LGB) adults.* https://www.samhsa.gov/data/sites/default/files/reports/rpt37929/2020NSDUHLGBSlides072522.pdf

SAMHSA. (2022b). Key substance use and mental health indicators in the United States: Results from the 2021 National Survey on Drug Use and Health (PEP22-07-01-005, NSDUH Series H-57). Center for Behavioral Health Statistics and Quality, Substance Abuse and Mental Health Services Administration. https://www.samhsa.gov/data/

SAMHSA. (2023). *2021 NSDUH detailed tables.*https://www.samhsa.gov/data/report/2021-nsduh-detailed-tables

SAMHSA. (2024). *Key substance use and mental health indicators in the United States: Results from the 2023 National Survey on Drug Use and Health (HHS Publication No. PEP24-07-021, NSDUH Series H-59).* Center for Behavioral Health Statistics and Quality, Substance Abuse and Mental Health Services Administration. https://www.samhsa.gov/data/report/2023-nsduh-annual-national-report

Wiginton, K. (2023). *What is dissociation?* https://www.webmd.com/mental-health/dissociation-overview

Yen, S., Peters, J. R., Nishar, S., Grilo, C. M., Sanislow, C. A., Shea, M. T., Zanarini, M. C., McGlashan, T. H., Morey, L. C., & Skodol, A. E. (2021). Association of borderline personality disorder criteria with suicide attempts: Findings from the collaborative longitudinal study of personality disorders over 10 years of follow-up. *JAMA Psychiatry, 78*(2), 187–194. https://doi.org/10.1001/jamapsychiatry.2020.3598

Zablotsky, B., & Terlizzi, E. P. (2020). *Mental health treatment among children aged 5–17 years: United States, 2019.* Centers for Disease Control and Prevention (CDC), National Center for Health Statistics. https://www.cdc.gov/nchs/products/databriefs/db381.htm#ref1

3 Mental Health Treatment as Usual

Treatment of mental health disorders has traversed an evolution of varied theories and models. To fully understand the many twists and turns of our current mental healthcare system it helps to know the context within which these theories were formed. Mental healthcare is part of a healthcare system that has changed over time offering new treatment options guided by emerging research that enables viewing health from different perspectives.

CHANGES IN HEALTHCARE

One of the key factors that has changed the healthcare system has been the shift in the primary cause of death over the last century. In the early 1900s, most adults died from either traumatic injury or infectious diseases such as pneumonia and tuberculosis. As the field of medicine grew, it made huge strides in reversing these life-threatening events. By the 1950s, following the development of antibiotics, the tables were beginning to turn (Penn Wharton, 2016). Traumatic injuries were treated by setting broken bones and sewing up torn soft tissue. Infectious diseases (including potential infections associated with surgery) were treated by identifying the problematic pathogen, be it bacteria, virus, fungi, or parasite, and administering a medication targeted to kill that specific pathogen while hopefully not damaging the body in the process. With the invention of antibiotics, anti-fungal, and anti-parasitic medications, doctors were able to effectively treat many known diseases of the time with tremendous success. Thus, a shift occurred in the healthcare system, as more adults recovered from injuries and infections and went on to live for several more decades before dying of a different type of disease.

Chronic disease became the leading cause of death in the U.S. Mortality rates decreased for infectious diseases and increased for chronic diseases such as heart disease, cancer, stroke, Alzheimer's disease, and diabetes mellitus. The impact of lifestyle has become an increasing area of interest and a growing area in determining a person's long-term health and quality of life. Smoking, obesity, chronic insomnia, environmental toxins, and a sedentary lifestyle all began to be identified as major contributors to the likelihood of developing a chronic disease over an expanded lifespan, while still leading to diseases that could eventually kill you. Still more difficult in determining the impact of lifestyle on disease, was the fact that often these diseases began quietly with symptoms that most people cannot feel, so that without medical tests, the body has been damaged, sometimes by more than one disease, by the time a person feels any physical discomfort (Brannon et al., 2022; Kochanek et al., 2019).

The healthcare system has been slow to recognize how whole-body health and multiple-body systems become affected during this decline and conventional (allopathic) medicine often still approaches illness from an infectious disease model, focused on one primary cause of disease. Practitioners develop a diagnosis and then look for a medication to treat that diagnosis. Unfortunately, chronic disease is a complicated affair that requires a dynamic, multi-faceted approach to care and is not generally solved by taking a pill. The concept of a "pill for every ill" usually does not work for these types of diseases (Busfield, 2010).

A MEDICATION APPROACH TO MENTAL HEALTH TREATMENT

Mental illness falls into the camp of chronic disease in that it can last a lifetime with no clear pathogen (e.g., bacteria or virus) that causes the disease. Here too, the current trend is to make a diagnosis and prescribe a medication. With mental illness, there are no labs to run, no blood tests to take, to

 DOI: 10.1201/9781032647647-4

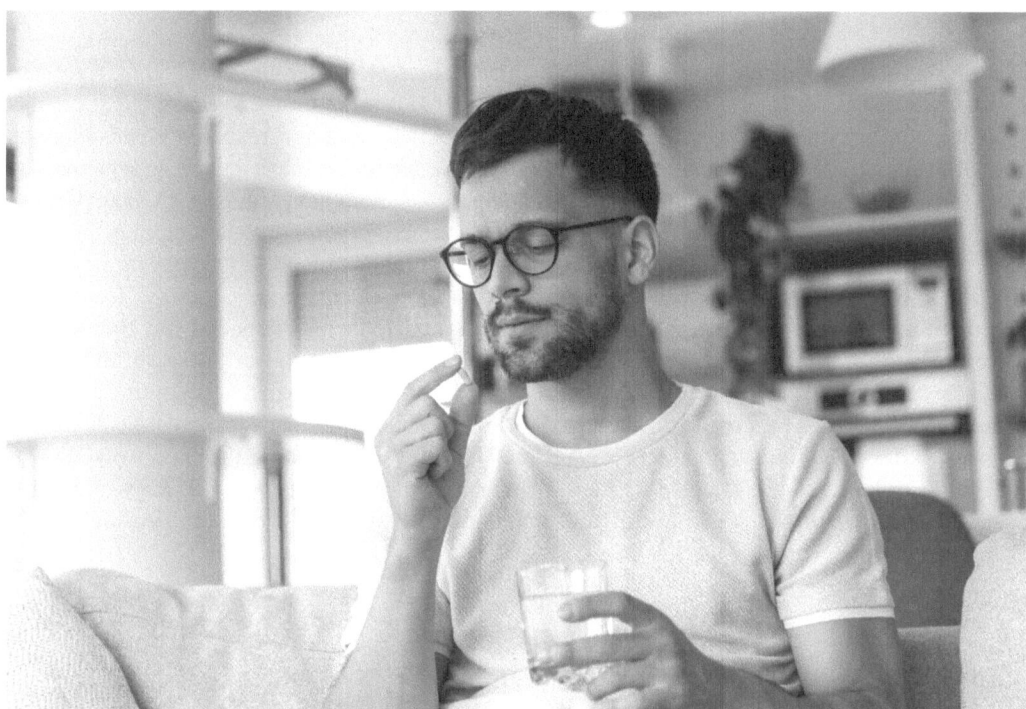

FIGURE 3.1 Man feeling concerned about taking psychotropic medication for his mental illness. Credit: Photoroyalty (Shutterstock).

determine a diagnosis, so we rely on interviewing patients to hear about their symptoms to determine a DSM diagnosis. Sometimes this includes a thorough evaluation by a mental health practitioner over several appointments, but not always. Medication is often the first-line treatment, which has raised concerns about patients being over-medicated without a clear diagnosis or follow-up to ensure the medication is working as expected during long-term use (Maust et al., 2017; Mojtabai & Olfson, 2011; Pagaduan, 2021; Safer, 2019).

The trend to quickly diagnose and medicate increased with the publication of the DSM-5 in 2013. This brought about criticism in the field that the DSM was written by psychiatrists with a financial stake in psychotropic medication and thereby a conflict of interest that caused the DSM-5 to over-emphasize the benefit of psychotropic medications to treat mental health disorders (Ericson, 2014). Many are concerned that well-meaning doctors are being overly influenced by the pharmaceutical corporations that develop the drugs to quickly prescribe medication without a thorough diagnosis and in a system that provides poor ongoing assessment and follow-up services to make sure the drugs are doing their job and helping people (Lembke, 2016).

PERSPECTIVES ON CAUSE OF MENTAL ILLNESS

There are many theories about the cause of mental illness characterized by varying facets depending on the type of mental illness, its origin, and the severity of the symptoms. How do you compare a person who is depressed and sleeps a lot to a person with obsessive-compulsive disorder who is having a hard time slowing down? What do those behaviors have in common and what makes the symptoms get worse or better? Human beings are complex beings with numerous factors that affect our wellbeing, including social connection, financial challenges, traumatic experiences, environmental toxins, family influences, and genetic vulnerabilities, which have been broadly grouped into the psychogenic perspective and the somatogenic perspective (Comer & Comer, 2024).

PSYCHOGENIC PERSPECTIVE

The *psychogenic perspective* focuses of psychological causes of mental illness including early family experiences, social factors, and trauma. Treatment protocols from this perspective might examine
thoughts, behaviors, and emotions to understand how and why a person responds to stressors with
mental health symptoms. Examination of past experiences often reveals ways that a person has become
stuck in certain ways of thinking and behaving that makes situations worse and causes them pain.

Learning new skills to better manage stress and to communicate more clearly often helps clients
to develop improved coping mechanisms so that they can function more effectively. For example,
if a person with depressive tendencies has not learned how to set good limits, they can feel helpless
and taken advantage of by other people. A therapist might help them understand why they struggle
to speak openly with their supervisor to set a limit such as declining to work overtime at their job
when they have other commitments. Perhaps the client has a history of a parent becoming angry and
critical of them for not wanting to do extra work beyond their share, so they learned (unconsciously)
to just shut down, go limp and become exhausted (i.e., depressed) to avoid the extra work. Now as
an adult with an employer, this same pattern of shutting down is their coping strategy rather than
speaking up and telling their employer that they do not want to work overtime and it should not be
demanded of them.

Of Note . . . SHAME AND ANGER

Two emotions often reveal themselves as powerful drivers of behavior: shame and anger. *Shame*
has been defined as, "The intensely painful feeling or experience of believing that we are flawed
and therefore unworthy of love and belonging" (Brown, 2012, p. 68). Shame is different from
guilt. With guilt, the focus is on a behavior and the idea that "I did something bad." With
shame, it defines you as a person with the belief that "I am bad" (Miceli & Castelfranchi, 2018).

Most clinicians agree that shame is neither helpful nor productive because it feeds our fear
of rejection and often becomes the source of destructive or hurtful behavior. Shame is a universal experience on a broad range of topics including appearance, money, parenting, physical
and mental health, addiction, sex, aging, and surviving a trauma. Psychotherapy often works
with clients to recognize unhelpful feelings of shame to move toward self-acceptance and self-
forgiveness; to differentiate that they can be unhappy about aspects of their life (guilt) without
the heavy verdict that, because of those aspects, they are therefore unlovable. That we are all
a work in progress, constantly learning and growing.

Shame therapist Jane Pennington (2015) uses a clever acronym for shame that reminds us
of the common misconception that it is not okay to make mistakes: SHAME = Should Have
Already Mastered Everything (Table 3.1). When we can embrace the universal truth that we
all make mistakes and are still good people even with those mistakes, it helps us feel closer
to humanity and to fully accept and like ourselves, even with all of our flaws.

TABLE 3.1
SHAME – Should Have Already Mastered Everything

S hould
H ave
A lready
M astered
E verything

The emotion of *anger* is another powerful feeling that people often struggle with. People often live in the extremes around anger, either feeling angry all of the time or feeling that anger is a bad emotion to be avoided. In the field of psychotherapy, emotions are respected as information and impulses to act, which are useful functions. Anger serves a protective function in that we are activated to change an unhealthy situation, to solve a problem, to protect ourselves from being hurt by others, or even to recognize our own contribution to creating or maintaining what is not working in our lives.

Anger is often referred to as a *secondary emotion* in response to a threat. We resort to anger to protect ourselves from vulnerable primary feelings like fear or hurt. At first, we feel afraid, attacked, offended, frustrated, disrespected, forced, trapped, or pressured. Even if we are not fully aware of these underlying feelings, we instinctually respond with anger as our mind and body gears up for a fight in our own defense. Developed by John and Julie Gottman, pioneers in couples therapy training, an *anger iceberg* (see Figure 3.2) is a metaphor often used to describe anger, where the emotion being expressed is anger (above the water line), but the driver or root of that anger is fear and hurt (below the water line) (The Gottman Institute, 2023).

Learning to recognize anger as a basic, valid emotion that serves an important purpose often helps people to be less afraid of that emotion. An important feature of psychotherapy is to help clients learn to see past the anger to the underlying feelings like hurt and rejection in themselves and in other people. When we can see and feel our hurt and sadness and not be blinded by our anger, it allows us to move the focus and communication to addressing the hurt and sad feelings and to move away from the drive to respond to our anger by fighting back and

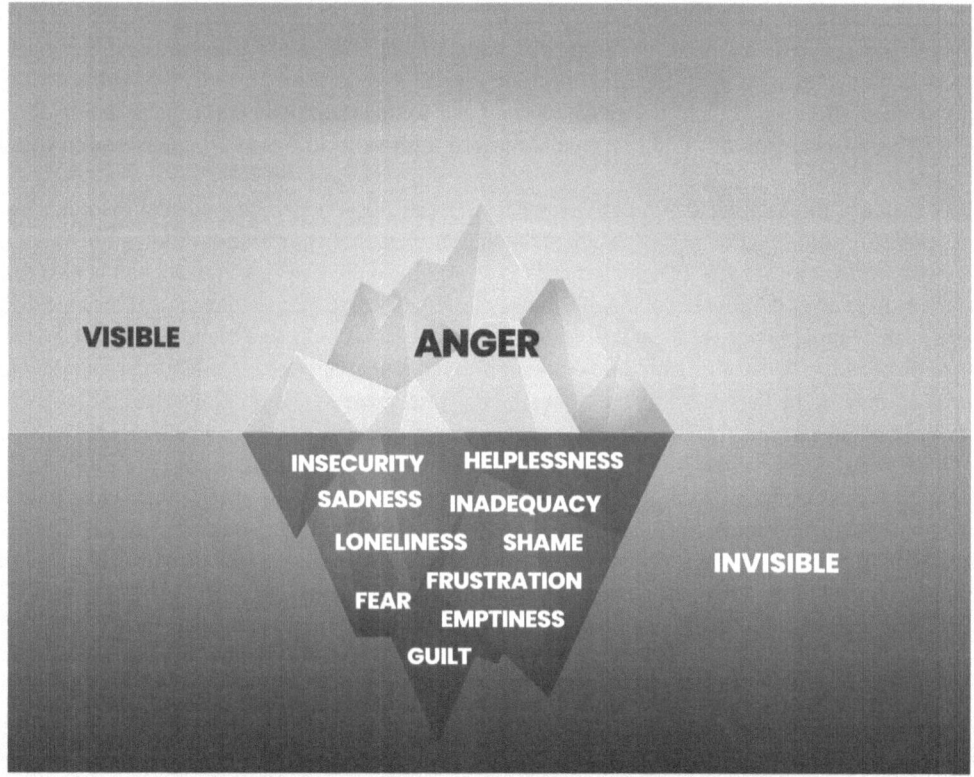

FIGURE 3.2   The anger iceberg. Adapted from Whale Design (Shutterstock).

saying or doing something hurtful. It is an act of courage to sit with the hurt feelings, whereas anger makes us feel safe. For example, if a person is angry that their partner forgot their birthday, when examined more closely, the underlying feelings are hurt, sadness, and fear that their partner does not really care enough about them to remember their birthday. It is from this vulnerable place of hurt and sadness that honest communication can be most effective at creating real changes in the relationship. Rather than yelling at your partner for forgetting and calling them names, you could say, "I was really sad when you forgot my birthday. It makes me feel like you don't really care about me. Do you know why you forgot or what would help you remember in the future?"

Healthy anger includes observing but not necessarily reacting to our anger. It is important to see anger as a signal to explore our feelings, thoughts, and bodily sensations in order to better identify our core desires, needs, and values. When we better understand what we want and need, we can learn how to communicate assertively with others to figure out how to meet those needs and desires. This is not an easy process, but it is one where we can develop skills and get better at it as long as we maintain some compassion for ourselves and others, recognizing that we are all struggling to get our needs met and that it is often confusing and difficult to make that happen.

SOMATOGENIC PERSPECTIVE

A *somatogenic perspective* on mental illness focuses on the physical causes of mental health such as genetics, brain chemistry, environmental toxins, hormone imbalances, chronic low-level infections (often overgrowths of bacteria and fungi), and nutritional deficiencies. Treatment protocols from this perspective focus on changing the state of the body, including prescribing medications that change neurotransmitter and hormone levels, genetic testing to identify vulnerabilities, detoxification methods to help the body to clear out toxins, supplements to help remove bacterial and fungal overgrowths, and dietary changes to remove food-based allergens and to provide adequate nutrients.

The primary mechanism to support psychotropic medication use to treat mental disorders is the *brain chemistry* model of mental illness. This model implies that your brain is broken due to a brain chemistry imbalance because of your genetics (i.e., you have the bad luck to have bad genes) therefore the only course of treatment is long-term use of medication to maintain chemical balance. Many people with a family history of mental illness receive a diagnosis in their 20s and end up taking medication for decades. Clearly this model favors a pharmaceutical approach to treating mental illness, which continues to be the predominant model in many healthcare systems. However, new research is pushing back against this model and questioning some of the research upon which it is based.

A new focus for an underlying mechanism that causes mental illness is the impact of inflammation on the brain. Depression, in particular, has received a lot of attention in this area of study. Inflammation is an immune system response that activates the healing process by cueing the release of different chemicals in the body, such as lymphocytes and macrophages. Inflammation is often measured by detection of biomarkers like cytokines or C-reactive protein (CRP) (Miller et al., 2009).

Inflammation is often a response to an infection and can exist in the body for a long time in response to a chronic low-level infection. Research shows a clear association between chronic body inflammation and depressive symptoms (Bullmore, 2018). For example, in a large study of over 70,000 adults, elevated levels of CRP were associated with an increased risk for psychological distress and depression (Wium-Andersen et al., 2013). When we help the body to heal and reduce inflammation, often depressive symptoms will clear up (Kohler et al., 2016). One treatment approach is to increase the consumption of anti-inflammatory foods to help the body cool the inflammation and decrease depressive symptoms (Firth et al., 2019).

CASE STUDY: COLLABORATION TO TREAT PTSD

Dr. Champion worked with a female firefighter who spent the past ten years carrying around the trauma of seeing a person hanging from a bridge after shooting himself in the head. She was in therapy. She tried everything she could think of and the only solace she found was in the bottom of a daily bottle of vodka. Her spouse was ready to leave her. She was only able to hold it together at work due to the adrenaline coursing through her veins every moment of her 24-hour shift, wondering if she would see a situation as horrible as the one that haunted her every time she closed her eyes.

A nutrition intake and exam were the first steps to assessing her nutritional status. From these Dr. Champion determined that both adrenal and sex hormones needed to be assessed. The client's test results showed reduced estrogen, progesterone, and cortisol, with testosterone and DHEA within normal range. Oftentimes, when there is extreme stress or trauma present, a woman's estrogen and progesterone levels will fall, and those who had low estrogen or progesterone before the stressful experience are more likely to develop PTSD (Biddle & Knox, 2023; Miedl, 2018). Typically, short bursts of stress increase cortisol, but for those with chronic or sustained stress, the cortisol production eventually flattens to a greatly reduced level, depleted from overuse, which also signals a reduction of progesterone production. Insomnia, anxiety, and depression are inversely related to estrogen, progesterone, and cortisol levels in that low hormone levels are associated with an increased risk of sleep and mood issues.

Over the next several months, Dr. Champion worked with the client to increase sex hormone levels and restore proper cortisol function. Since sleep was an issue for this client, it became the primary focus between the therapist, the client, and Dr. Champion. Typically, Dr. Champion recommends up to ten hours of sleep nightly to help restore the adrenal glands to optimal functioning. However, since this client also presented with a history of night terrors, working with the therapist was essential to increase the sleep duration.

For the next six months, the client worked on improving her sleep while also supporting her nutritional needs with a balanced macronutrient diet that included complex carbohydrates. Healthy, whole-food carbohydrates such as fruits and vegetables provide the body with the necessary nutrients to build up serotonin levels which are important to restore restful sleep (Wurtman & Wurtman, 1996). Therefore, a low carbohydrate diet would not have been ideal for helping this client get the sleep she needed and to help keep her blood glucose out of the "panic" level that could have been contributing to her night terrors and waking her due to hypoglycemia during sleep.

The body works diligently to ensure that blood glucose is kept at a steady level. When glucose levels drop too low or too quickly, it triggers the release of stress hormones including cortisol. When complex carbohydrates are consumed, it reduces cortisol levels by maintaining steadier glucose levels. For someone like this client with depleted cortisol levels, healthy dietary carbohydrates and increased sleep allow the body periods of rest to build the cortisol savings account. Dr. Champion suggested a diet robust in complex carbohydrates such as beets, plantains, sweet potatoes, lentils, legumes, parsnips, turnips, rutabaga, quinoa, wild or brown rice, buckwheat, and steel-cut oats. These complex carbohydrates were less likely to send the client's blood glucose on a roller coaster ride.

The client was able to increase her sleep from four hours per night to nearly nine hours per night and to balance her blood sugar. At the time of publication, the client's weight had dropped 22 pounds, her estrogen and progesterone moved into the optimal ranges, and her cortisol had improved significantly.

MEDICATION BENEFITS AND CHALLENGES

The somatogenic perspective has been powerfully entwined in promoting the use of medication to treat mental health disorders. Drug therapy is by far the most popular first-line approach to treating mental health symptoms. Beginning in the 1950s, researchers discovered certain drugs that affect people's emotions and thought processes and began using them both alone and in combination with other treatment approaches such as psychotherapy. For example, there has been consistent evidence that antidepressant medication can be helpful for people with chronic severe depressive symptoms, especially when used in combination with psychotherapy (Barkham & Lambert, 2021). It appears that the medication gives clients the energy and focus necessary to fully engage in psychotherapy progressing the ability to make important changes in their life. We discuss more about psychotherapy in the next section of this chapter.

While the psychotropic drug revolution has helped some people it has also produced some major problems. As introduced earlier in this chapter, many are concerned that the drugs are overprescribed and overused and are continued long-term with little supervision or confirmation that the drugs are still benefitting the client enough to warrant the negative side effects that often go along with these medications.

There are five major psychotropic drug groups used in mental health treatment. *Antianxiety drugs*, also known as minor tranquilizers or anxiolytics, help people feel calm and reduce symptoms of anxiety such as muscle tension, restlessness, and insomnia. *Mood stabilizers* are generally used to even out the high and low mood swings experienced by people with bipolar disorder to decrease their symptoms of mania and depression. *Antidepressant drugs* help to energize people with depressive symptoms and to quell negative thinking and feelings of intense sadness. *Antipsychotic drugs* help to quiet psychotic symptoms associated with schizophrenia and other psychotic disorders, such as hallucinations, delusions, and confusion. *Stimulant drugs* are prescribed primarily to treat ADHD and help increase focus and attention and decrease impulsivity and restlessness.

IMPACT OF PSYCHOTROPIC MEDICATION

Many mental health professionals are concerned that the current structure of the healthcare system promotes prescribing medication over other forms of treatment which has led to an over-medicated population. Psychotropic drugs (especially antidepressants for depression, anxiolytics for anxiety, and stimulants for ADHD) are often prescribed in a primary care medical office after a very brief (sometimes five to ten minutes) assessment by a medical doctor. There are often minimal follow-up visits to assess if the drug is being taken correctly and is having the desired effect, and little discussion about adjunctive treatment such as psychotherapy or a plan to eventually get the patient off the drug. Psychotropic drugs often cause withdrawal symptoms when the drug is removed, so a careful discontinuation plan with clinical monitoring is essential to avoid distressing and possibly dangerous withdrawal effects (Breggin, 2012), recognizing that the taper and withdrawal process can take as much as half the time the person was on the medication (e.g., on medication 12 months, withdrawal six months) (Korn, 2016).

There is particular concern about the steady increase in prescriptions of psychotropic drugs for children and adolescents up to age 21 in the U.S. Increasingly, youth are prescribed one medication or a combination of medications (known as polypharmacy) to manage their mental health symptoms, for example, a stimulant for ADHD at the same time as an antidepressant for depression. This is problematic since there is minimal research about the impact of polypharmacy on the developing brain of a young person (Girand et al., 2020; Horace et al., 2020; Zito et al., 2021).

SEROTONIN THEORY OF DEPRESSION

The serotonin theory of depression argues that the driver of depressive symptoms is low levels of serotonin in the brain. This chemical imbalance of the brain is the result of genetics that causes a person to become depressed and as such, continues as a chronic illness. Depressive symptoms can be relieved by taking medication that allows the body to hang on to more of the serotonin it produces, thereby increasing overall levels of serotonin in the brain. Thus, the argument is laid for the long-term use of antidepressants to balance the brain chemistry and maintain appropriate serotonin levels. Unfortunately, after many decades of research and hope that we have finally found a cure for depression, the evidence is still not there.

In 2022, a study performed by Moncrieff et al. did a deep analysis of the research to understand the evidence behind the serotonin theory of depression that low levels of serotonin in the brain cause a person to have depressive symptoms such as fatigue, low mood, insomnia, and anhedonia (lack of pleasure in life) (Moncrieff et al., 2022). This study was an umbrella review that analyzed 17 large studies that were themselves systematic reviews and metanalyses of multiple studies. Their conclusion was that the research provided "no consistent evidence of there being an association between serotonin and depression, and no support for the hypothesis that depression is caused by lowered serotonin activity or concentrations." Even more confusing was the fact that there was some evidence that long-term antidepressant use reduces serotonin levels, which is surprising since the premise of antidepressants is that they raise serotonin levels.

Yet antidepressants work well for some people, so researchers continue to explore what other mechanisms of change in the brain might be the real healing benefit of taking an antidepressant. One hypothesis that has gathered interest is the *neurotrophic model of mood disorders*. There is a growing body of evidence that chronic stress negatively impacts the brain by decreasing the production of brain-derived neurotrophic factor (BDNF) in the parts of the brain that control mood (i.e., the limbic system), which interferes with the brain's ability to grow new cells (i.e., neurons) and cell connections (i.e., synapses) known as neurogenesis. Research into the brains of depressed people demonstrated low levels of BDNF compared to people who were not depressed (Castrén & Monteggia, 2021). In addition to depression, low levels of BDNF are linked to other disorders including Alzheimer's disease, anorexia nervosa, and schizophrenia (Gliwińska et al., 2023). Antidepressants increase the release of BDNF in the limbic system that may reverse the effects of stress on this area of the brain (Duman & Monteggia, 2006; Malberg et al., 2021). This hypothesis may help to account for the fact that people who begin taking an antidepressant show an immediate rise in serotonin levels yet do not report feeling better for a few weeks after they began the medication. This timing aligns with the amount of time it takes for the increased BDNF levels produced by the antidepressant to stimulate neurogenesis in the brain with its healing benefits.

Publication Bias

There continues to be intense controversy in the clinical field that antidepressant drugs may not be as effective as previously thought. One key reason for this shift in perspective was research done in the early 2000s to explore the impact of publication bias. *Publication bias* is the tendency of professional journals to publish studies that have positive findings versus neutral or negative findings, that is, this drug works (positive) versus this drug might work (neutral) or this drug does not work (negative). To better understand if publication bias had inflated the reported efficacy of antidepressants, researchers compared the efficacy rates for studies that were published versus efficacy rates for antidepressant research studies that were never published. They found that when you included the unpublished studies, antidepressants were less effective compared to placebo than previously proclaimed (Turner et al., 2008). A more recent analysis performed in 2020 reports that, while recent literature has been more transparent about research demonstrating neutral or negative findings which has decreased the magnitude of bias, there continues to be bias in the literature that overstates the efficacy of antidepressant medications (Turner et al., 2020). Irving Kirsch at Harvard Medical School argues that "most (if not all) of the benefits of antidepressants in the treatment of depression and anxiety are due to the placebo response" and that other treatments such as psychotherapy and physical exercise produce the same benefits as antidepressants without the side effects and with a lower rate of relapse where the intense depressive symptoms return (Kirsch, 2019).

Some of the concern about the lack of efficacy of antidepressants is that it must be weighed against the risk of adverse side effects. For some people, the small positive effect produced by taking an antidepressant is outweighed by the risk of harmful effects including nausea, insomnia, weight gain, dry mouth, low libido, and headache (Jakobsen et al., 2017). Of particular concern is the evidence that antidepressants increase the risk of suicidal thoughts, especially in children and adolescents (Kwon, 2016; Sharma et al., 2016). In 2018, the FDA reported, "Antidepressants increase the risk of suicidal thinking and behavior (suicidality) in children and adolescents with MDD [major depressive disorder] and other psychiatric disorders" as an appropriate topic to be included in their boxed warning for antidepressants (FDA, 2018).

There is also concern that we do not have sufficient evidence to support long-term use of antidepressants. In a landmark study in the international journal *The Lancet*, the authors report that, while antidepressants are helpful for some people, the research results may be skewed by the short duration of the studies (median duration was eight weeks). "Depressive symptoms tend to spontaneously improve over time and this phenomenon contributes to the high percentage of placebo responders in antidepressant trials" (Cipriani et al., 2018, p. 7). Meaning that we might be confusing the efficacy of the medications with the natural progression of the disorder and that people who are struggling with depression will naturally pull out of it over time with or without medication. So, there is a question about the long-term need for antidepressants.

A large qualitative study performed in New Zealand noted significant diversity in how clients responded to taking an antidepressant. They reported that 54 percent had a positive experience and saw antidepressants as "necessary" and "a steppingstone" to accessing additional treatment support such as psychotherapy. In comparison, 16 percent had a negative response and 28 percent had a mixed response to taking an antidepressant. Those with a negative response described antidepressants as being "ineffective," having "unbearable side effects," and "masking real problems," while those with a mixed response "felt calmer but less like themselves" and "felt stuck with continuing on antidepressants when they wished to stop" (Gibson et al., 2016).

ANTIDEPRESSANT DISCONTINUATION SYNDROME

Some of the confusion about the efficacy of antidepressants is also due to the sometimes-significant impact of stopping the medication. Initially, it can be difficult to determine if a person is experiencing an increase in their original depressive symptoms, or just having a response to no longer ingesting the antidepressant medication (Carey & Gebeloff, 2018). Often referred to as *antidepressant discontinuation syndrome* or *antidepressant withdrawal*, approximately 20 percent of people who stop taking an antidepressant after being on it for at least six weeks experience a month or two of symptoms including insomnia, nausea, dizziness, irritability, fatigue, and nightmares, with increased risk of mania and suicide (Cleveland Clinic, 2023; Fava et al., 2015; Warner et al., 2006). Patients assume that the medication was working because when they stop taking it they feel so terrible, however, this is an inaccurate assumption. When a person chooses to stop taking an antidepressant, it is important to create a discontinuation plan to slowly taper off of the medication with minimal discomfort and adverse symptoms. (Cartwright et al., 2016). Then it takes time away from the medication for a person to reassess the nature of their depressive symptoms and the status of their disorder when they are medication free.

SIMILAR CONCERNS FOR OTHER PSYCHOTROPIC MEDICATIONS

While this has been a deep dive into concerns about antidepressants, the same can be said for many psychotropic medications. Concerns about overprescribing and prescribing off-label have grown. Off-label use of medication means prescribing it to a patient whose situation is outside the evidence-based approved use of that medication based on the current research. For example, there is real concern that antipsychotic medications are being prescribed to older adults in assisted-living facilities not because the person has been evaluated and diagnosed with a psychotic disorder, but because the drugs often have a sedating effect that makes the patients easy for the staff to manage. When patients are quickly prescribed a psychotropic medication with a minimal evaluation or a broader-than-intended application and then expected by their doctor to stay on that medication for years, important considerations may be overlooked or entirely missed. Each drug has its list of adverse side effects which can range from uncomfortable to debilitating, which can be worse for some people than their psychiatric symptoms.

In addition to overprescribing and off-label use, we are also beginning to understand the negative impact of taking psychotropic medication on eating behavior and nutrition. For example, side effects for stimulants prescribed for ADHD include stomach upset and loss of appetite which can lead to weight loss and nutritional deficiencies that, among other things, can contribute to increased anxiety and difficulty sleeping (WebMD, 2023). Antipsychotics and antidepressants also impact eating behavior and nutrition in that they commonly cause constipation and weight gain, which can contribute to the development of metabolic issues such as high cholesterol and diabetes. Psychotropic medications can also deplete the body of micronutrients such as vitamins B, D, and E, calcium, selenium, the antioxidant CoQ10, and Omega-3 fatty acids (Korn, 2016).

PSYCHOTHERAPY BENEFITS AND CHALLENGES

Psychotherapy involves communication between therapists and clients to help clients experience relief from emotional distress, explore solutions to problems in their lives, and find ways to modify behaviors and thoughts that interfere with productivity and relationships. Often it begins with an initial assessment where the therapist gathers information about the client's background and current concerns and then uses that information to create a treatment plan for how they will work together. The treatment goals may include reducing the number, severity, or frequency of negative thoughts, finding new ways to interpret events, recognizing and accepting emotions, and developing new and more productive coping strategies to manage stress. A therapist is educated and experienced in understanding psychological problems and coping strategies that help relieve suffering and improve overall health. This relationship is different from a friendship in that the psychotherapy time is devoted entirely to the client's needs versus a friendship where the relationship is mutual and balanced, and the needs of both people need to be met (American Psychological Association, 2023).

PSYCHOTHERAPY TREATMENT MODELS

There are a variety of different styles of psychotherapy (known as therapy modalities) used by mental health clinicians depending on their training and theoretical outlook (known as theoretical orientation) about what causes people to become mentally ill and what most helps them to feel better. A survey of over 2200 North American psychotherapists found the most popular modalities to be cognitive-behavioral therapy (CBT), family systems therapy, psychodynamic and psychoanalytic therapies, and acceptance/mindfulness-based therapies such as acceptance and commitment therapy (ACT), dialectical behavior therapy (DBT), and mindfulness-based stress reduction (MBSR) (Cook et al., 2010). Most therapists describe their orientation as *eclectic*, meaning they use a combination of different modalities when treating clients based on the client's needs and desires in psychotherapy.

Most of the treatment provided is individual therapy where the therapist works alone with a single client. Other treatment formats are couples, families, and groups where the therapist meets with more than one person at a time. Couples and family therapy can include any combination of children and adults that make up a family system, generally focusing on people who live together and take care of each other. Group therapy models range in their level of structure. A process group is focused on clients exploring current challenges and interactions establishing a safe environment to share fears and concerns. In contrast, a structured or manualized therapy group (manualized because there is a written manual that guides the therapist about how to lead each group) has an agenda for each group, has a defined structure, and is focused on helping clients learn different ways of thinking about and approaching problems by building new skills and coping strategies.

PSYCHOTHERAPY EFFECTIVENESS

Psychotherapy, in its many forms, has been rigorously studied to see if it is effective in reducing psychiatric symptoms. Repeatedly, research done both in lab and in clinical settings has found psychotherapy to be effective, with positive effects that tend to last over time (Lambert, 2013). In fact, new technology using functional magnetic resonance imaging (fMRI) and positron emission tomography (PET) has demonstrated that psychotherapy changes the structure and activity of the brain in positive ways associated with improved mental health (Dichter et al., 2009).

While there is general agreement that one therapy modality has not risen above the others to be more effective across the board, some researchers have made the case that certain psychotherapies are superior for addressing specific problems and diagnoses. They argue that an evidence-based or prescriptive approach should be taken that matches psychotherapy modalities to specific diagnoses based on existing research studies that demonstrate positive outcomes. Along these lines, the Clinical Psychology Division 12 of the American Psychological Association has developed a website that documents research support for using a particular psychotherapy modality to treat a specific disorder (Society of Clinical Psychology, 2015). For example, it lists *CBT for substance use disorders* and *ACT for psychosis*.

The prescriptive approach has gained some traction and there continues to be general consensus that the research evidence continues to support the perspective that no one psychotherapy modality (e.g., CBT, family systems, psychodynamic) stands out as better than the others overall. They are all consistently beneficial for different populations and different diagnoses (Barkham & Lambert, 2021). Exploration into what is similar across psychotherapy modalities has led to the concept that psychotherapy models all share some fundamental components or *common factors* that are essential for psychotherapy to be effective. The common factors focus on the quality of the therapeutic relationship or therapeutic alliance, which is the quality of the relationship between the therapist and the client. These common factors are not merely present in good therapy, they are essential and at their core, intended to be therapeutic. Therapist qualities such as empathy, positive regard, genuineness, and collaboration are among the key common factors found in an effective psychotherapy relationship. Other important elements are the therapist's ability to form a feeling of cohesion with individual clients and between group therapy clients, the ability to provide constructive feedback to clients, and the capacity to inspire hope and positive expectations that the therapy will help the client to feel better (Elkins, 2022; Gallagher et al., 2020; Wampold, 2015).

In an effort to better understand the key elements essential to effective psychotherapy, the American Psychological Association Task Force on Evidence-Based Relationships and Responsiveness studied the existing research on this topic and came up with some clear conclusions (Norcross & Lambert, 2018). First and foremost, "The psychotherapy relationship makes substantial and consistent contributions to outcome independent of the type of treatment." The quality of the client-therapist relationship is as or more important than the particular treatment method. Therefore, the therapist should be able and willing to adapt and tailor the psychotherapy to best match client characteristics such as culture and client preferences to best support the therapeutic alliance.

FOOD FOR THOUGHT: MOTIVATIONAL INTERVIEWING AND THE STAGES OF CHANGE MODEL

As mentioned at the beginning of this chapter, the 21st century brought a shift in healthcare. Treatment for infectious disease and traumatic injury has improved dramatically over the years with new medications, surgical procedures, and technology. Our current societal struggle must expand beyond the disease model to find modern interventions and answers. Research clearly shows a significant link between chronic diseases and lifestyle factors, especially nutrition, stress, movement, sleep, and isolation. Therefore, the entirety of the healthcare field has been paying considerable attention to how to help people make better lifestyle choices and behavior changes that can improve their health. Making dietary and eating behavior changes is at the heart of nutritional psychology. The stages of change model rely on gaining knowledge to understand the process of how to make these life-altering changes. *Motivational interviewing (MI)* stands out as a clear leader in how to approach clients about making positive lifestyle changes.

The concept of MI was first introduced in 1983 by clinical psychologist William Miller as a brief psychotherapy treatment for alcohol overuse problems. In 1991, together with clinical psychologist Stephen Rollnick, they published the first book on MI (Miller & Rollnick, 1991) as a contemporary variation of humanistic therapy that is both person-centered and goal-oriented. The focus of this approach is to explore clients' *ambivalence* about making major lifestyle changes.

Most people are aware of behaviors they can engage in to improve their health, such as eating less sugar and exercising more frequently, yet they find themselves struggling to both activate and then to maintain these positive behaviors for any period of time. MI helps clients look at their reasons for change and the obstacles that stop them, examining the discrepancies between their core values (i.e., what is most important to them) and their behaviors (what they actually do). *Ambivalence* is the experience of having mixed feelings or contradictory ideas. When it comes to physical and mental health, most people want to be healthy and agree to complete some behaviors that will improve their health. However, people are also comfortable with their familiar routines. Many find change to be difficult and the process of giving up something in favor of something that could be better to be uncomfortable. A telltale sign of ambivalence is the *but* in the middle of their statements.

- "I need to lose some weight, *but* I hate exercising."
- "I should quit smoking, *but* I just can't seem to do it."

MI works by activating clients' motivation for change and commitment to treatment. It is *not* a technique for tricking people into doing what we think they should do. Rather it is a clinical style that helps clients clarify their *why* for making lifestyle changes, and then supports their intrinsic motivation to make behavior changes by examining and overcoming obstacles. The focus is more on guiding than directing, more on listening than telling. The work has been described as collaborative, evocative (activates resources for change), and honoring patient autonomy so there is no coercion on the part of the therapist. It is important for the therapist to accept client choices and detach from the outcomes. You can't want it more for your client than they want it. The therapist can inform and advise, but ultimately it is the client who decides what to do and it is the therapist's role to listen to the client, attempt to understand their motivations, and empower the client to make changes.

MI works well when paired with the Transtheoretical Model (also known as the Stages of Change Model) developed by Prochaska and DiClemente (1983). This model studied people who attempted to quit smoking cigarettes to better understand why some people were capable of quitting and others were not. They developed a model that helps clarify the status of a person's intention to make a behavior change in their life. The model identifies five stages that people go through:

- *Precontemplation stage* – No intention to change
- *Contemplation stage* – Aware a problem exists, considering doing something to address it, but not ready to commit
- *Preparation stage* – Intending to take action within a short time (e.g., weeks, a month)
- *Action stage* – Actively changing behavior and making notable efforts to overcome problems
- *Maintenance stage* – Preventing relapse and retaining gains made during action stage

MI helps clients to recognize their current level of intention or readiness to make lifestyle changes, and then helps guide them toward the action and maintenance stages if that matches their goals and values.

There is impressive empirical data that supports the efficacy of MI for treating not just substance abuse, but for a wide range of psychological and physical problems, including anxiety, depression, weight loss, fitness, blood pressure, and diabetes management (Naar & Suarez, 2021; Pomerantz, 2019). The research evidence also demonstrates that MI can be integrated into other forms of treatment (Marker & Norton, 2018) including emotion-focused therapy for depression and anxiety (Greenberg & Goldman, 2019), positive psychology interventions (Csillik, 2015), and treatment of eating disorders (Macdonald et al., 2012).

REFERENCES

American Psychological Association. (2023). *What is psychotherapy?* American Psychological Association.

Barkham, M., & Lambert, M. J. (2021). The efficacy and effectiveness of psychological therapies. In M. Barkham, W. Lutz, & L. G. Castonguay (Eds.), *Bergin and Garfield's handbook of psychotherapy and behavior change: 50th anniversary edition* (7th ed., pp. 135–189). John Wiley & Sons, Inc.

Biddle, M., & Knox, D. (2023). The role of estrogen receptor manipulation during traumatic stress on changes in emotional memory induced by traumatic stress. *Psychopharmacology*, *240*(5), 1049–1061. https://doi.org/10.1007/s00213-023-06342-6

Brannon, L., Updegraff, J. A., & Feist, J. (2022). *Health psychology: An introduction to behavior and health* (10th ed.). Cengage Learning.

Breggin, P. R. (2012). *Psychiatric drug withdrawal: A guide for prescribers, therapists, patients and their families*. Springer Publishing Company.

Brown, B. (2012). *Daring greatly: How the courage to be vulnerable transforms the way we live, love, parent, and lead*. Penguin Publishing Group, Avery Division.

Bullmore, E. (2018). *The inflamed mind: A radical new approach to depression*. Picador.

Busfield, J. (2010). 'A pill for every ill': Explaining the expansion in medicine use. *Social Science & Medicine*, *70*(6), 934–941. https://doi.org/10.1016/j.socscimed.2009.10.068

Carey, B., & Gebeloff, R. (2018). Many people taking antidepressants discover they cannot quit. *New York Times*. https://www.nytimes.com/2018/04/07/health/antidepressants-withdrawal-prozac-cymbalta.html

Cartwright, C., Gibson, K., Read, J., Cowan, O., & Dehar, T. (2016). Long-term antidepressant use: Patient perspectives of benefits and adverse effects. *Patient Preference and Adherence*, *10*(null), 1401–1407. https://doi.org/10.2147/PPA.S110632

Castrén, E., & Monteggia, L. M. (2021). Brain-derived neurotrophic factor signaling in depression and antidepressant action. *Biological Psychiatry*, *90*(2), 128–136.

Cipriani, A., Furukawa, T. A., Salanti, G., Chaimani, A., Atkinson, L. Z., Ogawa, Y., Leucht, S., Ruhe, H. G., Turner, E. H., & Higgins, J. P. (2018). Comparative efficacy and acceptability of 21 antidepressant drugs for the acute treatment of adults with major depressive disorder: A systematic review and network meta-analysis. *The Lancet*, *391*(10128), 1357–1366.

Cleveland Clinic. (2023). *Antidepressant discontinuation syndrome*. https://my.clevelandclinic.org/health/diseases/25218-antidepressant-discontinuation-syndrome

Comer, R. J., & Comer, J. S. (2024). *Psychopathology: Science and practice* (12th ed.). Worth Publishers.

Cook, J. M., Biyanova, T., Elhai, J., Schnurr, P. P., & Coyne, J. C. (2010). What do psychotherapists really do in practice? An internet study of over 2,000 practitioners. *Psychotherapy: Theory, Research, Practice, Training*, *47*(2), 260.

Csillik, A. (2015). Positive motivational interviewing: Activating clients' strengths and intrinsic motivation to change. *Journal of Contemporary Psychotherapy*, *45*(2), 119–128.

Dichter, G. S., Felder, J. N., Petty, C., Bizzell, J., Ernst, M., & Smoski, M. J. (2009). The effects of psychotherapy on neural responses to rewards in major depression. *Biological Psychiatry*, *66*(9), 886–897.

Duman, R. S., & Monteggia, L. M. (2006). A neurotrophic model for stress-related mood disorders. *Biological Psychiatry*, *59*(12), 1116–1127. https://doi.org/10.1016/j.biopsych.2006.02.013

Elkins, D. N. (2022). Common factors: What are they and what do they mean for humanistic psychology? *Journal of Humanistic Psychology*, *62*(1), 21–30.

Ericson, J. (2014). A pill for every ill. *Newsweek Magazine.* https://www.newsweek.com/2014/02/07/pill-every-ill-245476.html

Fava, G. A., Gatti, A., Belaise, C., Guidi, J., & Offidani, E. (2015). Withdrawal symptoms after selective serotonin reuptake inhibitor discontinuation: A systematic review. *Psychotherapy and Psychosomatics, 84*(2), 72–81. https://doi.org/10.1159/000370338

FDA. (2018). *Suicidality in children and adolescents being treated with Antidepressant medications.* U.S. Food & Drug Administration. https://www.fda.gov/drugs/postmarket-drug-safety-information-patients-and-providers/suicidality-children-and-adolescents-being-treated-antidepressant-medications

Firth, J., Veronese, N., Cotter, J., Shivappa, N., Hebert, J. R., Ee, C., Smith, L., Stubbs, B., & Sarris, J. (2019). What is the role of dietary inflammation in severe mental illness? A review of observational and experimental findings. *Frontiers in Psychiatry, 10*, 443755.

Gallagher, M. W., Long, L. J., & Phillips, C. A. (2020). Hope, optimism, self-efficacy, and posttraumatic stress disorder: A meta-analytic review of the protective effects of positive expectancies. *Journal of Clinical Psychology, 76*(3), 329–355.

Gibson, K., Cartwright, C., & Read, J. (2016). 'In my life antidepressants have been…': A qualitative analysis of users' diverse experiences with antidepressants. *BMC Psychiatry, 16*(1), 135. https://doi.org/10.1186/s12888-016-0844-3

Girand, H. L., Litkowiec, S., & Sohn, M. (2020). Attention-deficit/hyperactivity disorder and psychotropic polypharmacy prescribing trends. *Pediatrics, 146*(1). https://doi.org/10.1542/peds.2019-2832

Gliwińska, A., Czubilińska-Łada, J., Więckiewicz, G., Świętochowska, E., Badeński, A., Dworak, M., & Szczepańska, M. (2023). The role of brain-derived neurotrophic factor (BDNF) in diagnosis and treatment of epilepsy, depression, schizophrenia, anorexia nervosa and Alzheimer's disease as highly drug-resistant diseases: A narrative review. *Brain Sciences, 13*(2). https://doi.org/10.3390/brainsci13020163

Greenberg, L. S., & Goldman, R. N. (2019). *Clinical handbook of emotion-focused therapy.* American Psychological Association.

Horace, A. E., Golchin, N., Knight, E. M. P., Dawson, N. V., Ma, X., Feinstein, J. A., Johnson, H. K., Kleinman, L., & Bakaki, P. M. (2020). A scoping review of medications studied in pediatric polypharmacy research. *Paediatric Drugs, 22*(1), 85–94. https://doi.org/10.1007/s40272-019-00372-4

Jakobsen, J. C., Katakam, K. K., Schou, A., Hellmuth, S. G., Stallknecht, S. E., Leth-Møller, K., Iversen, M., Banke, M. B., Petersen, I. J., Klingenberg, S. L., Krogh, J., Ebert, S. E., Timm, A., Lindschou, J., & Gluud, C. (2017). Selective serotonin reuptake inhibitors versus placebo in patients with major depressive disorder. A systematic review with meta-analysis and trial sequential analysis. *BMC Psychiatry, 17*(1), 58. https://doi.org/10.1186/s12888-016-1173-2

Kirsch, I. (2019). Placebo effect in the treatment of depression and anxiety. *Frontiers in Psychiatry, 407.*

Kochanek, K. D., Murphy, S. L., Xu, J., & Arias, E. (2019). Deaths: Final data for 2017. *National Vital Statistics Reports, 68*(9), 1–77.

Kohler, O., Krogh, J., Mors, O., & Eriksen Benros, M. (2016). Inflammation in depression and the potential for anti-inflammatory treatment. *Current Neuropharmacology, 14*(7), 732–742.

Korn, L. E. (2016). *Nutrition essentials for mental health: A complete guide to the food-mood connection* (1st ed.). W.W. Norton & Company. https://search.library.wisc.edu/catalog/9912234502802121

Kwon, D. (2016). The hidden harms of antidepressants: Data about the true risks of suicide and aggression for children and teens taking these drugs have been suppressed. *Scientific American.* https://www.scientificamerican.com/article/the-hidden-harms-of-antidepressants/

Lambert, M. J. (2013). Outcome in psychotherapy: The past and important advances.

Lembke, A. (2016). *Drug dealer, MD: How doctors were duped, patients got hooked, and why it's so hard to stop.* Johns Hopkins University Press.

Macdonald, P., Hibbs, R., Corfield, F., & Treasure, J. (2012). The use of motivational interviewing in eating disorders: A systematic review. *Psychiatry Research, 200*(1), 1–11.

Malberg, J. E., Hen, R., & Madsen, T. M. (2021). Adult neurogenesis and Antidepressant treatment: The surprise finding by Ron Duman and the field 20 years later. *Biological Psychiatry, 90*(2), 96–101. https://doi.org/10.1016/j.biopsych.2021.01.010

Marker, I., & Norton, P. J. (2018). The efficacy of incorporating motivational interviewing to cognitive behavior therapy for anxiety disorders: A review and meta-analysis. *Clinical Psychology Review, 62*, 1–10.

Maust, D. T., Sirey, J. A., & Kales, H. C. (2017). Antidepressant prescribing in primary care to older adults without major depression. *Psychiatric Services, 68*(5), 449–455. https://doi.org/10.1176/appi.ps.201600197

Miceli, M., & Castelfranchi, C. (2018). Reconsidering the differences between shame and guilt. *Europe's Journal of Psychology, 14*(3), 710–733. https://doi.org/10.5964/ejop.v14i3.1564

Miedl, S. F., Wegerer, M., Kerschbaum, H., Blechert, J., & Wilhelm, F. H. (2018). Neural activity during traumatic film viewing is linked to endogenous estradiol and hormonal contraception. *Psychoneuroendocrinology*, *87*, 20–26. https://doi.org/10.1016/j.psyneuen.2017.10.006

Miller, A. H., Maletic, V., & Raison, C. L. (2009). Inflammation and its discontents: The role of cytokines in The pathophysiology of major depression. *Biological Psychiatry*, *65*(9), 732–741.

Miller, W., & Rollnick, S. (1991). *Motivational interviewing: Preparing people to change addictive behavior.* Guilford Press.

Mojtabai, R., & Olfson, M. (2011). Proportion of antidepressants prescribed without a psychiatric diagnosis is growing. *Health Affairs*, *30*(8), 1434–1442. https://doi.org/10.1377/hlthaff.2010.1024

Moncrieff, J., Cooper, R. E., Stockmann, T., Amendola, S., Hengartner, M. P., & Horowitz, M. A. (2022). The serotonin theory of depression: A systematic umbrella review of the evidence. *Molecular Psychiatry*. https://doi.org/10.1038/s41380-022-01661-0

Naar, S., & Suarez, M. (2021). *Motivational interviewing with adolescents and young adults.* Guilford Publications.

Norcross, J. C., & Lambert, M. J. (2018). Psychotherapy relationships that work III. *Psychotherapy*, *55*(4), 303.

Pagaduan, M. (2021). America's epidemic of antidepressants. *Berkeley Political Review.* https://bpr.berkeley.edu/2021/11/07/americas-epidemic-of-antidepressants/

Penn Wharton. (2016). *Mortality in the United States: Past, present, and future.* University of Pennsylvania. https://budgetmodel.wharton.upenn.edu/issues/2016/1/25/mortality-in-the-united-states-past-present-and-future

Pennington, J. R. (2015). *Shame: Should have already mastered everything: How unresolved shame gets in the way of our humanity (and what to do about it).* Wiseselfpublications.

Pomerantz, A. M. (2019). *Clinical psychology: Science, practice, and diversity.* Sage Publications.

Prochaska, J. O., & DiClemente, C. C. (1983). Stages and processes of self-change of smoking: Toward an integrative model of change. *Journal of Consulting and Clinical Psychology*, *51*(3), 390.

Safer, D. J. (2019). Overprescribed medications for US adults: Four major examples. *Journal of Clinical Medicine and Research*, *11*(9), 617–622. https://doi.org/10.14740/jocmr3906

Sharma, T., Guski, L. S., Freund, N., & Gøtzsche, P. C. (2016). Suicidality and aggression during antidepressant treatment: Systematic review and meta-analyses based on clinical study reports. *BMJ*, *352*, i65. https://doi.org/10.1136/bmj.i65

Society of Clinical Psychology. (2015). *Psychological treatments.* Division 12. American Psychological Association. https://div12.org/treatments/

The Gottman Institute. (2023). *The anger iceberg.* https://www.gottman.com/blog/the-anger-iceberg/

Turner, E. H., Alavi, S., Cipriani, A., Furukawa, T., Ivlev, I., McKenna, R., & Ogawa, Y. (2020). An update on reporting bias in the antidepressant literature: An FDA-controlled examination of drug efficacy. *International Congress on Peer Review and Scientific Publication.* https://peerreviewcongress.org/abstract/an-update-on-reporting-bias-in-the-antidepressant-literature-an-fda-controlled-examination-of-drug-efficacy/

Turner, E. H., Matthews, A. M., Linardatos, E., Tell, R. A., & Rosenthal, R. (2008). Selective publication of antidepressant trials and its influence on apparent efficacy. *New England Journal of Medicine*, *358*(3), 252–260.

Wampold, B. E. (2015). How important are the common factors in psychotherapy? An update. *World Psychiatry*, *14*(3), 270–277.

Warner, C. H., Bobo, W., Warner, C., Reid, S., & Rachal, J. (2006). Antidepressant discontinuation syndrome. *American Family Physician*, *74*(3), 449–456.

WebMD. (2023). *Stimulant medications for ADHD.* https://www.webmd.com/add-adhd/adhd-stimulant-therapy

Wium-Andersen, M. K., Ørsted, D. D., Nielsen, S. F., & Nordestgaard, B. G. (2013). Elevated C-reactive protein levels, psychological distress, and depression in 73 131 individuals. *JAMA Psychiatry*, *70*(2), 176–184. https://doi.org/10.1001/2013.jamapsychiatry.102

Wurtman, R. J., & Wurtman, J. J. (1996). Brain serotonin, carbohydrate-craving, obesity and depression. *Advances in Experimental Medicine and Biology*, *398*, 35–41, https://doi.org/10.1007/978-1-4613-0381-7_4

Zito, J. M., Zhu, Y., & Safer, D. J. (2021). Psychotropic polypharmacy in the US pediatric population: A methodologic critique and commentary. *Frontiers in Psychiatry*, *12*, 644741, https://doi.org/10.3389/fpsyt.2021.644741

Section II

Foundations of Nutrition

4 Nutrition Basics

The field of nutrition is forever growing and changing. Nutrition scientists are rapidly expanding our understanding of how the human body processes the foods we eat and the impact that food makes on our health. There are amazing discoveries. There are mistakes. There are recommended changes that many of us want to make. And there is also lots of confusion with differing opinions and directions given. In this chapter, we discuss nutrition fundamentals, including the definitions and roles of macronutrients and micronutrients, phytonutrients and antioxidants, common dietary habits, whole foods, and the role of sugar in the diet.

MACRONUTRIENTS

The starting place for almost any discussion of nutrition is *macronutrients*, which are focused on the three main types of food: proteins, fats, and carbohydrates. While there is a lot of conversation about when and how many grams of each of the macronutrients is ideal to eat, there needs to be in-depth conversations about what each of these macronutrients is and what they do in the body.

PROTEINS

Protein provides the building blocks of the body. In many ways, it is an integral part of all living organisms. Protein is a nutrient found mainly in animal sources such as meat, milk, and eggs, and in smaller amounts in plant-based foods such as legumes, grains, and vegetables. Chemically speaking, proteins consist of large molecules made of one or more long chains of amino acids connected by peptide bonds. Our muscles, hormones, hair, collagen, enzymes, and antibodies are all made from protein. In addition to being an essential part of body structure, adequate protein intake is also essential to the function and maintenance of tissues and organs.

According to most research, protein deficiency is uncommon in the U.S. However, the quality of our protein sources must also be considered. When we look at the frequent occurrence of sarcopenia (muscle wasting), hormonal imbalances, and blood sugar dysregulation in the U.S. associated with chronic illnesses including insulin resistance, metabolic syndrome, and diabetes, we can see that the *quality* of the protein consumed is an often missed and important distinction.

There is growing evidence that points to the value of sourcing wild-caught, organic, and grass-fed animal protein as opposed to conventionally grown feedlot animal protein sources that make up most of the current U.S. protein food supply. The majority of diets in the U.S. tend to be focused on carbohydrates, especially processed carbohydrates which are more readily available and often more affordable. Unfortunately, a diet that is high in carbohydrates can lead to spikes in our blood sugar levels and over time, an increased risk of metabolic disorders, which can result in an inability to metabolize cells properly. Simply increasing the amount of protein can help, but increasing the quality of protein is even more critical.

There are approximately 20 *amino acids* that build protein molecules. These amino acids are alanine, arginine, asparagine, aspartic acid, cysteine, glutamine, glutamic acid, glycine, histidine, isoleucine, leucine, lysine, methionine, phenylalanine, proline, serine, threonine, tryptophan, tyrosine, and valine. Each of these amino acids is categorized into *essential* (we must obtain the amino acid through our diet) and *non-essential* (the body can manufacture these amino acids from other materials). When what we eat lacks the essential amino acids, we begin to see the deterioration of our muscles, organs, and other tissues, as well as a negative impact on our ability to think, filter emotions and feelings (think hangry!), and, if not corrected, an overall decline in wellbeing.

DOI: 10.1201/9781032647647-6

Proteins are crucial to the function and repair of every cell in the human body – from hair to fingernails to each organ – all comprised of amino acids. Therefore, the amount and quality of the proteins we ingest are directly linked to how we function.

FATS

Fat is sometimes overshadowed by the carb/protein debates and has gotten such a bad rap over the last 40 years! In the 1980s, the fat-free, cholesterol-free movement took over the media and the grocery shelves. Heart disease, chronic obesity, and strokes were making the news headlines every other hour. The shelves in the grocery stores became filled with products touting that they were "heart healthy" with their enriched grains and colorful packaging, promising a slimmer, more convenient life with less heart attack risk. Most people quickly bought into the marketing ploys. It has taken us four decades to recognize that heart disease, obesity, cancer, and stroke rates have not declined since the removal of fat and cholesterol from our diets. In fact, it has been quite the opposite. Fast forward 40 years and we have more cancer, heart disease, strokes, and autoimmune conditions (some of which did not even exist in the 1980s), and the rate of obesity has more than tripled. In an inverse relationship, the above-mentioned conditions have increased as the average daily consumption of fat decreased. As a society, we haven't gained health from removing fat and cholesterol from our diets. We have gotten sicker.

The driving mantra of the low-fat movement focused on correcting medical concerns associated with eating a high-fat diet (e.g., heart disease and obesity), with little regard for the impact of a low-fat diet (which often has increased sugar) on mental health. Unfortunately diets low in fats and proteins and high in sugar disrupt brain health in a number of ways that will be discussed in later chapters. Healthy fats play an important role in brain health as well as helping with the all-important feelings of satiety so you know when to quit eating.

Dietary fats provide essential *fatty acids* which the body cannot make for itself. Incorporating healthy fats into our diets is necessary to help with the absorption and utilization of the fat-soluble vitamins A, D, E, and K. Without adequate dietary fat consumption, we have trouble absorbing these vitamins, many of which are vital to overall health and to mental health in particular. In addition, the body must have an adequate energy source to function. Fat serves as a stabilizing energy source, protects our organs, supports cellular regeneration, helps with hormonal balance, and keeps cholesterol and blood pressure within healthy ranges. With the seductive health claims in packaged low-fat foods promising a fat-free and cholesterol-free lifestyle, we have also seen a rise in hormonal imbalances, mental health diagnoses, and overall morbidity and mortality.

CARBOHYDRATES

Carbohydrates are the body's other energy source. Carbohydrates are found in plant foods and include leafy green and cruciferous vegetables such as kale and broccoli, starchy vegetables such as carrots and potatoes, legumes such as lentils, beans, and peas, and grains such as rice, wheat, and corn, and fruits from apples to watermelon. Diet trends have varying and often conflicting recommendations about how many carbohydrate grams to eat daily, however, most Americans consume far too many grams of carbohydrates daily. The Food Pyramid from the 1980s and the Plate from the early 2000s perpetuated the belief that we need massive amounts of carbohydrates in our diet. But unless you are an elite athlete, you probably consume many more than you need.

An important distinction to make with carbohydrates is whether they are *simple or complex carbohydrates*. Carbohydrates include fiber, starches, and sugars, but the amounts of each can vary widely depending on the specific type of carbohydrate you are eating. Fiber and starches are complex carbohydrates because it takes the body longer to break them down and digest them into smaller food particles. Simple carbohydrates are high in sugars and break down and enter the blood stream quickly in what some describe as a "sugar rush" followed by tiredness.

Foods that are high in *fiber* include fruits, vegetables, and whole-grain products. Animal products have no fiber. There are two types of fiber: insoluble and soluble. *Insoluble fiber* is hard to chew and includes things like celery strings and whole corn kernels. *Soluble fiber* forms a gel when it absorbs water and includes oats, lentils, and apples. The body does not break down fiber for its nutrients, but fiber is essential for digestion to build bulk in the stool which helps it move smoothly through the intestines, stimulating and aiding digestion of the other foods. Fiber also takes longer to digest than simple carbohydrates, so when fiber and simple carbohydrates are eaten together (e.g., raspberries and toast), the fiber slows down the rate the food particles enter the bloodstream, which helps regulate blood sugar and decreases the sugar high/fatigue roller coaster. It also helps you feel full longer.

Starches are complex carbohydrates that the body can break down for their vitamins and minerals and which are slower to enter your bloodstream than sugars. You can find starchy carbohydrates in beans and legumes, fruits, whole grains like brown rice, and vegetables, like corn, peas, and potatoes. For people who are sensitive to carbohydrates or working to manage their blood sugar, starchy vegetables can enter their blood stream more quickly than desired and cause a glucose spike (more on this later), so they may need to limit their starchy vegetables.

Sugars can either be naturally occurring or added sugars in foods. Examples of naturally occurring sugars are lactose in dairy products and fructose in whole fruit. Added sugars are those found in sweets like brownies, candy bars and ice cream, canned fruit, fruit juice, and soda. They are generally processed from their original form such as sugar cane or sugar beets to create white table sugar, which removes the fiber and water found in the original plant form. Removal of the fiber is one of the main reasons simple carbohydrates quickly move through the stomach and intestines to rapidly enter the blood stream. For example, when you eat a whole apple it takes longer to digest than an apple in a smoothie that has already been partially broken down or "pre-chewed" by the blender. Faster still to digest is when the apple is made into fruit juice where all of the fiber has been removed, and the body responds to it as a simple sugar that is quickly absorbed.

The *glycemic index* (GI) is a measure of how drastically a food makes your blood sugar rise in the two to three hours after eating. Foods are ranked on a scale of 0 to 100, with pure sugar receiving a value of 100. The lower the score, the slower your blood sugar is likely to rise after eating that food. In general, the higher the level of processing of a food, the higher the GI, and the more fiber and fat in a food, the lower the GI. However, the GI does not give the full picture. The *glycemic load* (GL) also takes into account the normal serving size of a food. For example, carrots have a moderately high GI of 47, but a low GL of 4 due to their high amounts of fiber and water, and a normal serving offers relatively few carbohydrates compared to a serving of pasta which has a GI of 45 and a GL of 33.

One of the main problems with eating too many simple or refined carbohydrates is the effect on blood sugar (known as *glucose*). The fast absorption of sugars into the bloodstream causes a surge or spike of glucose. The body is not designed for this type of influx. As hunter-gatherers, foods always came in their whole form including the fiber, which had to be chewed to release the sugars slowly into the bloodstream. It has only been in our recent agricultural era that we began mechanically breaking down or removing the fiber from foods to make them easier to eat, digest, and store. Glucose spikes cause a rapid release of the hormone insulin and when repeated throughout the day nearly every day can cause significant health problems which we discuss more in Chapter 6.

CASE STUDY: LIPID THERAPY FOR PTSD

Dr. Champion's client, John, a 53-year-old Army veteran, presented with complex PTSD, chronic fatigue, chronic pain so debilitating that he was unable to complete simple tasks, and irritable bowel syndrome with diarrhea (IBS-D). His condition severely impacted his quality of life, leaving him unable to perform everyday activities like yard work, housework, and even his beloved pastime of riding his motorcycle. John had no energy to complete even the most basic tasks and would find himself sleeping for long periods of time, often losing days of his life to sleep.

Due to the wide range of his symptoms, Dr. Champion suspected that the root cause of John's symptoms was improper cellular function, and that treatment focused on improving cell function was an important first step. Nutrient deficiencies can weaken cellular walls and disrupt their proper function. Research on lipid therapy, which includes healthy dietary fats such as fat extracted from soybeans, began in the 1950s, but like most things, it was abandoned after the next great thing came along. Lipid therapy targets improving cellular structure and function. Impaired cellular walls, the site of lipid therapy action, allow the nutrients to leak out of the cells, making the nutrients unusable by the mitochondria. When using lipid therapy, the goal is to heal the structure of the cellular walls to increase nutrient retention.

After extensive consultations, John began a regimen of a lipid therapy supplement at a high dosage to help repair the cellular structure. Remarkably, within just one month, he experienced a 50 percent reduction in pain; by six months, his pain had reduced by 75 percent. This significant improvement allowed him to resume yardwork, housework, and motorcycle riding. Additionally, John made substantial changes to his diet, focusing on an anti-inflammatory diet devoid of grains, dairy, and legumes, and increased his water intake. These combined efforts not only alleviated his chronic pain but also improved his overall wellbeing and mental health, marking a dramatic turnaround in his health and lifestyle.

MICRONUTRIENTS

While less focus is given to them by the media and many health providers, the micronutrients within our foods are even more significant to our health than the proportions of macronutrients (proteins, fats, carbohydrates) that we eat. Twenty-eight micronutrients acquired through diet include iron, magnesium, iodine, selenium, vitamin E, manganese, phosphorus, the B vitamins (B1, B2, niacin, B5, folate, biotin, B6, B12), zinc, vitamin A, sulfur, vitamin C, calcium, vitamin D, potassium, vitamin K, choline, and beta carotene. These micronutrients are all food components essential for us to acquire at the appropriate levels for the body to function efficiently, which is very individual. We are all predisposed to have certain micronutrients that we either do not manufacture well in the body or for which we struggle to supply from our food, which causes us to become nutrient deficient.

When these nutrients are scarce in our soil, they become scarce in the body, thus leading to a myriad of diseases and mental health challenges. With the advent of industrial agricultural practices, we have lost soil integrity and nutrient concentration, resulting in lower nutrient density in the food being harvested, leading to a nutrient deficit in the food that we eat. This general lack of nutrients leaves our bodies craving more micronutrients, which we often confuse as signals to consume more food. We continue to eat and then wonder why we are not feeling better, while also witnessing a rise in our blood pressure, cholesterol, insulin levels, and overall risk of all-cause morbidity and mortality.

SELENIUM, ZINC, AND MAGNESIUM

While all micronutrients are critical, some play a more direct role in optimal mental health. Selenium, zinc, and magnesium all play significant roles in mental health (Ferreira de Almeida et al., 2021; Wang et al., 2018). For example, thyroid hormone imbalances, which may be exacerbated by iodine and selenium deficiencies, can contribute to mental health challenges like depression. When we strive to get to the bottom of conditions from which our bodies need healing, we must include the body's various organ systems. Research demonstrates that, for some people with iodine and/or selenium deficiencies, thyroid hormones can be balanced, and depression symptoms can be reduced through dietary changes that increase consumption of these micronutrients (Sánchez-Villegas et al., 2018).

PHYTONUTRIENTS AND ANTIOXIDANTS

We cannot have a robust conversation about micronutrients without mentioning phytonutrients and antioxidants. A *phytonutrient* (also known as a phytochemical) is a chemical compound found in various plants believed to be beneficial to prevent or reverse various health conditions. There are hundreds of phytonutrients, the most common include the carotenoids such as lutein, flavonoids, coumarins, indoles, isoflavones, lignans, plant sterols, and organosulfur. According to research by Gupta and Prakash, phytonutrients are critical nutrients in preventing and reversing numerous diseases (Gupta & Prakash, 2014).

Antioxidants are a particular class of micronutrients whose function is scavenging for and neutralizing *free radicals*, which are unstable molecules that can harm your cells. Free radicals serve a positive function to help fight infections, however when there are a higher number of free radicals than antioxidants, it can lead to a state of *oxidative stress* which damages cells and increases the risk for cancer. Lifestyle factors that promote oxidative stress include cigarette smoke, environmental toxins, and high blood sugar levels.

Vitamins C, E, and melatonin are prime examples of antioxidants that can remove potentially harmful substances in the body. Sadly, with the loss of nutrient-rich soil over the last hundred years or so, the decline in bioavailable food sources for antioxidants in the Standard American Diet has impacted the optimal health of our population. Overall consumption and absorption of fat-soluble vitamins have declined as we moved away from eating organ meats and dietary fats. Vitamin E deficiency symptoms include numbness and tingling, muscle pain and weakness, vision problems, and lackluster immune system functioning.

As we dive further into specific mental health conditions, the connections between macronutrients, micronutrients, phytonutrients, and antioxidant deficiencies can be the missing puzzle piece in many mental health approaches. While reading, look at the mental health conditions as puzzles with many different pieces that may be present (and don't forget to look under the couch, too, for that stray piece).

NUTRITION SCIENCE IDEOLOGY

Now that you have a basic understanding of the foundational components of food, it is time to tease apart some of the ideology behind nutrition science. While many theories have advanced the study of nutrition regarding mental health, many reductionistic ideas are embedded in the educational system and mainstream information which led people down a well-meaning path of "health." As an example, despite widely shared evidence that dietary fat and cholesterol are linked to chronic disease, it is still far too easy to walk down the aisles in a grocery store and see "nonfat, low fat, low cholesterol" labels splashed across the packages of processed food products that all promise you better health. But without more understanding of how macro and micronutrients work together in providing optimal nutritional support, a general "health" claim is often based more on marketing than actionable advice.

NUTRITIONISM

Nutritionism is a term that describes the model of reducing foods to their basic macronutrient, micronutrient, or ingredient. The term coined by Gyorgy Scrinis (2013) was popularized by Michael Pollan, and is met with mixed reviews. Proponents of nutritionism argue that it creates more of a scientific, research-based approach to nutrition that allows us to take more control of our health by understanding the impact of specific aspects of food. Opponents of nutritionism say that this approach to nutrition has distorted our way of seeing whole foods because it disregards the complex interplay between the nutrients within a whole-food item. The concern is that this model has been used to promote the health benefits of processed foods, which makes the benefits of whole foods less obvious by comparison. A whole orange does not have a flashy health label that says, "High in Vitamin C!"

With whole foods, the nutrients work together in concert with one another to support, balance, and correct absorption and utilization. When we disregard this and eat processed foods that focus on individual ingredients, we can create deficiencies in some nutrients and excesses in others. For many, looking at the nutrition labels to find out how many grams of fat, protein, and carbohydrate leaves them feeling like they have mastered their nutrition. Unfortunately, the bigger picture may be missed.

Enrichment is the industrial process of removing core nutrients from a food and then adding back in one or two key nutrients so that the food item can be marketed as having higher nutritional value. Food labels can then include that their product has been *fortified* with the key nutrient that was added during the enrichment process. For example, cereal grains are often highly processed, so by the time they are put in the cereal box an extremely limited nutritional value is present. As the push toward whole-grain consumption and the awareness of nutrition overall increased, food producers started adding individual nutrients to their food products to increase sales. Vitamin B12 and folic acid are commonly added to cereals to enrich their nutrient content. What about the other vitamins and minerals like zinc and thiamine? Those are often lost in the cereal manufacturing process, which leaves those foods without a full complement of the core nutrients found in the whole grains. Manufacturers remove these parts of the whole grains, so the product stays intact for a longer time, increasing the shelf life of the product. Shelf life is an important aspect of processed foods since preserving foods long enough for people to buy and eat them has not always been easy. Developing foods that can be stored without refrigeration opens more options to get those foods to consumers. However, sometimes the level of processing required to extend the shelf life results in food that has lost many of its valuable micronutrients.

Imagine for a moment that you are walking through a major city park at night, and you are approached by someone demanding all of your clothes, money, wallet, hat, jacket, and gloves. As you strip down and feel the cold air on your skin, the assailant shows slight mercy and hands you back your jacket. Suddenly, you are "enriched" even if you are still missing the rest of what was yours. Just like you not feeling comfortable without the rest of your belongings, the food item lacks nutritional stability, which may create discomfort in those who consume it.

Nutritionism also tends to favor those with the financial resources that allow them to choose to live that way. For those who live in a food desert, it is not always about choosing the healthiest options. It is about choosing what will fit in the budget or by what is actually available and at what cost. This tends to leave out a significant population of people who often need and want quality nutrition but have limited access to in their community. We dive more into food insecurity in Chapter 14, but for now, know that the critical nutrients emphasized in nutritionism may be more difficult for some to obtain than others.

Of Note . . . NOVA SCALE OF WHOLE, PROCESSED, AND ULTRA-PROCESSED FOODS

Whole foods, processed foods, and ultra-processed foods represent three distinct categories within the *NOVA classification system*, which is widely used to assess the degree of food processing. Whole foods, categorized as Group 1 in the NOVA scale, include minimally processed items like fruits, vegetables, nuts, seeds, grains, and unprocessed animal products. Whole foods retain their natural structures and nutritional profiles and are typically consumed in their original state or with minimal alterations, such as washing, cutting, or lightly steaming. In contrast, *ultra-processed foods*, classified as Group 4, are industrial formulations made from substances extracted or derived from whole foods, such as oils, fats, sugars, starches, and proteins, along with additives like preservatives, emulsifiers, and colorings. These foods are designed to be hyper-palatable, convenient, and shelf-stable but often lack the nutritional quality of whole foods.

Hyper-palatable foods are energy dense (high in calories) and contain ingredients that stimulate our brain reward system, especially fat, sugar, and sodium (e.g., fast food, fried food, desserts) (Fazzino et al., 2019). Shelf-stable foods can be safely stored at room temperature because they have been treated by heat and/or dried to destroy foodborne microorganisms that can cause illness or spoil food, and are generally packaged in sterile, airtight containers (USDA, 2015). Shelf-stable foods have traditionally included canned and bottled foods, rice, pasta, flour, and sugar. They are now expanded to include processed foods such as MREs (meal, ready-to-eat) where you add water and heat, nutrition bars and powders, chips, dips, and a variety of snack foods. Since many oils and fats become rancid relatively quickly if not refrigerated, many food manufacturers have replaced them with hydrogenated oils to delay the onset of rancidity, which increases the product's shelf life. Unfortunately, hydrogenated oils are high in *trans fats*, which are pro-inflammatory and have been linked to an increased risk of obesity, diabetes, heart disease, and depression, particularly among our most vulnerable socio-economic groups (Ejtahed et al., 2024; Remig et al., 2010), which is why many countries have policies in place to reduce consumption of foods with hydrogenated or partially hydrogenated oils (Downs et al., 2017). See Chapter 14 for more details about trans fats.

Ultra-processed foods have also been linked to negative health outcomes, including obesity, metabolic syndrome, and other chronic diseases, making the differentiation between these whole foods and ultra-processed foods crucial for informed dietary choices. Between these two category extremes lies a middle ground, Groups 2 and 3, where the foods start as whole foods and are then turned into something else. For example, whole wheat berries are ground into flour to be baked into bread and other baked goods. The whole wheat flour is processed, but the nutrients remain since the bran and hull were ground instead of removed. Continuing on with the example of the wheat flour, Group 3 would be a complete removal of the hull and bran during processing, with nutrients added back in for enrichment.

U.S. DIETARY GUIDELINES AND NUTRITION LABELS

The first *Dietary Guidelines for Americans* was published in 1980. Since 1990, the Secretaries of Agriculture (USDA) and Health and Human Services (HHS) are required by law to publish the Dietary Guidelines for Americans every five years (USDA, n.d.-a; USDA & HHS, 2023). The goal was to synthesize nutrition science into simple guidelines that could be utilized by government food programs, healthcare institutions, public health programs, and professional societies to educate the public about healthy eating. The guidelines are in place both to advise the public as well as to guide decisions pertaining to food that is distributed or sold in public institutions like hospitals, prisons, and schools.

THE FOOD PYRAMID

The *1992 Food Guide Pyramid* (Figure 4.1) identifies what proportion of the diet should include each of the food groups (USDA, n.d.-a). The largest portion of the diet, the base of the pyramid, recommended 6–11 servings of bread, cereal, rice, and pasta per day. Fruits, vegetables, protein (meat, eggs, beans), and dairy, were in the middle of the pyramid, and the tip of the pyramid recommended consuming fats and oils sparingly (i.e., eat very little).

MYPLATE: A GUIDE

In 2011, the USDA introduced *MyPlate: A Guide* (see Figure 4.2) to help people visualize what to eat in a healthy typical meal (USDA, 2023). The basics of *MyPlate* are:

- Make half your plate fruits and vegetables. Focus on whole fruits and vary your veggies.
- Make half your grains whole grains.

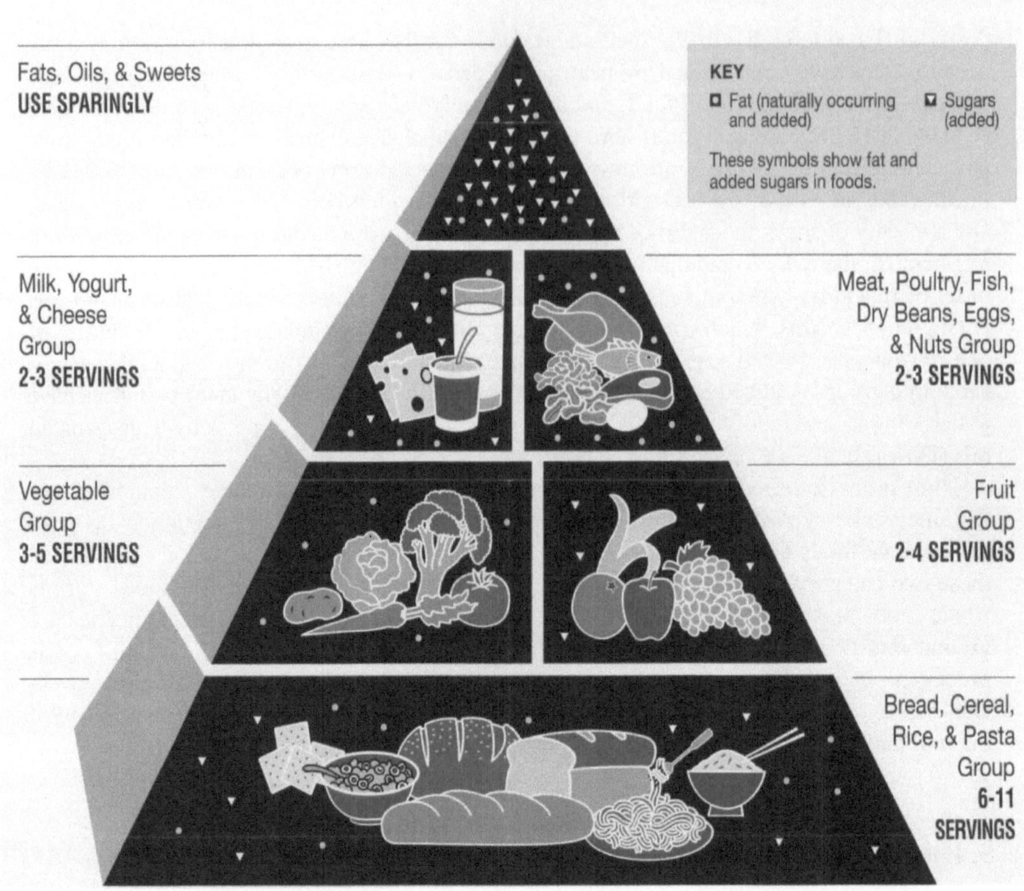

Fats, Oils, & Sweets
USE SPARINGLY

KEY
☐ Fat (naturally occurring and added)   ☐ Sugars (added)

These symbols show fat and added sugars in foods.

Milk, Yogurt, & Cheese Group
2-3 SERVINGS

Meat, Poultry, Fish, Dry Beans, Eggs, & Nuts Group
2-3 SERVINGS

Vegetable Group
3-5 SERVINGS

Fruit Group
2-4 SERVINGS

Bread, Cereal, Rice, & Pasta Group
6-11 SERVINGS

FIGURE 4.1   1992 USDA Food Guide Pyramid. (Courtesy of the U.S. Department of Agriculture.)

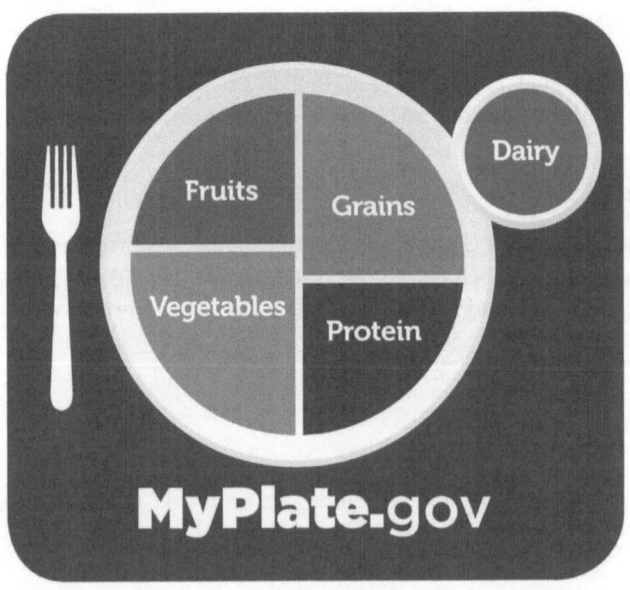

FIGURE 4.2   My plate: A guide. (Courtesy of the U.S. Department of Agriculture.)

- Vary your types of protein.
- Move to low-fat or fat-free dairy milk or yogurt (or lactose-free dairy or fortified soy versions)

The current *Dietary Guidelines for Americans, 2020–2025*, has four overarching guidelines (USDA, n.d.-b):

1. Follow a healthy dietary pattern at every life stage.
2. Customize and enjoy nutrient-dense food and beverage choices to reflect personal preferences, cultural traditions, and budgetary considerations.
3. Focus on meeting food group needs with nutrient-dense foods and beverages, and stay within calorie limits.
4. Limit foods and beverages higher in added sugars, saturated fat, and sodium, and limit alcoholic beverages.

The guidelines also recommend:

- Limiting added sugars to less than 10 percent of calories per day for ages two and older and to avoid added sugars for infants and toddlers
- Limiting saturated fat to less than 10 percent of calories per day starting at age two
- Limiting sodium intake to less than 2300 mg per day (or even less if younger than 14)
- Limiting alcoholic beverages (if consumed) to two drinks or less a day for men and one drink or less a day for women

Nutrition Labels

Understanding how to read a nutrition label is important for making informed food decisions. A nutrition label (see Figure 4.3) shows the key nutrients that impact health. Fats, for example, are listed in total and types, such as saturated and trans fats, which can affect heart health. Carbohydrates are broken down into total carbs, fiber, and sugars, each playing a different role in energy production, glucose regulation, and digestive health. Fiber is essential for maintaining a healthy gut and promoting satiety, while sugars, especially added sugars, can contribute to weight gain and other health issues when consumed in excess. Protein is vital for muscle repair, providing amino acids for mental health and overall body function. When you read a nutrition label, be sure to keep the serving size in mind. Sometimes the servings are smaller than people expect, like a candy bar that is listed as two servings instead of one.

Besides the nutritional breakdown, reading the ingredients list is equally important. The first five ingredients listed are the most prominent in the product, providing insight into the true composition of the food. By avoiding chemicals and additives, mental health can improve, and the body can heal. Consideration of the nutrition facts and the ingredient list allows an individual to make informed food choices that support optimal health.

To put this into perspective, the nutrition label provided in Figure 4.4 shows that there are 12 grams of fat, 34 grams of carbohydrates, and 11 grams of protein. Next to these figures are the percentage of Daily Value (DV) figures which calculate the percentage recommended for daily intake with a 2000 calorie per day diet. So, 12 grams of fat represents 14 percent of the recommended daily consumption of 86 grams of fat if you are consuming 2000 calories per day. There are 4 grams of Added Sugars, which is 8 percent of the total recommended amount of 50 grams or 12 teaspoons of added sugar per day.

COMMON FOOD MYTHS AND MISPERCEPTIONS

One of the struggles within the nutrition industry is all the misinformation out there. Between the variety of available diets, it is no wonder there is confusion! One day the news or social media says that the best way to eat is low-fat, and the next, it is ketogenic (high fat) with options ranging from vegan to carnivore. The confusion level increases every time the news airs.

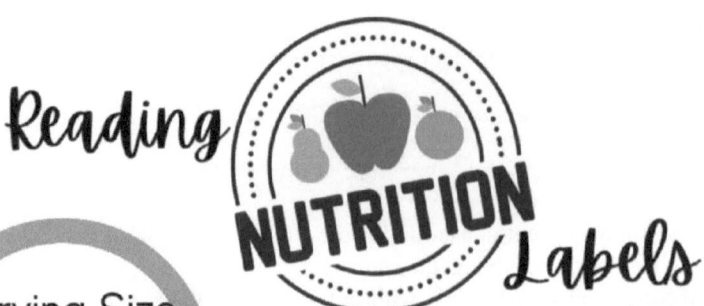

Reading Nutrition Labels

Serving Size
Refers to how much of that food is recommended

Fat
How much fat is included in a single serving

Sugar
Refers to how much sugar is in one serving. Watch for added sugars, which is often refined sugar

Carbohydrates
Total carbohydrate includes sugar and fiber in a single serving

Fiber
Fiber helps to slow glucose absorption and improve bowel movements

Protein
This shows how much protein is in a single serving

Nutrition Facts

Serving Size oz.
Serving Per Container

Amount Per Serving:

Calories	Calories From Fat
	% Daily value*
Total Fat	%
Saturated Fat	%
Trans Fat	
Cholesterol	%
Sodium	%
Total Carbohydrate	%
Dietary Fiber	%
Sugars	
Protein	

*Percent Daily values are based on a 2000 calorie diet. Your daily values may be higher or lewer depending on you calorie needs.

FIGURE 4.3 Reading nutrition labels. (Created by Jennifer Champion.)

Part of the issue is that we are always searching for the latest and greatest. We are a society searching for solutions that provide immediate gratification, even when it comes to our nutrition. We try one way of eating, thinking that the promises of weight loss or gain, more energy, more stamina, etc., will magically appear after just a few days. When it does not, we shift gears and move to another without realizing what we're doing to our bodies. Our metabolism works best when we are consistent and eat real food.

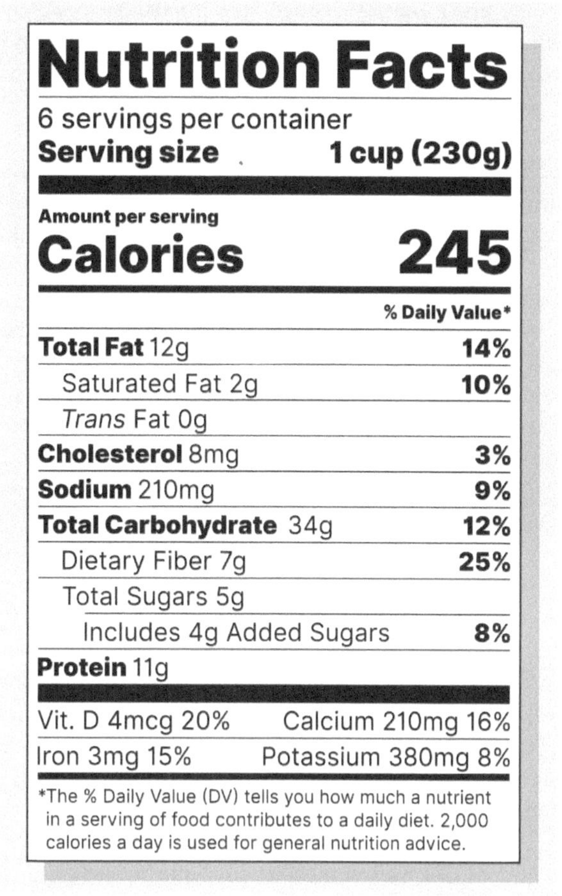

Nutrition Facts

6 servings per container

Serving size   1 cup (230g)

Amount per serving

Calories   245

	% Daily Value*
Total Fat 12g	**14%**
Saturated Fat 2g	**10%**
Trans Fat 0g	
Cholesterol 8mg	**3%**
Sodium 210mg	**9%**
Total Carbohydrate 34g	**12%**
Dietary Fiber 7g	**25%**
Total Sugars 5g	
Includes 4g Added Sugars	**8%**
Protein 11g	

Vit. D 4mcg 20%	Calcium 210mg 16%
Iron 3mg 15%	Potassium 380mg 8%

*The % Daily Value (DV) tells you how much a nutrient in a serving of food contributes to a daily diet. 2,000 calories a day is used for general nutrition advice.

FIGURE 4.4   A sample nutrition facts label. Credit: Maradaisy (ShutterStock).

AN INDIVIDUALIZED APPROACH TO NUTRITION

While no single diet will fit everyone, when we eat real food that is limited in processing and is high in nutrients and color, we begin to feel better. (See Chapter 8 for a detailed discussion of popular diets.) However, after years of eating a diet high in refined carbohydrates, salt, and sugar, it takes time to build our levels of nutrients. Therefore, our bodies do not immediately respond to changing how we eat over a few days; it's a process that requires patience and commitment.

Depending on the level of activity, muscular build, and genetic predispositions, what we need to eat for balance and optimal health varies from person to person. Let's examine some of the latest dietary crazes that are out there. As mentioned earlier, the low-fat diet hit the shelves and TV screens in the 1980s. However, over the last five to ten years, the ketogenic diet, a high-fat/low-carbohydrate diet, gained popularity. The ketogenic diet (described in more detail in Chapter 8) dates back to the 1920s as a treatment for epilepsy. It was developed as an alternative to long-term fasting, which was another established treatment for epilepsy. However, once anticonvulsant medications hit the market, many doctors quit recommending the ketogenic diet, despite its efficacy. However, the medications left about 20 percent to 30 percent of people with epilepsy without resolution; for those people, the ketogenic diet was often resumed.

Currently, the ketogenic diet is used for weight loss, as well as a treatment for those with diabetes, polycystic ovarian syndrome, reactive hypoglycemia, morbid obesity, and more recently, psychiatric issues. Like any major dietary change, it is important to weigh the pros and cons. For some, it elevates liver enzymes, causes digestive upset, and can create an improper gut microbial balance. For others, it decreases inflammation, improves non-alcoholic fatty liver disease, resolves cognitive issues, and improves mood (Anekwe et al., 2020; Chrysafi et al., 2024; Danan et al., 2022; Luukkonen et al., 2020; Newport, 2024; Volek et al., 2005).

Another closely related and currently popular diet is the carnivore diet. Essentially, the Carnivore diet omits all carbohydrates, including vegetables, fruit, grains, legumes, nuts, and seeds. All that is left is meat, fish, and eggs. It can improve mood, increase weight loss, and regulate blood sugar. Yet it lacks phytonutrients and antioxidants, many of which are beneficial for optimal mental health, gastrointestinal health, and cardiovascular health.

On the opposite end of the dietary spectrum is the vegan diet. Unlike the carnivore or ketogenic diet, the vegan diet omits all animal products from the diet, down to honey and white sugar (which is processed with animal bone char to make it white). Purportedly, the vegan diet incorporates more fiber, phytonutrients, and antioxidants through the increased consumption of vegetables and fruit. However, the vegan diet, much like the others we have discussed thus far, can also lead to nutrient deficiencies. The vegan diet lacks B12, an essential nutrient in neurological health, and is often a low-fat diet due to the lack of animal fats.

Which style of eating is better? While there is no simple answer to this question, we know that the human body needs a balance of critical macronutrients to function. Not enough fat in the diet will lead to a lack of absorption of the fat-soluble vitamins (A, D, E, and K) and cognitive and hormonal problems. Low-fat diets are often riddled with ultra-processed foods filled with sugar and chemicals to hold the food products together and provide flavor, since removing the fats tends to also remove much of the flavor. High-fat diets can also be problematic depending on the source of the fats. Trans fats, oxidized fats, and too many saturated fats can be problematic. In addition, if the gallbladder has been removed, the ability to break down and utilize fats has been reduced – too much dietary fat for someone without a gallbladder can lead to gastrointestinal upset.

While there is a great deal of disagreement about what it means to consume a healthy diet, most experts agree that we have far too much sugar in our diet. From the moment we wake up, with our lattes and waffles to our evening desserts of ice cream, the average American consumes about 17 teaspoons (71 grams) of sugar daily (CDC, 2024). This extra sugar raises blood sugar levels, increases insulin, and causes a decrease in magnesium entering the receptor sites, which leads to the kidneys excreting more magnesium. While researchers elucidated the impact sugar had on insulin sensitivity dating back to 1968 (Kahil et al., 1968), the push to add sugar to the food supply has continued to make foods more addictive. When food producers removed fat and cholesterol from their offerings, they exchanged them for sugar. Unfortunately, like many other drugs (see Chapter 13), sugar addiction (including needing to eat increasing amounts to feel satisfied due to tolerance) began to set in. To keep sales going, the manufacturers kept increasing the sweetness to satisfy the increasingly sugar-craving American palate to create a large population of "sugar junkies." As one can imagine, the gradual increases in sugar consumption led to increased demand for insulin. Over time, the body no longer recognizes the insulin naturally produced and becomes insulin resistant (see Chapter 6 for more details). As this process continues, the individual can develop diabetes. Long-term blood sugar imbalance decreases magnesium levels, which interferes with brain function properly, and emotional lability (moodiness) may develop.

In addition to wreaking havoc on blood glucose levels, sugar creates inflammation in the body (Stewart et al., 2022). If this inflammation progresses, the body will increase cholesterol production to protect the arteries from damage. Hence, sugar can raise cholesterol levels, which increases the risk of heart attack and stroke (Van Rompay et al., 2015). Current research continues to make clear the connections between body and brain inflammation (see Chapter 9 for more details), as well as common mental health issues such as depression.

A Return to Whole Foods

Over the last decade, an emphasis has been placed on eating whole foods. From the Whole30® to the Paleo diet, the focus is on eating whole foods, meaning foods with less processing and more closely matching their natural state at harvest. This is quite different from the convenience era that rolled out in the decades following World War II as families started to need two incomes to make ends meet. The promises of ease and simplicity moved the American population away from using natural and homegrown ingredients for canning, preserving, and cooking meals from scratch to frozen TV dinners and packaged meals – all coming with a hefty dose of salt, fat, and sugar.

After decades of meals made up primarily of packaged and prepared ingredients, we are seeing people returning to their kitchens and cooking with whole food ingredients. Grocery stores offer greater options of produce and fresh meats, some big box stores now feature fresh produce, there is increased access to farmer's markets, and more individuals and families are growing or raising their food. More recipes are showing up online on how to make foods from scratch with the promise of higher nutrient concentrations.

Myths and Facts about Dietary Fats

High-fat, low-fat, or no-fat, which is correct? The truth is that it depends on a person's genetics and health circumstances. For some people, a diet high in fat is the best route, such as a diet with a higher proportion of foods that are high in healthy fat, like butter and olive oil, compared to foods low in fat, like rice and cereal. For others, a more moderate to low-end fat consumption would be a better choice. A lower-fat diet will alleviate some digestive issues for those who have fat maldigestion issues. Whereas, for those who can digest fat well, a high-fat diet can help with cognitive, neurological, and endocrine imbalances. As we move away from the one-size-fits-all diet approach, we see that for many people, following a low-fat diet has led to negative health repercussions. There has been a steady increase in adults with hormonal imbalances, a rise in neurological disorders, and an overall lack of proper cellular functioning that are potentially all attributed to a lack of adequate quality fat in the diet.

The evidence continues to mount that including healthy, anti-inflammatory fats in the diet, like avocado, coconut, olives, and nuts, while avoiding vegetable, corn, soybean, canola, and seed oils, improves overall health (Bartimoccia et al., 2022; Muller et al., 2003). The low-fat craze is slowly being replaced by the low-carbohydrate movement, which seeks to reduce the overall consumption of foods high in starch and sugars and replace them with quality fats. In fact, diets higher in SMASH fish (sardines, mackerel, anchovies, salmon, and herring) can help to lower inflammation and LDL cholesterol levels while increasing HDL levels. Our bodies are designed to process and utilize fats for hormonal and cognitive benefits and padding for our internal organs.

Alongside the fat debate is the cholesterol debate. *Cholesterol* is a sterol molecule found in most body tissues, and its derivatives are integral components of cell membranes throughout the body. Cholesterol synthesizes steroid hormones (sex, adrenal, and thyroid), vitamin D, bile acids, and neurological function. In addition, cholesterol also regulates cellular function. Without sufficient cholesterol, the cells cannot function properly, digestion of fats is impaired, hormones become imbalanced, and the immune system is compromised.

When we talk about cholesterol, the discussion includes both the dietary cholesterol that we ingest when we eat animal products and the cholesterol that the body manufactures. Too much cholesterol in the bloodstream is associated with "clogging of the arteries" and an increased risk of heart attack and stroke. Mainstream medicine looks at cholesterol as an evil and deadly player in the health game, yet cholesterol is necessary for proper brain and hormone function. In many Integrative and Functional Medicine realms, cholesterol is a messenger conveying information about overall inflammation in the body. Greater levels of cholesterol indicate more inflammation is present in the body. When medicine focuses exclusively on reducing cholesterol levels without addressing the inflammation, it creates a greater risk of that inflammation doing irreparable damage to the arteries and heart.

Mainstream medical ideology states that healthy foods high in dietary cholesterol, such as ghee, lard, and coconut oil, can raise blood cholesterol levels. However, these foods typically do not raise blood cholesterol levels when eaten as part of a diet lower in processed, packaged foods, takeout foods, deep-fried foods, and sugar. How we cook food is also an important factor. Not all fats are created equally, and some should never be consumed. Much funding has been put forth to encourage the use of canola, corn, soy, and vegetable oils, touting that they are significantly healthier than other oils. Unfortunately, the increased oxidation in these highly refined oils (a change because of extra oxygen) contributes to systemic inflammation. Choose coconut oil, avocado oil, or ghee as a better option. What about olive oil? Olive oil can be used if the cooking temperature is below 400 degrees Fahrenheit. Otherwise, keep it cold-pressed and in dressing and dips, or drizzled on foods after they have been cooked!

NUTRITIONAL SUPPLEMENTS

The supplement industry is an area that has seen an immense amount of growth, and rightfully so! Our soil is depleted after decades of short-sighted agricultural practices. As discussed in Chapter 15, some of the newer farming practices such as organic farming include methods to return nutrients to the soil to better support more nutrient-dense fruits and vegetable products. In the meantime, conventional produce may have lower nutrient levels. Many feel their best option is to add supplements to make up for the lackluster quality of our nation's soil that results in plant harvests with reduced nutrient density.

Supplements are designed to supplement the diet, but not to replace proper nutrition. Supplements can be a good adjunct to a well-rounded diet but are not a replacement for it. Whenever possible, it is important to buy fresh local organic products and to get to know your farmers and their agricultural practices. For many people, the addition of supplements has been shown to improve symptoms related to nutrient deficiencies, however, not all supplements are created equal. Many contain fillers and stabilizers that have some evidence of being problematic. If you are going to use supplements, it is helpful to consult with a knowledgeable nutrition professional who can provide information about higher-quality supplements with transparency about where the raw materials are sourced and the manufacturing process.

FOOD FOR THOUGHT: SCOPE OF PRACTICE AND EDUCATION PATHWAYS IN NUTRITION

The nutrition industry's evolution led to many new and revised pathways to educate the American population. There are three primary groups of nutrition professionals in the United States: Certified Nutrition Specialist (CNS®) and Certified Clinical Nutritionist (CCN®), both of which are referred to as *Nutritionists*, and Registered Dietitian (RD), which are referred to as *Dietitians*. Depending on the state where they provide services, the scope of practice may differ between these three groups. One of the key differences between Nutritionists and Dietitians is which states will recognize that licensure for practice. The training between the CNS and the RD has a great deal of overlap, while the CCN pathway has less rigorous life sciences studies and no supervised internship, making it ineligible for licensure in most states. The RD license allows practice anywhere in the U.S., while the CNS license is more limited. Currently, there are 20 states or jurisdictions that allow CNSs to practice. Unfortunately, in several states, the training requirements are less clear for those who can call themselves a nutritionist, so it is important to check if a person is licensed as a CNS or other state-recognized license to ensure they have completed a thorough training program.

Having a pathway to state recognition is critical to ensure the person is qualified to give sound nutrition recommendations. State recognition helps to prevent an individual who is self-educated in nutrition from using the title "nutritionist." Self-identification as a nutritionist can be problematic, as there is a great deal of nuance to the art, science, and practice of helping people improve their nutrition. An RD and a CNS take extensive chemistry, biology, anatomy, physiology, and nutrition sciences coursework to fully understand the mechanisms for how nutrition impacts the body. The RD and CNS educational backgrounds prepare them to work with a diverse client population with many health concerns. Let us look at each of these pathways individually.

A CNS is a professional who has graduated with an advanced nutrition degree, such as a masters or doctorate from a fully accredited university, plus has a minimum of 1000 hours of supervised internship and passed a rigorous national board exam. The CNS is the only non-dietitian credential widely recognized in state nutrition laws. The CNS approach is often "root cause" and focuses mainly on prevention. This type of training is most in alignment with Functional or Integrative Medicine, where practice is focused on individual patient care. For this reason, you are not as likely to see a CNS managing food systems for a large organization, such as working in a hospital, which is a role generally filled by an RD.

A CCN is a nutritionist who has at least a four-year bachelor's degree coupled with a minimum of 56 hours of post-graduate study in clinical nutrition. The CCN focuses on digestion, absorption, assimilation, and how foods affect the body biochemically. CCNs must also pass a national board exam, however, there is no practicum or internship.

The RD is a food and dietary professional with at least a bachelor's degree and 900 to 1200 hours in a dietetic internship through an accredited program. An RD must also pass a national dietetics registration exam. Dietetics education typically focuses on calories, quality and freshness of food, food hygiene practices, and specific diets for medical conditions. Dietitians often work in clinics, schools, prisons, and hospitals, but some also work in private practice.

Each of the training programs offers certain benefits and drawbacks. While more job opportunities are available for RDs, if you fancy a career with a "root cause" approach to healthcare, the CNS pathway may be a better match. If you prefer consistency and a variety of job opportunities, then the RD approach may suit you. Of the three types of certifications, the CCN is the least accepted state-to-state and may pose additional professional restrictions.

The three licenses discussed thus far (CNS, CCN, and RD are all considered college-educated nutritionists or dietitians with the CNS being a master's degree-specific training. Both the CCN and RD pathways offer a bachelor's pathway. Beyond that, there are options for earning a doctorate. As of 2024, two options exist for a doctorate in clinical nutrition: a Ph.D. and a DCN. A Ph.D. is a Doctor of Philosophy. To achieve a Ph.D. in Nutrition, a student must complete the curriculum and produce significant and original research. The second doctoral degree in clinical nutrition is a Doctor of Clinical Nutrition (DCN), which is less research-focused than the Ph.D. and more focused on expanding clinical practice. Both programs offer a deeper understanding of nutrition science research, and their graduates are prepared to work with multidisciplinary teams in various health and wellness programs in conventional and holistic settings. Both the CNS and RD are eligible for a doctoral degree in nutrition.

For those who do not wish to seek a formal degree but wish to support those trying to change their health and wellness, certification as a *health coach* may be a better fit. A health coach is not a licensed professional, nor have they undergone the rigorous training that a certified nutritionist or dietitian has. A health coach supports the client by helping them sort through the recommendations or prescriptions made by degreed practitioners in the client's healthcare team. However, health coaches do not have the scope of practice to advise or tell a client what nutrition changes to make or which supplements to use and must be careful not to overstep. Their role is to learn each client's unique and individual circumstances and environment, actively listen as the client processes and incorporates the nutrition and lifestyle recommendations made by their healthcare team and provide ongoing support and accountability as these changes are made.

REFERENCES

Anekwe, C. V., Chandrasekaran, P., & Stanford, F. C. (2020). Ketogenic diet-induced elevated cholesterol, elevated liver enzymes and potential non-alcoholic fatty liver disease. *Cureus*, *12*(1), e6605. https://doi.org/10.7759/cureus.6605

Bartimoccia, S., Cammisotto, V., Nocella, C., Del Ben, M., D'Amico, A., Castellani, V., Baratta, F., Pignatelli, P., Loffredo, L., Violi, F., & Carnevale, R. (2022). Extra virgin olive oil reduces gut permeability and metabolic endotoxemia in diabetic patients. *Nutrients*, *14*(10). https://doi.org/10.3390/nu14102153

CDC. (2024). *Get the facts: Added sugars.* https://www.cdc.gov/nutrition/php/data-research/added-sugars.html

Chrysafi, M., Jacovides, C., Papadopoulou, S. K., Psara, E., Vorvolakos, T., Antonopoulou, M., Dakanalis, A., Martin, M., Voulgaridou, G., Pritsa, A., Mentzelou, M., & Giaginis, C. (2024). The potential effects of the ketogenic diet in the prevention and co-treatment of stress, anxiety, depression, schizophrenia, and bipolar disorder: From the basic research to the clinical practice. *Nutrients*, *16*(11), 1546.

Danan, A., Westman, E. C., Saslow, L. R., & Ede, G. (2022). The ketogenic diet for refractory mental illness: A retrospective analysis of 31 inpatients [Original research]. *Frontiers in Psychiatry*, *13*. https://doi.org/10.3389/fpsyt.2022.951376

Downs, S. M., Bloem, M. Z., Zheng, M., Catterall, E., Thomas, B., Veerman, L., & Wu, J. H. (2017). The impact of policies to reduce trans fat consumption: A systematic review of the evidence. *Current Developments in Nutrition*, *1*(12), cdn.117.000778.

Ejtahed, H. S., Mardi, P., Hejrani, B., Mahdavi, F. S., Ghoreshi, B., Gohari, K., Heidari-Beni, M., & Qorbani, M. (2024). Association between junk food consumption and mental health problems in adults: A systematic review and meta-analysis. *BMC Psychiatry*, *24*(1), 438. https://doi.org/10.1186/s12888-024-05889-8

Fazzino, T. L., Rohde, K., & Sullivan, D. K. (2019). Hyper-palatable foods: Development of a quantitative definition and application to the US food system database. *Obesity (Silver Spring)*, *27*(11), 1761–1768. https://doi.org/10.1002/oby.22639

Ferreira de Almeida, T. L., Petarli, G. B., Cattafesta, M., Zandonade, E., Bezerra, O., Tristao, K. G., & Salaroli, L. B. (2021). Association of selenium intake and development of depression in Brazilian farmers, *Frontiers in Nutrition*, *8*, 671377, https://doi.org/10.3389/fnut.2021.671377

Gupta, C., & Prakash, D. (2014). Phytonutrients as therapeutic agents. *Journal of Complementary & Integrative Medicine*, *11*(3), 151–169. https://doi.org/10.1515/jcim-2013-0021

Kahil, M. E., Simons, E. L., & Brown, H. (1968). Magnesium deficiency and sugar transport in muscle. Effect of acute insulin deficiency. *Diabetes*, *17*(11), 673–678. https://doi.org/10.2337/diab.17.11.673

Luukkonen, P. K., Dufour, S., Lyu, K., Zhang, X. M., Hakkarainen, A., Lehtimäki, T. E., Cline, G. W., Petersen, K. F., Shulman, G. I., & Yki-Järvinen, H. (2020). Effect of a ketogenic diet on hepatic steatosis and hepatic mitochondrial metabolism in nonalcoholic fatty liver disease. *Proceedings of the National Academy of Sciences*, *117*(13), 7347–7354. https://doi.org/doi:10.1073/pnas.1922344117

Muller, H., Lindman, A. S., Blomfeldt, A., Seljeflot, I., & Pedersen, J. I. (2003). A diet rich in coconut oil reduces diurnal postprandial variations in circulating tissue plasminogen activator antigen and fasting lipoprotein (a) compared with a diet rich in unsaturated fat in women. *The Journal of Nutrition*, *133*(11), 3422–3427. https://doi.org/10.1093/jn/133.11.3422

Newport, M. T. (2024). Ketogenic strategies for Alzheimer's disease and other memory impairments: History, rationale, and 288 caregiver case reports. *Medical Research Archives*, *12*(4). https://doi.org/10.18103/mra.v12i4.5316

Remig, V., Franklin, B., Margolis, S., Kostas, G., Nece, T., & Street, J. C. (2010). Trans fats in America: A review of their use, consumption, health implications, and regulation. *Journal of the American Dietetic Association*, *110*(4), 585–592. https://doi.org/10.1016/j.jada.2009.12.024 .

Sánchez-Villegas, A., Pérez-Cornago, A., Zazpe, I., Santiago, S., Lahortiga, F., & Martínez-González, M. A. (2018). Micronutrient intake adequacy and depression risk in the SUN cohort study. *European Journal of Nutrition*, *57*(7), 2409–2419. https://doi.org/10.1007/s00394-017-1514-z

Scrinis, G. (2013). *Nutritionism: The science and politics of dietary advice.* Columbia University Press.

Stewart, K. L., Gigic, B., Himbert, C., Warby, C. A., Ose, J., Lin, T., Schrotz-King, P., Boehm, J., Jordan, K. C., Metos, J., Schneider, M., Figueiredo, J. C., Li, C. I., Shibata, D., Siegel, E., Toriola, A. T., Hardikar, S., & Ulrich, C. M. (2022). Association of sugar intake with inflammation- and angiogenesis-related biomarkers in newly diagnosed colorectal cancer patients. *Nutrition and Cancer*, *74*(5), 1636–1643. https://doi.org/10.1080/01635581.2021.1957133

USDA. (2015). *Shelf-stable food safety.* https://www.fsis.usda.gov/food-safety/safe-food-handling-and-preparation/food-safety-basics/shelf-stable-food

USDA. (2023). *Learn how to eat healthy with MyPlate.* https://www.myplate.gov/

USDA. (n.d.-a). *History of dietary guidance development in the United States and the dietary guidelines for Americans – a chronology.* Dietary Guidelines for Americans. https://www.dietaryguidelines.gov/about-dietary-guidelines/history-dietary-guidelines/summary-dietary-guidance-development

USDA. (n.d.-b). *Top 10 things you need to know about the dietary guidelines for Americans, 2020-2025.* Dietary Guidelines for Americans. https://www.dietaryguidelines.gov/2020-2025-dietary-guidelines-online-materials/top-10-things-you-need-know

USDA & HHS. (2023). *Dietary guidelines for Americans.* https://www.dietaryguidelines.gov/about-dietary-guidelines

Van Rompay, M. I., McKeown, N. M., Goodman, E., Eliasziw, M., Chomitz, V. R., Gordon, C. M., Economos, C. D., & Sacheck, J. M. (2015). Sugar-sweetened beverage intake is positively associated with baseline triglyceride concentrations, and changes in intake are inversely associated with changes in HDL cholesterol over 12 months in a multi-ethnic sample of children. *The Journal of Nutrition, 145*(10), 2389–2395. https://doi.org/10.3945/jn.115.212662

Volek, J. S., Sharman, M. J., & Forsythe, C. E. (2005). Modification of lipoproteins by very low-carbohydrate diets. *The Journal of Nutrition, 135*(6), 1339–1342. https://doi.org/10.1093/jn/135.6.1339

Wang, J., Um, P., Dickerman, B. A., & Liu, J. (2018). Zinc, magnesium, selenium and depression: A review of the evidence, potential mechanisms and implications. *Nutrients, 10*(5). https://doi.org/10.3390/nu10050584

5 Microbiome and Mental Health

Now that we have discussed psychology and nutrition basics, we can begin to examine how they interact. Let us take a trip through your digestive system to explore how we digest food, what can go wrong in that process, and what that all has to do with mental health. We have all heard the phrase, "You are what you eat." This takes us to the next level by focusing on the process of how we digest food and the mechanisms that impact how that process impacts our thoughts and emotions.

WELCOME TO YOUR DIGESTIVE TRACT

From the moment we smell (and sometimes think about) food, our body prepares for digestion. It is the sensation we feel as we prepare food or wait for its arrival at our door or table. Aromas and thoughts can begin to trigger the physiological processes of digestion. The stronger the allure of the aroma, the stronger the response can be. Typically, the first reaction is that your mouth starts to salivate. *Saliva* combines sodium, potassium, calcium, magnesium, bicarbonate, and phosphates. When the brain has signaled your pancreas to join the fun, the salivary glands and pancreas begin to secrete amylase. Both amylases – salivary and pancreatic – are necessary as they code for different levels of digestive activity to prepare for the breakdown of starches.

Digestion begins in the mouth as enzymes and saliva prepares the body for digestion. The stomach is signaled to increase stomach acid production, and the small intestine prepares to receive the *chyme* (the partially digested food that passes from the stomach to the small intestine) from the stomach to extract the key nutrients needed to sustain life and better body functioning. Every cell in the body requires nutrients to perform its duties. Nutrients are vital components and cofactors for every process, from building muscles to reproduction.

As the food enters the mouth, the *tongue* begins communicating with the brain, each portion of the tongue features taste buds registering different flavors. Each tongue section is mapped to receive and convey flavor messages to the brain. The most posterior portion of the tongue registers bitter tastes, such as vinegar. The sides of the tongue register sour flavors, like lemons (this is why your cheeks may pucker when eating a lemon). The center portion of the tongue registers sweets, and the forward edges of the tongue register salty whereas umami flavors combine tastes such as those found in fermented foods like kimchi, meat broths, aged cheeses, and mushrooms. The sweet and salty flavor centers can easily trigger us to crave more of those foods. In contrast, the bitter and sour centers are more cautionary. They are often considered somewhat protective to keep us from eating the wrong things, especially during Paleolithic times when humans had to forage for their food, and eating the wrong food could mean death.

Chewing (known as *mastication*) triggers the rest of the enzymes, prepares the digestive tract to receive food, breaks it into its nutritional components, and then sends it to the small intestine for nutrient extraction and absorption. Without proper processing signaled by chewing, the digestive tract, especially the stomach and small intestines, has to work significantly harder to get nutrients into the body. So really good mastication is essential for nutrient extraction and breakdown of food.

THE HIGHS AND LOWS OF STOMACH ACID

After each swallow, the food *bolus* (food that has been chewed and mixed with saliva) travels from the mouth through the esophagus and into the stomach. The stomach acid is released here to help break the food into chyme. Most people produce sufficient stomach acid when they are

DOI: 10.1201/9781032647647-7

young. However, stomach acid level production can decline as people age when they are under stress, or if they chronically engage in poor dietary habits. Low stomach acid creates problems breaking down protein into individual amino acids. Amino acids are the building blocks of all cells and are necessary for proper functioning, so when we do not properly digest and break down protein, the body may not be able to absorb the important amino acids that it needs. In addition to breaking down protein, stomach acid is essential to maintaining a healthy microbiome by managing the levels of opportunistic bacteria. Opportunistic bacteria live in the body and proliferate when the body's natural systems for keeping them in check are knocked off balance. Stomach acid normally kills most of the opportunistic bacteria to prevent them from getting down into the intestines where they can grow. Low stomach acid allows opportunistic bacteria to get through where their numbers can multiply, which can play a significant role in mental health and will be discussed in more detail later in the chapter.

It is easy to understand why many people suffer from reduced stomach acid as a result of chronic stress, fast eating, and poor mastication. This may seem confusing since many people are diagnosed with elevated stomach acid. However, this is often a misdiagnosis typically based on symptoms alone and not through diagnostic testing such as an endoscopy. The reality is that, for the most part, stomach acid levels have declined over the years due to the increased stress demand and improper diet. We hear you screaming, "But what about those with acid reflux?" That is a great question!

While the conventional theory of acid reflux is that the body is producing too much stomach acid, there is another perspective that it is actually due to insufficient stomach acid levels and the resulting buildup of opportunistic bacteria. As an analogy, take a moment to imagine that your intestinal tract is an elevator at a busy international airport. As you eagerly await the elevator's opening, you stand there with your luggage. As the door opens, you see suitcases piled on top of one another, and everyone crammed in so tightly that you know there is no way to get in. Unfortunately, you may miss your flight if you miss this elevator, so you attempt to cram in. The people and luggage push against you blocking your way and then the door closes. There was simply no room! As you stand there waiting for the next elevator, you notice even more people showing up to catch the next elevator.

Much like this all too frequent airport scenario, when there is an overgrowth of opportunistic bacteria in the small intestine, the chyme sits in the stomach, waiting for the next elevator. In this case, the elevator is the sphincter between the bottom of the stomach and the small intestine. The stomach is supposed to move the chyme into the small intestine but does not because it senses the small intestine is already full due to the bacteria. When the stomach does not empty properly (known as gastric emptying) and the food sits too long, the stomach secretes more stomach acid. After doing this for a while, the stomach acid has only one direction to go because it cannot get into the small intestine where it is supposed to go. The stomach acid goes up through the lower esophageal sphincter and into the esophagus and throat, and acid reflux ensues. If sufficient stomach acid had been originally present, the opportunistic bacteria (think crowded elevator) would have been more balanced, and the chyme could have progressed naturally into the small intestines.

An example of the impact of an opportunistic bacterial overgrowth is the development of a stomach (gastric) ulcer that forms as a result of *Helicobacter pylori (H. pylori)* bacteria overgrowth. These bacteria live within the human digestive tract at all times. Once stomach acid levels decline, the door is open for overgrowth of *H. pylori*. From this point, the population of *H. pylori* will embed itself in the stomach lining, creating irritation as it eats into the lining, which also increases stomach acid levels as the body attempts to eradicate the *H. pylori*. This overgrowth accounts for approximately 80 percent of stomach ulcers and 90 percent of duodenal ulcers and is active in as much as 40 percent of the population (Zamani et al., 2018).

The condition of *dysbiosis*, which is the state of microorganism imbalance in the gut, with conditions like *small intestinal bacteria overgrowth (SIBO)* has made their presence known in our healthcare system. Dysbiosis can create bowel discomfort, such as gas, bloating, constipation, and diarrhea. The greater the imbalance or overgrowth, the higher the risk of losing critical nutrients due to the food not being broken down and absorbed properly. Dysbiosis and SIBO can also impact the gut–brain axis (see more below), leading to cognitive issues such as brain fog, anxiety, depression, mood swings, and irritability (Rogers et al., 2016).

Dysbiosis also includes fungal or yeast overgrowth in the body, such as candidiasis. A diet with excess sugar consumption can encourage fungal overgrowth, which can contribute to depression, anxiety, and other mental health symptoms. Dietary changes can reduce fungal overgrowth by consuming foods with naturally anti-fungal properties, such as coconut oil or coconut milk, which contains monolaurin and help reduce yeast proliferation throughout the body (Nitbani et al., 2022).

Stomach Acid Reflux

A common misconception is in play when people begin experiencing stomach acid reflux associated with dysbiosis, and mistakenly think it is due to having too much stomach acid rather than too little. Acid reflux medication is one of the most prescribed medications. Many people seek relief from their acid reflux or GERD (gastroesophageal reflux disease) and are given a *proton pump inhibitor (PPI)* medication to reduce stomach acid production. PPIs generally provide some initial relief from their acid reflux; however, it is often temporary, requiring additional medication and that comes at a price. Side effects of PPIs include weakened bones, pneumonia, and other lung infections, stroke, headaches, rashes, dizziness, nausea, abdominal pain, constipation, and diarrhea. Those diagnosed with non-alcoholic fatty liver disease (NAFLD) or any other liver disease should avoid using these medications as the PPIs can potentially damage the liver. PPIs can also create nutrient malabsorption, particularly calcium, magnesium, iron, potassium, and zinc, which interferes with the function of the gut–brain axis. This is an example of a pathway that contributes to nutrient deficiencies in the body that diminish both physical and mental health (Herreros Valenzuela, 2020; Urbas et al., 2016).

THE GUT–BRAIN AXIS

The *enteric nervous system (ENS)*, is a mesh-like system of nerves that governs the function of the *gastrointestinal (GI) tract* from the esophagus to the rectum. Structurally and neurochemically the ENS is now recognized "as a complex, integrated brain in its own right" and is referred to as the *second brain* (Gershon, 1999, p. 1). Similar to the brain, the ENS is filled with neurons and driven by many of the same neurotransmitters, including acetylcholine, dopamine, and serotonin, which enable the ENS to do some of its own "thinking" separate from the brain in your head. Science has finally found an explanation for the power of having a "gut feeling" about something and offers recognition that the gut provides valuable information when we can slow down and listen to it.

The communication between the ENS and the brain via the vagus nerve is known as the *gut–brain axis*. In addition to signaling from the gut organs (e.g., stomach, small intestine), there is evidence that the bacteria that live in the gut (the microbiome) communicate with the brain by releasing different chemicals such as GABA and short-chain fatty acids which profoundly influences our mental state and emotional regulation (Appleton, 2018; Dicks, 2024). Gut metabolites and the microbiome send signals directly to the brain asking for what it needs to function. Unfortunately, in our fast-paced society, we have learned to disregard or ignore the signals from our gut and instead opt for the convenience of fast food, the drive-thru, and processed packaged foods instead. The urgency of gut messaging gets over-ridden by whatever food is on hand rather than heard as a signal to guide us to eat what the body needs to provide key nutrients to function. This is one reason there has been so much emphasis on meal preparation and whole food availability. Often if better foods are not readily available to us, we favor urgency over quality.

THE CHEMISTRY OF THE GUT–BRAIN AXIS

Carbohydrates, fats, and proteins are broken down to release stored energy through a chemical reaction called the *Krebs cycle*. One of the essential nutrients for the Krebs cycle to function properly is riboflavin (vitamin B2). When the body is deficient in riboflavin due to a poor diet, inadequate functioning of the Krebs cycle can lead to nutritional deficiencies due to the food not being fully digested. This mechanism helps explain a potential pathway for the association between riboflavin deficiency and depression symptoms (Wu et al., 2022). This is especially true for our adolescent population, which typically consumes a diet high in processed, packaged foods that lacks critical nutrients (Herbison et al., 2012).

Essential fatty acids (EFAs) perform multiple functions in the brain, helping to regulate both the immune system and the inflammatory responses. These inflammatory responses can and often do occur in the brain. Chronic brain inflammation can contribute to psychiatric illness, cognitive decline, delirium, brain fog, and mental confusion. (See more about brain inflammation in Chapter 7.) Over the years, our modern Western diet has demonstrated decreased consumption of EFAs, which is likely a major contributor to chronic brain inflammation in the mentally ill. There is evidence that providing the body with EFAs in a supplement can make a dramatic difference for those with EFA deficiencies. In a 2002 study on young adult prisoners with antisocial behavior, those who received supplemental EFAs along with vitamins and minerals committed 26.3 percent fewer offenses than those who received the placebo. This study highlights the importance of nutrients and dietary intake in mental illness and behavioral disorders (Bernard et al., 2002).

EFAs are the building materials for the phospholipid membrane surrounding each cell, including those in the brain. This membrane can suffer irreparable damage when insufficient healthy fatty acids are consumed, which causes the cell membrane to leak. Here again, supplementing EFAs can be beneficial to improve cell membrane health. Without proper fatty acid intake, cell membranes suffer and communication between cells declines, leading to mental illness. In 1996, Horribon found that those diagnosed with schizophrenia were more likely to have leaky cell membranes (Horrobin, 1996). While the researchers at that time claimed that damaged cell membranes due to poor nutrition is a "novel field," it was actually Eugene Kennedy and his team of researchers in the 1950s who discovered the phospholipid membrane of the cells and the ability of supplements to strengthen this membrane and allow for proper communication between the cells (van der Veen et al., 2017).

HEALTHY ELIMINATION

Trying to figure out if the gut is healthy can be a challenge from an empirical perspective. One of the most common indicators of gut health is the frequency and consistency of bowel movements. Ideally, we should have two to four well-formed bowel movements (elimination) daily without black, blood, or food particles. Most people deal with mild-to-moderate constipation daily and are told that it is entirely normal to have a single bowel movement every three to four days. This allows for bacteria overgrowth, putrefaction, and an increased toxic burden on our bodies. Fecal matter is the body's primary tool to eliminate food waste, toxins, chemicals, and metabolic waste, such as unused hormones and neurotransmitters. When we do not have consistent and complete bowel movements, these chemicals get backed up in our systems and cause problems including increased inflammation.

NEUROTRANSMITTERS AND THE GUT

A *neurotransmitter* is a chemical messenger that carries a signal from a nerve cell (neuron) to another neuron, muscle cell, or gland. Many neurotransmitters are synthesized from amino acids, the molecules that make proteins, such as tyrosine and tryptophan. Common neurotransmitters include acetylcholine, dopamine, and serotonin.

SEROTONIN

Serotonin is a neurotransmitter primarily associated with mood regulation, happiness, and wellbeing. Within the last 10–15 years, the scientific and medical research communities have worked to ascertain the role and function of the microbiome and GI tract in serotonin production. Surprisingly, it turns out that serotonin is primarily synthesized and stored in the intestinal tract, not in the brain where our study of neurotransmitters has typically focused (Bornstein, 2012). They found that up to over 90 percent of serotonin production occurs in the distalmost portion of the intestinal tract (Banskota et al., 2019; Jones et al., 2020). Researchers now believe serotonin may also help regulate GI functioning, including regulating *gut motility* (movement of food through the intestines at the correct rate), which decreases constipation, helps regulate blood sugar, and improves gut health (Keating & Spencer, 2019). This is intriguing when we ponder the association between serotonin and mood and encourages us to consider that gut health may be an important factor in their connection.

The serotonin hypothesis was first developed in 1967, the same year that the first antidepressant hit the market as a cure for depression. As discussed in Chapter 3, the serotonin theory of depression became the predominant model for understanding that disorder. Over time, the serotonin deficiency hypothesis has been refined and now faces more scrutiny as deeper study is being done on serotonin deficiency as the source of depression (Möller & Falkai, 2023).

Serotonin communicates with the brain through the gut–brain axis, and research on autism spectrum disorder indicates that gut–brain dysfunction can increase serotonin dysfunction while potentially leading to social anxiety and awkwardness (Israelyan & Margolis, 2019). Serotonin has been the primary focal point of mental health treatment as it is implicated in several disorders, including depression, anxiety, schizophrenia, and attention-deficit hyperactivity disorder (ADHD) (Lin et al., 2014). In addition, those who are diagnosed with a mental health disorder also tend to struggle with glucose regulation. Serotonin helps to regulate blood glucose by improving gut motility. For those who struggle with fluctuating serotonin, self-care activities such as diet, meditation, and improved sleep can help regulate serotonin levels (see Figure 5.1). Eating a diet that helps

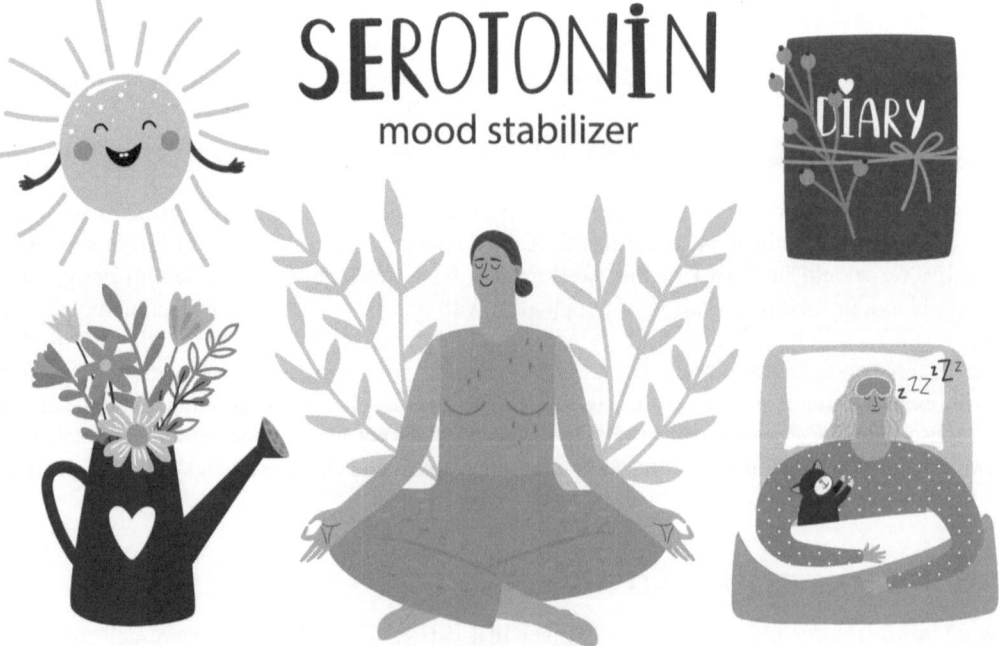

FIGURE 5.1   Self-care activities help regulate serotonin levels which improves mood. Credit: StockSmartStart (ShutterStock).

stabilize blood glucose and supports healthy serotonin production with adequate protein intake is critical (Martin et al., 2019).

Dopamine

If we think of serotonin as the happiness molecule, we can think of dopamine as the impulse and desire molecule. *Dopamine* gives us the desire to do something, to find pleasure and passion in the things we do, and to plan. It is a key player in the brain reward pathways and is often discussed as an important driver of the addiction process including cravings and withdrawal symptoms (see Figure 5.2). It also plays a significant role in learning, motivation, cardiovascular health, kidney function, sleep, mood, attention, and pain response, and helps to control nausea and vomiting. Dopamine must remain in homeostasis, not too high and not too low, or else the imbalances can lead to mental health struggles. Some mental health disorders are attributed to too little dopamine, such as ADHD, and others, such as schizophrenia, are attributed to too much dopamine (Howes et al., 2017).

Similar to serotonin, historically we associated dopamine only with the brain and then found the gut plays an integral role in the production and processing of dopamine. In fact, 50 percent of all dopamine found in the body is produced by the gut (Eisenhofer et al., 1997) and an integral part of that production is performed by the bacteria in the gut. The gut microbiome helps to facilitate dopamine synthesis and metabolite breakdown. Specific bacteria such as *Prevotella*, *Bacteroides*, *Lactobacillus*, *Bifidobacterium*, *Clostridium*, and *Enterococcus* all affect dopamine production and balance (Hamamah et al., 2022). Opportunistic (aka "bad") bacteria in the gut can dysregulate dopamine levels by crowding out the beneficial bacteria necessary for dopamine equilibrium. For example, overgrowths of bacteria such as *Bacillus*, *Staphylococcus*, *Proteus vulgaris*, and even *Escherichia coli (E. coli)* can cause excess dopamine levels to occur, leading to symptoms of increased aggression and poor impulse control (Sittipo et al., 2022).

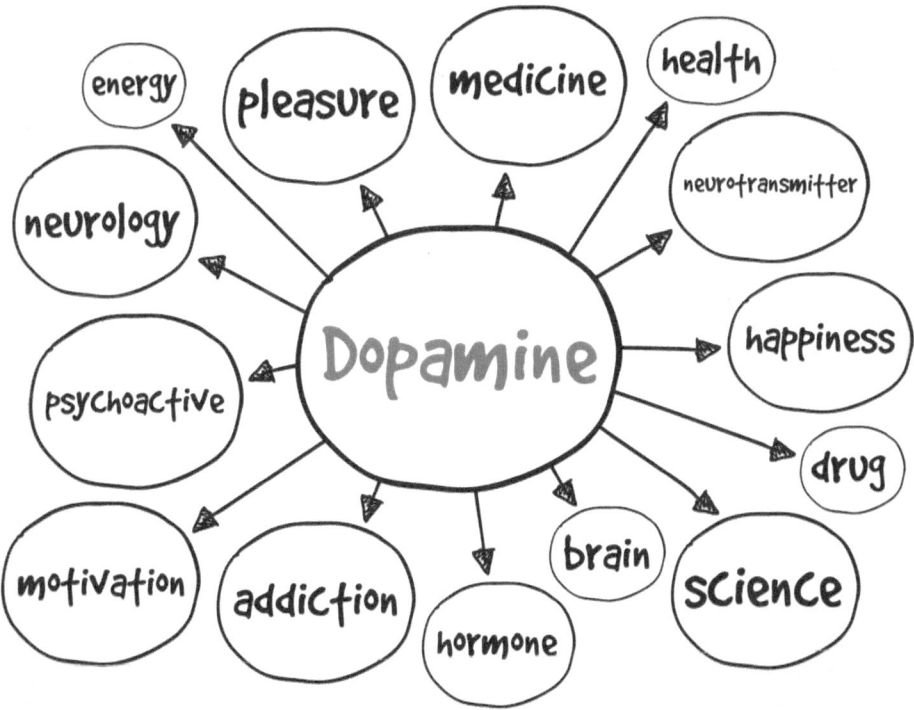

FIGURE 5.2 Dopamine. Credit: dizain (Shutterstock).

Parkinson's disease, ADHD, restless leg syndrome, depression, and schizophrenia may develop as a result of dysregulated dopamine production. Specific nutrients such as tyrosine, L-theanine, vitamins D, B5, and B6, magnesium, and omega-3 fatty acids can help regulate dopamine production. However, if the integrity of the gut is diminished, even if these nutrients are consumed, absorption of these essential nutrients may not yield as much benefit as anticipated.

LINKING GUT HEALTH TO MENTAL HEALTH

Gut health and the gut microbiome are currently an area of great interest in the healthcare system. We are just discovering the many intricate interconnections the gut has with the rest of the body. Newer in that exploration is the link between the gut and mental health. We are now beginning to understand the ways the gut influences mental health and factors that impair mental health by damaging the gut.

INTESTINAL PERMEABILITY

Intestinal permeability (IP or leaky gut) has recently earned medical recognition. While no current diagnosis code exists for this condition, many doctors recognize the intestinal tract's role in various health conditions (Bischoff et al., 2014). The intestinal tract has an inner lining of epithelial cells that are coated with a layer of mucus. IP denotes that the inner lining of the intestinal tract (known as the intestinal barrier) has been compromised and, therefore, cannot function properly. The cells of the intestinal barrier are designed to fit tightly together, but those tight junctions between cells are loosened with IP.

IP can occur as a result of food allergies, physical or emotional trauma, nutrient imbalances, substance abuse, medications, and infections (Bischoff et al., 2014). Diets high in sugar can damage the mucosal layer which also contributes to loosening the tight junctions of the intestinal barrier (Halverson & Alagiakrishnan, 2020). The permeable gut lining allows larger undigested food particles to get through the intestinal barrier and into the bloodstream where the immune system responds to them as pathogens to be destroyed rather than nutrients to be distributed to the cells, which leads to increased inflammation. Current research has demonstrated the harmful impact of IP on anxiety disorders, schizophrenia, alcoholism, ADHD, and autism spectrum disorders largely due to increased inflammation in the body (Wasiak & Gawlik-Kotelnicka, 2023).

LEAKY BLOOD–BRAIN BARRIER

The *blood–brain barrier (BBB)* is a highly selective semipermeable layer of cells that regulates which substances can pass from the bloodstream to the brain. It protects the brain from harmful substances like bacteria, viruses, and chemical toxins while allowing in critical nutrients. Some substances can get through the BBB if they are small enough such as alcohol, caffeine, and antidepressant medications.

When there is a leaky gut, there is also a significant chance of a leaky BBB being present. This leaky BBB will allow chemicals, hormones, and other substances to cross through the typically non-permeable BBB (Persidsky et al., 2006). These harmful substances can also include our body's metabolic waste products not designed to make contact with the brain. It is not only intruders from the outside world but also toxic by-products from our inside world that make this barrier one of the most integral protectors of the human body.

The BBB is lined with epithelial cells and a mucosal layer comparable to that found in the intestinal lining, with similar cells and functions. It is designed to keep the outside world (foods, chemicals, etc.) separate from the inside world. Whether it be the BBB or the mucosal layer of the intestines, once a substance crosses either one and enters a place where it does not belong, be it the bloodstream or the brain, inflammation ensues. Initially, inflammation serves to wall off the intruder, but when an expansion of inflammation occurs, it can overload the body's defenses. This inflammation can create pain in our bodies. It can also create chemical or nutrient imbalances which we do not recognize due to its gradual changes, which can lead to mental health disorders.

One substance that readily crosses the BBB is *monosodium glutamate (MSG)*. The MSG chemical goes by many names, including but not limited to yeast extract, glutamic acid, glutamate, autolyzed yeast, autolyzed plant protein, soy protein, maltodextrin, and monopotassium glutamate. MSG is an excitotoxin (meaning it is excitatory and stimulating) and a neurotoxin (meaning it damages nerve tissue) that readily crosses the BBB. Researchers knew as early as 1975 that MSG could cross the BBB and have negative effects if in large doses (Kazmi et al., 2017; Oser et al., 1975) and was considered safe to have in the food supply when consumed in reasonable doses. The research was based on finding safe levels based on staying below short-term high-dose intakes of MSG. This did not account for the cumulative effect of long-term ingestion of low levels of MSG over time. Currently, MSG is regularly added to fast food, restaurant food, and packaged foods to enhance flavor. People who regularly consume the foods end up with a high cumulative intake of MSG, exceeding the "safe" consumption limit (Rodgers, 2023).

Since it is both an excitotoxin and neurotoxin that passes through the BBB, MSG stimulates brain cells and eventually kills them. High levels of MSG have also been shown to produce brain lesions in children (Appaiah, 2010). There is some evidence that MSG has addictive properties (remember excitatory means it feels exciting so we want to do it more) and tricks the brain into thinking that what one consumes is delicious and increases cravings for that food. Glutamate functions as an excitatory neurotransmitter and has been associated with somatic and psychiatric disorders such as schizophrenia, psychosis, anxiety, and depressive disorders (Kraal et al., 2020; Kumar et al., 2021; Onaolapo & Onaolapo, 2021). In addition, MSG can impair cognition and worsen symptoms of cognitive decline (Kouzuki et al., 2019).

Of Note . . . FOOD DYES AND MENTAL HEALTH

Food dyes were initially made from coal tar but are now made from petroleum. (Yes, the same source your car's gasoline and oil are made from!) Many food dyes are banned in countries other than the U.S. Evidence is mounting that certain food dyes such as Red 3, Red 40, Yellow 5, and Yellow 6 have been found to cause cancer (Kobylewski & Jacobson, 2012; Wu et al., 2021). These food additives can induce IP and disrupt the gut–brain axis (Abiega-Franyutti & Freyre-Fonseca, 2021). With our brightly colored processed foods, we are disrupting the gut–brain axis and creating an environment for increased mental health disorder risk as these foods alter the gut microbiome (Cao et al., 2020).

One area of focus that has taken the spotlight concerning food dyes is the impact on ADHD. The diagnosis rates for ADHD have skyrocketed, right alongside the consumption of food dyes and additives. Researchers have found that diets that are low in or absent of food dyes tend to help those with ADHD (Kanarek, 2011; Nigg et al., 2012). There is also a potential link between certain food dyes (e.g., Yellow 5) and sleep disturbances, which often impact those with ADHD (Bakthavachalu et al., 2020).

GUT FUNCTION DISRUPTERS

By now it is clear that the gut is a multi-faceted, complex, and sensitive system that is core to our overall health. Numerous factors influence gut health and change how it functions. This in turn impacts the rest of the body primarily through malnutrition and activation of the immune system.

Immune System Function and Inflammation

The *immune system* functions to protect the body from the outside world by killing off and flushing out anything that may cause harm. Up to 85 percent of the immune system resides in the GI tract, with bacteria in the microbiome such as Firmicutes and Bacteroidetes playing a crucial role (Shi et al., 2017). Dysbiosis that reduces levels of Firmicutes impairs immune system function and increases the risk of disease development and depression (Huang et al., 2018; Methiwala et al., 2021). Bacteroidetes also contribute to the occurrence and worsening of depressive symptoms. The disrupted colonization of Bacteroidetes in the small and large intestines alters the essential amino acid tryptophan pathways, which interrupts their conversion to the neurotransmitter serotonin (Zhang et al., 2022). Therefore, when we protect gut microbiome health we also protect immune system health, which has many benefits for both physical and mental health (Järbrink-Sehgal & Andreasson, 2020).

Heavy Metal Toxicity

Heavy metals (e.g., mercury, arsenic, iron, lead, chromium) can disrupt the delicate microbiome of the GI tract as they reduce the population of beneficial bacteria while promoting the growth of opportunistic ("bad") bacteria (Jaishankar et al., 2014). This imbalance can lead to inflammation and impaired healing of the mucosal lining (Bist & Choudhary, 2022). As discussed, the gut–brain axis relays between the brain and gut, making the gut the "second brain." Heavy metals can disrupt the communication between the gut and the brain by increasing oxidative stress and inflammation (Ayuso-Álvarez et al., 2019). Sadly, the brain is not immune to oxidative stress and inflammation, as evidenced by decreased neurotransmitter production in the brain as a response to oxidative stress. As an example, cadmium, which is found in meats, shellfish, mushrooms, and the water supply, can be problematic at high doses where it can significantly increase the risk of depression development in young adults ages 20–39. Cadmium levels are often elevated in cigarette smokers, as is the rate of depression (Scinicariello & Buser, 2015; Wu et al., 2023).

As of 1978, lead-based paints were banned in the U.S. after studies demonstrated that lead toxicity decreases cognitive function in children and adults (Lee et al., 2022). While lead poisoning is much less of a risk these days, the risk still exists in old water systems where there are lead pipes in the plumbing that leach lead into the water. Community members who drink the water are often unaware until people start developing lead toxicity symptoms. Most notably in recent history was the public crisis in Flint, Michigan, that hit the news in 2014 when lead in the old water pipes exposed residents to elevated lead levels.

Lead does not limit its deleterious effects to cognitive function and the brain. It also impacts the GI tract by creating dysbiosis and destroying delicate homeostasis by increasing oxidative stress (an imbalance of free radicals and antioxidants in the body), inflammation, and IP (Yu et al., 2021). Lead also decreases the intestinal tract's ability to absorb amino acids, the building blocks of every cell, tissue, and organ within the body.

One of those vital organs that is heavily impacted by lead toxicity is the liver. It is of utmost importance since we cannot live without a healthy, functioning liver. The liver is the primary site of detoxification, which is the removal of any toxic substances from the body including heavy metals, unused neurotransmitters and hormones, broken down cells, and immune system waste from destroying pathogens like viruses. Lead impairs the liver's ability to metabolize lipids (fats). This has many repercussions. The brain is primarily comprised of fat and cholesterol and must have a steady lipid source for proper function. When the liver has been damaged, the brain can struggle to maintain adequate lipid levels for optimal function (Yu et al., 2021).

Mold and Mental Health

Environmental mold exposure in buildings in damp climates or with water leaks is increasingly being recognized as a major health threat for some people. Those who are more sensitive to mold in their home or at work can develop symptoms such as chronic sinus congestion, imbalanced gut bacteria, and cognitive issues. People who suffer from mold toxicity are also more likely to experience increased depression and anxiety symptoms, stress, emotion dysregulation, brain fog, and insomnia (Gatto et al., 2024; Potera, 2007). Since these mental health symptoms are not always accompanied by physical symptoms like difficulty breathing, fatigue, and headaches, it is easy to miss mold as the primary cause of a mental illness. Mold also can disrupt the tight junctions of the gut, which increases the incidence of IP, increases inflammation, and compounds the mental health struggle (Liew & Mohd-Redzwan, 2018).

FUNCTIONAL DISORDERS OF THE BOWEL

Over one-third of the American population suffers, often silently, with a functional digestive disorder. A functional digestive disorder means that there is no clear cause, and it cannot be attributed to a particular pathogen such as an *E. coli* or *Salmonella* bacterial infection. For example, functional dyspepsia is essentially chronic indigestion with bloating, gas, and bowel irregularities (diarrhea and constipation). However, it only sometimes happens, and the cause may be elusive. Those dealing with functional digestive disorders can still, for the most part, complete their regular tasks throughout the day except for when they are having an acute flare. According to a recent study done in 2023, those with functional dyspepsia were more likely to also suffer from anxiety and depression, which was associated with decreased occupational productivity and overall quality of life (Huang et al., 2023).

STRESS AND THE GUT

Stress can have a significantly negative impact on the gut. Stressful events are often associated with digestive symptoms including bloating, pain, nausea, and bowel irregularities. Chapter 9 discusses how stress, particularly chronic stress, impacts the body and gut health. Chronic stress changes neurotransmitter production which then impacts gut function. Remember that the neurotransmitter serotonin helps regulate gut motility, so changes in serotonin create changes in gut health. Without proper neurotransmitter production to regulate gut motility, increased bowel dysregulation increase the risk of developing a functional bowel disorder (Barry & Dinan, 2006). Some psychiatric medications and supplements can increase or decrease the rate of peristalsis (gut motility), which can help alleviate diarrhea or constipation and reduce abdominal pain. Anything that helps a person relax and move out of a fight or flight response encourages proper gut motility, which decreases pain and improves neurotransmitter function. Self-care strategies that decrease stress and improve gut health include quality sleep and exercise, employing relaxation techniques such as deep breathing, yoga, massage, and meditation. See Chapter 16 for more information about the importance of self-care strategies for physical and mental health.

CASE STUDY: GUT DISRUPTION DUE TO STRESS

Dr. Champion had a client with frequent unexplainable diarrhea. Thinking that the chronic diarrhea was likely due to something she was eating, the client sought treatment from a nutritionist. Notable findings from the client's stool sample indicated a potential gut bacteria overgrowth. Dr. Champion worked with this client, modulating diet and implementing supplement strategies to rebalance the client's microbiome. However, after three months of continued unrelenting diarrhea, Dr. Champion referred the client back to her primary care doctor and to a gastroenterologist to assess for anything structural that may be causing the symptoms. Both doctors were unsuccessful in finding the cause.

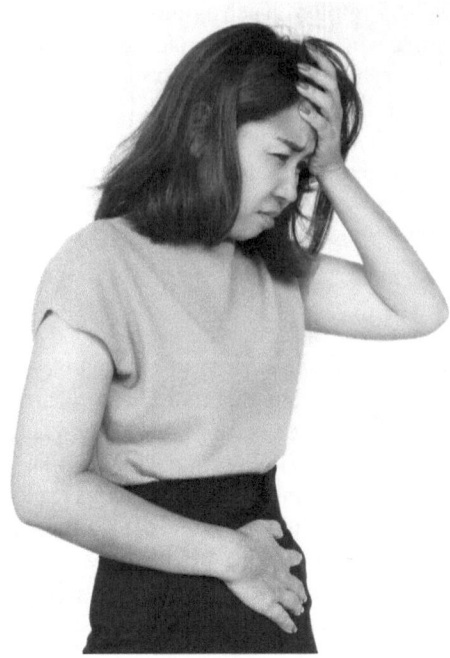

FIGURE 5.3 Stress and the gut. Credit: Doucefleur (Shutterstock).

Exploring other possible causes for the diarrhea, Dr. Champion encouraged the client to return to therapy with her psychiatrist, who suggested a temporary round of fluoxetine (an antidepressant). After two weeks on a low fluoxetine dosage, the client's diarrhea abated. It was also at that time the client revealed there had been a significant family altercation which had been weighing heavily on the client's mind and appeared to have lodged itself in her intestinal tract. Dr. Champion continued to work on the client's microbiome while the client explored the mental-emotional aspect of the healing process with her psychiatrist.

After six months of treatment, the client discontinued using fluoxetine while continuing to take her nutritional supplements, and the symptoms did not return. This case demonstrates how a nutritionist and therapist can collaborate to heal the gut, even when the symptoms appear to be only a physical health issue.

FOOD FOR THOUGHT: IMPACT OF ANTIBIOTICS ON THE GUT AND MENTAL HEALTH

Antibiotics are the most commonly prescribed medication. In 2022, over 230 million antibiotic prescriptions were dispensed in the U.S., which equates to seven prescriptions for every ten people (CDC, 2024). Most of us are familiar with the concerns around overuse of antibiotics and the risk of developing "superbugs" that no longer respond to an antibiotic during an infection. Superbugs are not the only problem associated with antibiotic use. They can also be very hard on the gut microbiome.

Many antibiotics work by altering the microbial balance in the intestinal tract. Unfortunately, antibiotics do not selectively kill only disease-causing bacteria but also commensal ("good") bacteria that help to regulate nutrient absorption, immune system functioning, and the gut–brain axis for mental health. One research study showed a dramatic increase in depressive symptoms after a single round of antibiotics. In addition, those who were prescribed one class of antibiotics (fluoroquino-lones) experienced an increase in anxiety symptoms, depression, insomnia, panic attacks, cognitive impairment, and schizophrenia-like symptoms (Dinan & Dinan, 2022).

While there is a time and place for emergency medicine and antibiotics, choosing a gentler way when possible, may be better for those who present with or are concerned about mental health struggles. Oregano oil is a potent antimicrobial, anti-fungal, antiviral, and anti-parasitic that provides many of the benefits found with an antibiotic. In addition to those health-boosting characteristics, oregano oil can elevate extracellular serotonin levels in the brain and induce behavioral changes characteristic of those created by antidepressants and anti-anxiety medications (Mechan et al., 2011). Food can be a powerful substance. Every bite is either fueling or discouraging disease, including mental illness. What we choose to put in our bodies makes a difference in our striving to maintain optimal mental health.

REFERENCES

Abiega-Franyutti, P., & Freyre-Fonseca, V. (2021). Chronic consumption of food-additives lead to changes via microbiota gut–brain axis. *Toxicology, 464*, 153001.

Appaiah, K. M. (2010). Monosodium glutamate in foods and its biological effects. In *Ensuring global food safety* (pp. 217–226). Elsevier.

Appleton, J. (2018). The gut–brain axis: Influence of microbiota on mood and mental health. *Integrative Medicine (Encinitas), 17*(4), 28–32.

Ayuso-Álvarez, A., Simón, L., Nuñez, O., Rodriguez-Blazquez, C., Martín-Méndez, I., Bel-Lán, A., Lopez-Abente, G., Merlo, J., Fernandez-Navarro, P., & Galan, I. (2019). Association between heavy metals and metalloids in topsoil and mental health in the adult population of Spain. *Environmental Research, 179*, 108784.

Bakthavachalu, P., Kannan, S. M., & Qoronfleh, M. W. (2020). Food color and autism: A meta-analysis. *Advances in Neurobiology, 24*, 481–504.

Banskota, S., Ghia, J. E., & Khan, W. I. (2019). Serotonin in the gut: Blessing or a curse. *Biochimie, 161*, 56–64.

Barry, S., & Dinan, T. G. (2006). Functional dyspepsia: Are psychosocial factors of relevance. *World Journal of Gastroenterology, 12*(17), 2701–2707.

Bernard, G. C., Hammond, S. M., Hampson, S. E., Eves, A., & Crowder, M. J. (2002). Influence of supplementary vitamins, minerals and essential fatty acids on the antisocial behaviour of young adult prisoners. *The British Journal of Psychiatry, 181*(1), 22–28.

Bischoff, S. C., Barbara, G., Buurman, W., Ockhuizen, T., Schulzke, J. D., Serino, M., Tilg, H., Watson, A., & Wells, J. M. (2014). Intestinal permeability–A new target for disease prevention and therapy. *BMC Gastroenterology, 14*(1), 25.

Bist, P., & Choudhary, S. (2022). Impact of heavy metal toxicity on the gut microbiota and its relationship with metabolites and future probiotics strategy: A review. *Biological Trace Element Research, 200*(12), 5328–5350.

Bornstein, J. C. (2012). Serotonin in the gut: What does it do? *Frontiers in Neuroscience, 6*, 16.

Cao, Y., Liu, H., Qin, N., Ren, X., Zhu, B., & Xia, X. (2020). Impact of food additives on the composition and function of gut microbiota: A review. *Trends in Food Science & Technology, 99*, 295–310.

CDC. (2024). *Outpatient antibiotic prescribing in the United States.* Antibiotic Prescribing and Use. https://www.cdc.gov/antibiotic-use/hcp/data-research/antibiotic-prescribing.html

Dicks, L. M. T. (2024). Our mental health is determined by an intrinsic interplay between the central nervous system, enteric nerves, and gut microbiota. *International Journal of Molecular Sciences, 25*(1), 38. https://www.mdpi.com/1422-0067/25/1/38

Dinan, K., & Dinan, T. (2022). Antibiotics and mental health: The good, the bad and the ugly. *Journal of Internal Medicine, 292*(6), 858–869.

Eisenhofer, G., Åneman, A., Friberg, P., Hooper, D., Fåndriks, L., Lonroth, H., Hunyady, B., & Mezey, E. (1997). Substantial production of dopamine in the human gastrointestinal tract. *The Journal of Clinical Endocrinology & Metabolism, 82*(11), 3864–3871. https://doi.org/10.1210/jcem.82.11.4339

Gatto, M. R., Mansour, A., Li, A., & Bentley, R. (2024). A state-of-the-science review of the effect of damp- and mold-affected housing on mental health. *Environmental Health Perspectives, 132*(8), 086001. https://doi.org/doi:10.1289/EHP14341

Gershon, M. D. (1999). The enteric nervous system: A second brain. *Hospital Practice*, *34*(7), 31–52. https://doi.org/10.3810/hp.1999.07.153

Halverson, T., & Alagiakrishnan, K. (2020). Gut microbes in neurocognitive and mental health disorders. *Annals of Medicine*, *52*(8), 423–443.

Hamamah, S., Aghazarian, A., Nazaryan, A., Hajnal, A., & Covasa, M. (2022). Role of microbiota-gut–brain axis in regulating dopaminergic signaling. *Biomedicines*, *10*(2), 436.

Herbison, C. E., Hickling, S., Allen, K. L., O'Sullivan, T. A., Robinson, M., Bremner, A. P., Huang, R. C., Beilin, L. J., Mori, T. A., & Oddy, W. H. (2012). Low intake of B-vitamins is associated with poor adolescent mental health and behaviour. *Preventive Medicine*, *55*(6), 634–638.

Horrobin, D. F. (1996). Schizophrenia as a membrane lipid disorder which is expressed throughout the body. *Prostaglandins, Leukotrienes and Essential Fatty Acids*, *55*(1-2), 3–7.

Howes, O. D., McCutcheon, R., Owen, M. J., & Murray, R. M. (2017). The role of genes, stress, and dopamine in the development of schizophrenia. *Biological Psychiatry*, *81*(1), 9–20. https://doi.org/10.1016/j.biopsych.2016.07.014

Huang, Y., Shi, X., Li, Z., Shen, Y., Shi, X., Wang, L., Li, G., Yuan, Y., Wang, J., & Zhang, Y. (2018). Possible association of Firmicutes in the gut microbiota of patients with major depressive disorder. *Neuropsychiatric Disease and Treatment*, 3329–3337.

Huang, Q., Yuan, H., Li, Q., Li, Y., Geng, S., & Jiang, H. (2023). Global trends in research related to functional dyspepsia and anxiety or depression over the past two decades: A bibliometric analysis. *Frontiers in Neuroscience*, *17*, 1218001.

Israelyan, N., & Margolis, K. G. (2019). Reprint of: Serotonin as a link between the gut–brain-microbiome axis in autism spectrum disorders. *Pharmacological Research*, *140*, 115–120.

Jaishankar, M., Tseten, T., Anbalagan, N., Mathew, B. B., & Beeregowda, K. N. (2014). Toxicity, mechanism and health effects of some heavy metals. *Interdisciplinary Toxicology*, *7*(2), 60.

Järbrink-Sehgal, E., & Andreasson, A. (2020). The gut microbiota and mental health in adults. *Current Opinion in Neurobiology*, *62*, 102–114.

Jones, L. A., Sun, E. W., Martin, A. M., & Keating, D. J. (2020). The ever-changing roles of serotonin. *The International Journal of Biochemistry & Cell Biology*, *125*, 105776.

Kanarek, R. B. (2011). Artificial food dyes and attention deficit hyperactivity disorder. *Nutrition Reviews*, *69*(7), 385–391.

Kazmi, Z., Fatima, I., Perveen, S., & Malik, S. S. (2017). Monosodium glutamate: Review on clinical reports. *International Journal of Food Properties*, *20*(sup2), 1807–1815.

Keating, D. J., & Spencer, N. J. (2019). What is the role of endogenous gut serotonin in the control of gastrointestinal motility? *Pharmacological Research*, *140*, 50–55.

Kobylewski, S., & Jacobson, M. F. (2012). Toxicology of food dyes. *International Journal of Occupational and Environmental Health*, *18*(3), 220–246.

Kouzuki, M., Taniguchi, M., Suzuki, T., Nagano, M., Nakamura, S., Katsumata, Y., Matsumoto, H., & Urakami, K. (2019). Effect of monosodium L-glutamate (umami substance) on cognitive function in people with dementia. *European Journal of Clinical Nutrition*, *73*(2), 266–275.

Kraal, A. Z., Arvanitis, N. R., Jaeger, A. P., & Ellingrod, V. L. (2020). Could dietary glutamate play a role in psychiatric distress? *Neuropsychobiology*, *79*(1), 13–19.

Kumar, P., Kraal, A. Z., Prawdzik, A. M., Ringold, A. E., & Ellingrod, V. (2021). Dietary glutamic acid, obesity, and depressive symptoms in patients with schizophrenia. *Frontiers in Psychiatry*, *11*, 620097.

Lee, H., Lee, M. W., Warren, J. R., & Ferrie, J. (2022). Childhood lead exposure is associated with lower cognitive functioning at older ages. *Science Advances*, *8*(45), eabn5164.

Liew, W. P. P., & Mohd-Redzwan, S. (2018). Mycotoxin: Its impact on gut health and microbiota. *Frontiers in Cellular and Infection Microbiology*, *8*, 60.

Lin, S. H., Lee, L. T., & Yang, Y. K. (2014). Serotonin and mental disorders: A concise review on molecular neuroimaging evidence. *Clinical Psychopharmacology and Neuroscience*, *12*(3), 196.

Martin, A. M., Yabut, J. M., Choo, J. M., Page, A. J., Sun, E. W., Jessup, C. F., Wesselingh, S. L., Khan, W. I., Rogers, G. B., & Steinberg, G. R. (2019). The gut microbiome regulates host glucose homeostasis via peripheral serotonin. *Proceedings of the National Academy of Sciences*, *116*(40), 19802–19804.

Mechan, A. O., Fowler, A., Seifert, N., Rieger, H., Wöhrle, T., Etheve, S., Wyss, A., Schüler, G., Colletto, B., & Kilpert, C. (2011). Monoamine reuptake inhibition and mood-enhancing potential of a specified oregano extract. *British Journal of Nutrition*, *105*(8), 1150–1163.

Methiwala, H. N., Vaidya, B., Addanki, V. K., Bishnoi, M., Sharma, S. S., & Kondepudi, K. K. (2021). Gut microbiota in mental health and depression: Role of pre/pro/synbiotics in their modulation. *Food & Function*, *12*(10), 4284–4314.

Möller, H. J., & Falkai, P. (2023). Is the serotonin hypothesis/theory of depression still relevant? Methodological reflections motivated by a recently published umbrella review. *European Archives of Psychiatry and Clinical Neuroscience*, *273*(1), 1–3.

Nigg, J. T., Lewis, K., Edinger, T., & Falk, M. (2012). Meta-analysis of attention-deficit/hyperactivity disorder or attention-deficit/hyperactivity disorder symptoms, restriction diet, and synthetic food color additives. *Journal of the American Academy of Child & Adolescent Psychiatry*, *51*(1), 86–97.e8.

Nitbani, F. O., Tjitda, P. J. P., Nitti, F., Jumina, J., & Detha, A. I. R. (2022). Antimicrobial properties of lauric acid and monolaurin in virgin coconut oil: A review. *ChemBioEng Reviews*, *9*(5), 442–461. https://doi.org/10.1002/cben.202100050

Onaolapo, A. Y., & Onaolapo, O. J. (2021). Glutamate and depression: Reflecting a deepening knowledge of the gut and brain effects of a ubiquitous molecule. *World Journal of Psychiatry*, *11*(7), 297–315. https://doi.org/10.5498/wjp.v11.i7.297

Oser, B., Morgareidge, K., & Carson, S. (1975). Monosodium glutamate studies in four species of neonatal and infant animals. *Food and Cosmetics Toxicology*, *13*(1), 7–14.

Persidsky, Y., Ramirez, S. H., Haorah, J., & Kanmogne, G. D. (2006). Blood–brain barrier: Structural components and function under physiologic and pathologic conditions. *Journal of Neuroimmune Pharmacology*, *1*, 223–236.

Potera, C. (2007). *Mental health: Molding a link to depression*. National Institute of Environmental Health Sciences.

Rodgers, E. (2023). *75+ fast food consumption statistics*. Drive Research. https://www.driveresearch.com/market-research-company-blog/fast-food-consumption-statistics/#:~:text=2%20in%203%20people%20consume,on%20fast%20food%20each%20month

Rogers, G., Keating, D. J., Young, R. L., Wong, M. L., Licinio, J., & Wesselingh, S. (2016). From gut dysbiosis to altered brain function and mental illness: Mechanisms and pathways. *Molecular Psychiatry*, *21*(6), 738–748.

Scinicariello, F., & Buser, M. C. (2015). Blood cadmium and depressive symptoms in young adults (aged 20–39 years). *Psychological Medicine*, *45*(4), 807–815.

Shi, N., Li, N., Duan, X., & Niu, H. (2017). Interaction between the gut microbiome and mucosal immune system. *Military Medical Research*, *4*(1), 7.

Sittipo, P., Choi, J., Lee, S., & Lee, Y. K. (2022). The function of gut microbiota in immune-related neurological disorders: A review. *Journal of Neuroinflammation*, *19*(1), 154.

Urbas, R., Huntington, W., Napoleon, L., Wong, P., & Mullin, J. (2016). Malabsorption-related issues associated with chronic proton pump inhibitor usage. *Austin Journal of Nutrition & Metabolism*, *3*(2), 1041.

van der Veen, J. N., Kennelly, J. P., Wan, S., Vance, J. E., Vance, D. E., & Jacobs, R. L. (2017). The critical role of phosphatidylcholine and phosphatidylethanolamine metabolism in health and disease. *Biochimica et Biophysica Acta (BBA)-Biomembranes*, *1859*(9), 1558–1572.

Wasiak, J., & Gawlik-Kotelnicka, O. (2023). Intestinal permeability and its significance in psychiatric disorders–a narrative review and future perspectives. *Behavioural Brain Research*, *448*, 114459.

Wu, L., Xu, Y., Lv, X., Chang, X., Ma, X., Tian, X., Shi, X., Li, X., & Kong, X. (2021). Impacts of an azo food dye tartrazine uptake on intestinal barrier, oxidative stress, inflammatory response and intestinal microbiome in crucian carp (Carassius auratus). *Ecotoxicology and Environmental Safety*, *223*, 112551.

Wu, Y., Zhang, L., Li, S., & Zhang, D. (2022). Associations of dietary vitamin B1, vitamin B2, vitamin B6, and vitamin B12 with the risk of depression: A systematic review and meta-analysis. *Nutrition Reviews*, *80*(3), 351–366.

Wu, Z., Yue, Q., Zhao, Z., Wen, J., Tang, L., Zhong, Z., Yang, J., Yuan, Y., & Zhang, X. (2023). A cross-sectional study of smoking and depression among US adults: NHANES (2005–2018). *Frontiers in Public Health*, *11*, 1081706.

Yu, L., Yu, Y., Xiao, Y., Tian, F., Narbad, A., Zhai, Q., & Chen, W. (2021). Lead-induced gut injuries and the dietary protective strategies: A review. *Journal of Functional Foods*, *83*, 104528.

Zamani, M., Ebrahimtabar, F., Zamani, V., Miller, W., Alizadeh-Navaei, R., Shokri-Shirvani, J., & Derakhshan, M. (2018). Systematic review with meta-analysis: The worldwide prevalence of Helicobacter pylori infection. *Alimentary Pharmacology & Therapeutics*, *47*(7), 868–876.

Zhang, Y., Fan, Q., Hou, Y., Zhang, X., Yin, Z., Cai, X., Wei, W., Wang, J., He, D., & Wang, G. (2022). Bacteroides species differentially modulate depression-like behavior via gut–brain metabolic signaling. *Brain, Behavior, and Immunity*, *102*, 11–22.

6 The Impact of Hormones on Mental Health

It is nearly impossible to have a robust conversation about the roots of mental health without involving the multitude of hormonal cascades that happen every day in the body. Hormones are chemical messengers produced by various glands in the body and distributed through the bloodstream to regulate different tissues like muscles and organs. Hormones differ from the neurotransmitters like serotonin and dopamine discussed in Chapter 5 in that they can impact parts of the body distant from the source or gland where they were released, whereas neurotransmitters are released into the synaptic gap between nerve cells transmitting a nerve signal from one nerve to its neighboring nerve. Hormones are part of the endocrine system, whereas neurotransmitters are part of the nervous system. Hormones regulate many physiological processes, including growth, metabolism, reproduction, and mood. In recent years, research has increasingly highlighted the intricate relationship between hormones and mental health. This chapter explores the role of hormones in influencing mood, cognition, and mental wellbeing.

HORMONES, APPETITE, AND STRESS

In the U.S., most people are overfed and undernourished. We have an abundance of calories readily available, and yet most of these calories come from processed and packaged food products. As mentioned in Chapter 4, ultra-processed foods generally come with a long ingredient list which usually includes chemicals, stabilizers, and fillers. These chemicals can disrupt key hormone-signaling within our bodies, especially for the hormones most associated with eating: leptin, ghrelin, and insulin.

LEPTIN

Leptin enables efficient cell communication that regulates the rest of our hormones, starting with ghrelin and insulin and then moving on to our thyroid, sex, and adrenal hormones. One of the key roles for leptin is that it helps the body realize when it has had enough food so that we feel satiated and full. It takes a little time for leptin to kick in after we have started eating. When we take the time to properly chew our food and pay attention to signals relayed from the stomach to the brain, we notice more quickly when we are full and avoid overeating. It takes about 20 minutes for our stomachs to relay to our brains that we are full and for the full release of leptin to take effect. Many of us chew-chew-swallow while watching TV, scrolling on our phones, or anything else that keeps us from paying attention to what and how we eat, which puts us at risk of over-eating and feeling over-full before the signal reaches us that it is time to stop eating.

GHRELIN

Ghrelin cues hunger signals when we need more fuel. Think of G for a growling stomach. Many things influence ghrelin production. One of the most problematic is the relationship between ghrelin release and sleep. Lack of sleep increases ghrelin hormone production, bolstering our desire to eat even when we are not in need of nutrients.

INSULIN

Insulin is another important hormone immediately involved in eating and digestion. Insulin is essential for signaling the cells to either immediately use glucose for energy or for the fat cells to store the

DOI: 10.1201/9781032647647-8

excess glucose in the blood stream. When the body is repeatedly flooded with glucose from eating simple carbohydrates like bread and sugar, the cells become *insulin resistant*, and it requires a higher production of insulin to get the cells to respond. When insulin resistance develops, the cells in the muscles, fat, and liver start ignoring the insulin and become less and less responsive to its effects. As a result, the body requires increasingly more insulin to keep blood sugar levels balanced. If this process continues, type 2 diabetes can develop. Those who are obese, lead a sedentary lifestyle, and eat a diet high in processed foods have an increased risk of developing insulin resistance.

This blood sugar instability can increase mental health struggles as well. Calkin et al. found that those diagnosed with bipolar disorder who had comorbid insulin resistance were more likely to experience stronger mood fluctuations (Calkin et al., 2015). Another 2019 study demonstrated a correlation between insulin resistance and adolescent mental health challenges (Scott et al., 2019). There appears to be a strong correlation between insulin resistance and depression, as multiple researchers have elucidated this connection (Bauermeister et al., 2023; Fernandes et al., 2022; Fryar et al., 2018).

Chronically high insulin levels are correlated with chronically high leptin levels, which is associated with obesity and leads to leptin resistance. *Leptin resistance* requires higher and higher levels of leptin production for the cells to respond, which can make it difficult to feel satiated and leaves you feeling constantly hungry. Blood sugar dysregulation due to insulin and leptin resistance can leave you hungry and depleted, especially magnesium depleted. As mentioned in Chapter 4, magnesium is an essential nutrient and is necessary for more than 300 biochemical reactions in the human body. Magnesium depletion occurs due to stress, sugar consumption, blood sugar dysregulation, and metabolic dysfunction. In addition, magnesium deficiency may contribute to mental health disorders such as depression, anxiety, bipolar, and schizophrenia (Misztak et al., 2015; Nechifor, 2011).

Diabetes mellitus is a chronic metabolic disorder characterized by impaired glucose regulation and insulin function that has been increasingly linked to an increased risk of mental health disorders. There are two types of diabetes. *Type 1 diabetes* is an autoimmune disease that begins early in life and results in inadequate insulin production by the pancreas. *Type 2 diabetes* is the result of a lifestyle with chronically high glucose levels that eventually damages the insulin production in the pancreas. The relationship between diabetes and mental health is bidirectional in that diabetes can have a negative impact on mood, and poor mental health increases the risk of poorly controlled diabetes. When a person has poorly managed diabetes, their hormones become dysregulated due to the frequent glucose spikes, which contributes to inflammation and increased mood issues (Holt et al., 2014). Conversely, those who are struggling with high or low moods typically make poor diet and lifestyle choices, often resorting to a diet high in refined, processed carbs for quick boosts of serotonin and dopamine, which makes their diabetes symptoms worse. *Hyperglycemia* (chronically high glucose levels) and insulin resistance, often the precursors to type 2 diabetes development, can lead to neuroinflammation and oxidative stress, which increases the symptoms of psychiatric disorders.

THYROID

Thyroid hormones, including thyroxine (T4) and triiodothyronine (T3), regulate metabolism and energy production. They also affect mood, cognition, and emotional wellbeing. Imbalances in thyroid hormones, such as hypothyroidism (low levels) or hyperthyroidism (high levels), can lead to symptoms of depression, anxiety, schizophrenia, bipolar disorder, cognitive impairment, and mood swings (Chakrabarti, 2011; Dayan & Panicker, 2013; Freuer & Meisinger, 2023). Untreated thyroid imbalances can exacerbate psychiatric conditions such as bipolar disorder and schizophrenia, and should be ruled out as part of the initial assessment of any treatment protocol (Baumgartner et al., 2000; Gau et al., 2010).

CORTISOL

Cortisol is a hormone produced by the adrenal glands in response to stress. It helps the body to cope with stressful situations by mobilizing energy and suppressing non-essential functions such as digestion and immune response. Prolonged exposure to high levels of cortisol can have detrimental effects on mental health, contributing to a broad range of mental health conditions.

In those with mental health challenges, there is an increased release of cortisol by the adrenal glands in response to stress or fear as part of our flight, fight, freeze, or fawn response (discussed more in Chapter 9). While short-term bursts of cortisol are helpful (think about the last exam or deadline that you had to meet), sustained production of cortisol can create a host of chemical imbalances in the body. Cortisol imbalances contribute to a range of health issues such as infertility, menstrual irregularities, thyroid dysfunction, reproductive disorders, and mood and behavior disorders (Ayuso-Álvarez et al., 2019; Caccappolo-van Vliet et al., 2002; Freire & Koifman, 2013).

Cortisol has an important relationship with blood sugar. Cortisol boosts blood sugar levels to provide immediate energy to help a person run from a threat, meet a deadline, or decide if they need to stand their ground and fight. Short-term cortisol boosts are helpful and designed for short sprints to meet a demand followed by an immediate return to normal levels. However, when cortisol remains elevated in the body due to chronic stressors, the body is continually instructed to release and utilize more glucose, which makes a constant demand and contributes to cravings for simple carbohydrates. Eating simple carbs can perpetuate the cycle, since rapid drops in glucose after an insulin spike cause the body to release stress hormones like cortisol to energize and motivate the person to find more food to maintain the glucose levels. Over consumption of simple carbohydrates, especially when they become the predominant food group consumed, directly impacts the rise and fall of our blood sugar levels, which then can drive elevated cortisol release. When we balance our blood sugar levels, as with a more balanced diet of whole foods, our cortisol levels can also become balanced.

Cortisol balance helps us be more mentally and emotionally resilient to the effects of stress. A diet rich in whole, nutrient-dense foods can support healthy cortisol levels. Complex carbohydrates, such as legumes, fruits, and vegetables, provide a steady energy source and help stabilize blood sugar levels. Foods high in vitamin C, such as citrus fruits, berries, kiwi, and bell peppers, support the adrenal glands' production of stress hormones like cortisol and reduce oxidative stress. Magnesium-rich foods like spinach, almonds, and avocados help the nervous system relax and modulate cortisol production. B vitamins in whole grains, leafy greens, and animal products help provide necessary co-factors for cortisol production.

OXYTOCIN

Oxytocin is a hormone that is associated with childbirth, breastfeeding, and mother-child bonding. Sometimes called the "love hormone," it is also involved in attraction, trust, cooperation, empathy, and sexual arousal. Oxytocin has a calming effect that lowers stress and anxiety, and motivates us to form social connections. Physical touch, social activities, and exercise all boost oxytocin levels.

Oxytocin impacts both physical and mental health. There is growing evidence that oxytocin decreases appetite, increases metabolism and energy expenditure, and improves insulin sensitivity and fat burning. Low oxytocin levels are associated with a higher BMI, larger waist circumference, increased blood glucose levels, and poor metabolic health (Ding et al., 2018; McCormack et al., 2020). In the mental health arena, deficiencies in the oxytocin brain mechanism have been associated with a childhood diagnosis of autism spectrum disorder, which is characterized by impairments in social interaction and communication (Moerkerke et al., 2021). There is even some early evidence that oxytocin stimulates serotonin release, and that oxytocin deficiencies may contribute to low serotonin levels and their associated depressive symptoms (Lefevre et al., 2017).

SEX HORMONES

Sex hormones can have a tremendous impact on mental health. The hormone system is intricate and complex. Each hormone interacts with and affects the production and function of the other hormones. The body works to keep hormones balanced and at the correct ratio with the other hormones

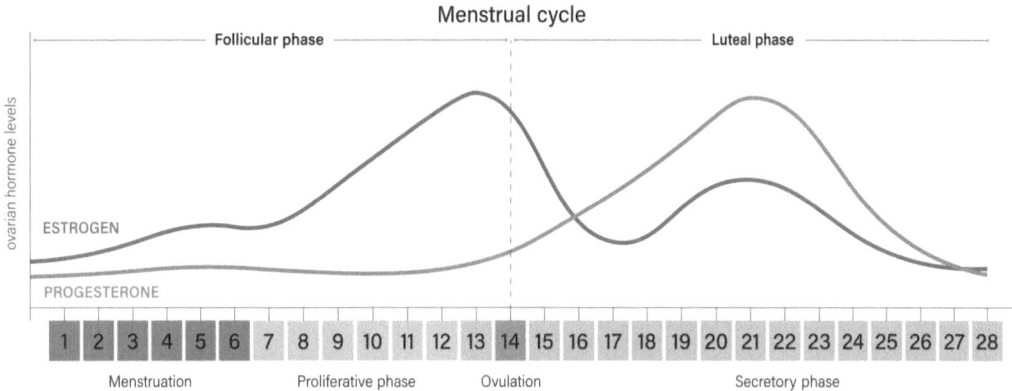

FIGURE 6.1   Menstrual cycle hormone fluctuations. Credit: Dee-sign (ShutterStock).

in the system. Dominance or deficiency of any one hormone can throw the whole system out of balance. Hormone imbalances contribute to a number of mental health issues including negative mood, low energy, and distorted thinking.

ESTROGEN AND PROGESTERONE LEVELS

Estrogen is known primarily as a female sex hormone, even though men also have estrogen, just at lower levels. *Progesterone* is a key hormone in regulating the menstrual cycle, fertility, and improving mood and sleep. During menstruation, the female body undergoes intricate hormonal fluctuations orchestrated by various hormones, notably estrogen and progesterone (see Figure 6.1). These hormonal shifts can profoundly affect the central nervous system, influencing mood, memory, and concentration. In particular, the luteal phase preceding menstruation is characterized by a decline in estrogen and progesterone levels, which may trigger alterations in neurotransmitter activity, specifically serotonin, gamma-aminobutyric acid (GABA), and dopamine.

Estrogen dominance, where estrogen levels are disproportionately high compared to progesterone levels, has been associated with an increased risk of developing mood disorders and exacerbating existing mental health conditions. Estrogen dominance can lead to a range of symptoms and health issues, including irregular menstrual cycles, heavy or painful periods, bloating, breast tenderness, mood swings, anxiety, and fatigue. Estrogen dominance can occur due to stress, environmental toxins, diet, certain medical conditions, and hormonal contraceptives. Women who are sensitive to hormonal changes need to be cautious about use of hormonal contraceptives if they are struggling with mental health issues. If left unaddressed, estrogen dominance may increase the risk of conditions such as endometriosis, fibroids, breast cancer, and thyroid dysfunction.

CASE STUDY: SEX HORMONES AND DEPRESSION

Dr. Champion had a female client we will call Beth, age 38, who presented with extreme emotional distress around the time of menstruation each month. Prior to having children, Beth reported she would have excruciating period cramps and some emotional lability (mood swings). Beth reported that after giving birth to each of her four children, she noticed an increase in the severity of her symptoms.

After the birth of her first child, Beth noticed that her cramps remained the same but that her emotions felt stronger. She reported this emotional increase to her OB/GYN, who stated that this would likely pass in time because her hormones would settle back into their standard patterns. Beth waited for a year but noticed that the symptoms persisted. Upon her next healthcare visit, she mentioned that her mood swings had not improved and she was put on an antidepressant.

Beth disclosed that the antidepressant only made her feel numb but did not stop the drastic mood swings around the time of menstruation. Within six months of starting her antidepressant, she became pregnant with her second child, and then about 14 months after delivering her second, she became pregnant again. She noticed her emotions improved slightly during her pregnancies, and then destabilized into what felt like she riding a rollercoaster when she was between pregnancies. After delivering her third child, she began struggling with depressive symptoms including suicidal ideation each month before she menstruated. By the time she gave birth to her fourth and final child, her symptoms became quite severe and met many of the DSM criteria for post-partum depression (see below). Beth felt significant amounts of shame and guilt because, according to her testimony, her family was falling apart due to her emotions.

It was clear that something had to be done. A series of lab tests were ordered including sex, adrenal, and thyroid hormone levels, blood glucose, lipids, and iron. The results showed Beth had significantly elevated estrogen and progesterone levels, low thyroid hormone levels (which often lead to depressive symptoms), cortisol insufficiency, and glucose dysregulation. An organic acids test revealed she was deficient in the amino acid tyrosine, an essential nutrient for the development and balance of dopamine.

Dr. Champion first suggested a diet filled with organic fruits and vegetables, and absent of any gluten, to support thyroid hormone production and glucose regulation. To improve her tyrosine levels, Beth was encouraged to consume adequate protein (at least 100 grams of quality protein daily) from organic, wild-caught, and pastured sources, while omitting dairy products since they often contain hormones from the cows that can impact hormones in the human body. At Beth's 6-week follow-up, she reported feeling about 40% better. They were on the right track!

TESTOSTERONE

Testosterone is often associated with male characteristics, but it is also present in females, albeit typically in lower levels, barring high-testosterone conditions like polycystic ovary syndrome. Testosterone is primarily produced in the testes in men and the ovaries and adrenal glands in women. Optimal testosterone levels, although different for men and women, respectively are associated with wellbeing, confidence, and motivation.

Testosterone influences cognitive function, including spatial abilities, memory, and emotion regulation (Tyagi et al., 2017). Low or fluctuating testosterone levels have been associated with symptoms of depression, anxiety, decreased cognitive function, and conditions like schizophrenia (Lodha & Karia, 2019). Understanding the intricate interplay between testosterone and mental health deserves continued evaluation and research.

SEX HORMONE CHANGES ACROSS THE LIFESPAN

Sex hormone levels naturally change throughout our life. Puberty is a period of significant hormonal changes marked by the onset of sexual maturation and the release of reproductive hormones such as estrogen, progesterone, and testosterone. These hormonal fluctuations impact adolescent mood, behavior, and mental health (Herpertz-Dahlmann et al., 2013; Vigil et al., 2011). The developing adolescent brain is more sensitive to environmental stressors than the adult brain, as it struggles to balance the daily hormonal fluctuations. Increased consumption of processed foods, chemical additives, and pesticide exposure has negatively impacted teen mental health. The addition of increased isolation through social media, chronic gaming, and limited outdoor time has decreased most teens' abilities to interact face-to-face with confidence and ease.

Continued hormonal changes occur as we transition from adolescence to adulthood. For women, dramatic shifts in hormone levels, including estrogen, progesterone, and oxytocin, characterize pregnancy and the postpartum period. While many women report feeling emotionally and mentally at their best during pregnancy which may be a function of more stable hormone levels without the monthly menstrual cycle, some women struggle with moodiness during pregnancy and an exacerbation of existing mood disorders (Van Bussel et al., 2006). After pregnancy, during the postpartum period, as the hormones begin rapidly trying to reset to pre-pregnancy levels, many women are distressed to find themselves feeling depressed.

Postpartum depression (PPD) is a complex and challenging condition that affects many women after giving birth. PPD is not to be confused with the "baby blues," which are common, less severe symptoms of low mood and fatigue. A combination of biological, psychological, and social factors, including hormonal changes, sleep deprivation, and physical recovery from childbirth, influence PPD. Additionally, a woman who has struggled with depression and anxiety before pregnancy is often most at risk. After giving birth, there is a significant drop in progesterone and estrogen with the release of the placenta. This significant drop in hormones, alongside the drop in thyroid hormones that is common postpartum, increases the risk of PPD (Hendrick et al., 1998).

As individuals age, hormone levels naturally decline (see Figure 6.2). This can have implications for mental health and cognitive function. For example, declining estrogen levels in postmenopausal women have been associated with an increased risk of depression and cognitive decline (Vivian-Taylor & Hickey, 2014). As men age, a decrease in testosterone puts them at a greater risk of mood disorders and mental health challenges. Exposure to environmental toxins such as pesticides, fungicides, herbicides, fluoride, heavy metals, plastics, fragrances, and air pollutants can interfere with the endocrine system, disrupting normal hormonal function, especially as we age

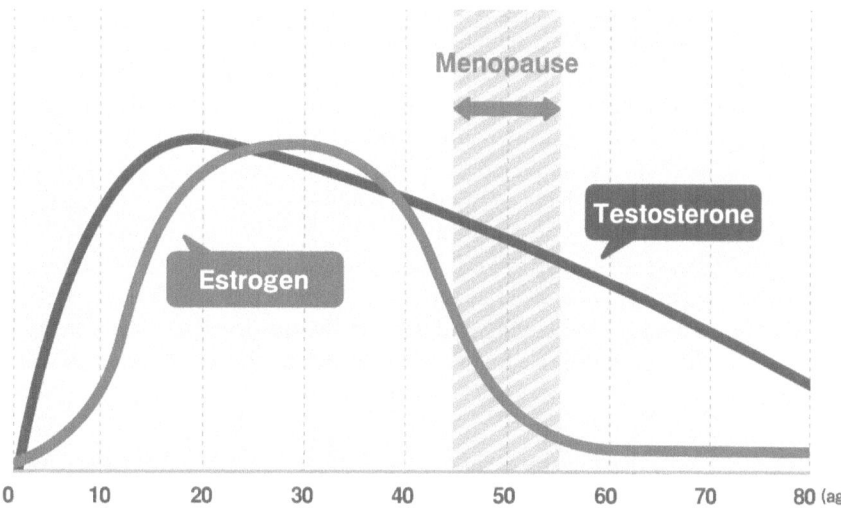

FIGURE 6.2 Sex hormones across the lifespan: Estrogen changes for women and testosterone changes for men. Credit: Barks (Shutterstock).

(Sakuragi et al., 2021). These toxins, known as endocrine-disrupting chemicals, can accumulate in the body over time and contribute to hormone imbalances that negatively impact mental health.

CONDITIONS OF HORMONE IMBALANCE AND THEIR IMPACT ON MENTAL HEALTH

HORMONAL CONDITIONS AFFECTING WOMEN

Hashimoto's thyroiditis (Hashimoto's) is an autoimmune disorder characterized by inflammation of the thyroid gland that is more commonly diagnosed in women than in men. When the immune system mistakenly attacks the thyroid gland in Hashimoto's, it can lead to an imbalance of vital hormones. This hormonal imbalance can disrupt the brain chemistry, affecting neurotransmitter function and increasing risk for symptoms of depression. Low thyroid hormone levels (hypothyroidism) can result from Hashimoto's and are associated with symptoms such as fatigue, weight gain, and cognitive impairment, all of which can contribute to or worsen depressive symptoms. Additionally, inflammation caused by the autoimmune response may directly impact the brain, triggering the neuroinflammatory processes that are implicated in depression and other mental health disorders.

Polycystic ovary syndrome (PCOS) is a complex endocrine disorder affecting reproductive-aged women. It is characterized by hormonal imbalance (generally elevated testosterone levels), menstrual irregularities, insulin dysregulation, infertility, and cyst formation on the ovaries, although not all women with PCOS will present with cysts, which has created some arguments within the research and medical communities to change the name of this condition. Beyond its reproductive implications, emerging evidence suggests a bidirectional relationship between PCOS and mental health. Women with PCOS often experience higher rates of depression, anxiety, and mood disorders compared to the general population (Damone et al., 2019; Dokras, 2012; Kolhe et al., 2022). The underlying mechanisms linking PCOS to mental health disturbances are multifaceted and may involve hormonal dysregulation, chronic inflammation, insulin resistance, and body image concerns.

The distress caused by irregular periods, acne, and hirsutism (excess hair growth, especially facial) can lead to body image issues and lowered self-esteem. Insulin resistance, a common feature of PCOS, further exacerbates the risk of mood disorders and may contribute to feelings of fatigue and irritability. The complex interplay between hormone imbalances, metabolic dysfunction, and psychological factors underscores the importance of a holistic approach to managing PCOS that addresses both physical and mental wellbeing.

Premenstrual dysphoric disorder (PMDD), a DSM diagnosis that is a severe form of premenstrual syndrome (PMS) characterized by debilitating mood changes and heightened emotional sensitivity, has been linked to high estrogen levels. PMDD can make a woman particularly vulnerable to the negative impact of trauma, which can intertwine in a complex relationship with PMDD, often exacerbating each other's effects on mental health (see more details about the impact of trauma in Chapter 9). Individuals who have experienced trauma may be more susceptible to the hormonal fluctuations that characterize PMDD, as trauma can sensitize the stress response system, including the HPA axis (Pilver et al., 2011). Consequently, the hormonal changes during the menstrual cycle may be incredibly challenging. Addressing the history of trauma concurrently with dietary and lifestyle changes can make a long-lasting, beneficial impact on a woman who struggles with PMDD.

HORMONAL CONDITIONS AFFECTING MEN

Erectile disorder (ED), a DSM diagnosis, is the persistent inability to achieve or maintain an erection sufficient for satisfactory sexual performance. There is an age-related prevalence, with the incidence going up as men age. The bidirectional relationship between ED and psychiatric symptoms is well established, with each condition potentially exacerbating the other (Corona et al., 2008; Quang et al., 2024; Saito et al., 2024). Psychiatric conditions such as depression, anxiety, and stress are frequently implicated in the development and progression of ED. The distress and loss of confidence resulting from ED can precipitate or worsen psychiatric symptoms, leading to a vicious cycle of psychological distress and sexual dysfunction. Furthermore, specific psychiatric medications used to treat mood disorders, such as selective-serotonin reuptake inhibitor (SSRI) antidepressants, may also contribute to ED as a side effect (Lipman et al., 2024).

From a physiological perspective, ED may be an early marker of metabolic syndrome and cardiovascular disease (Yao et al., 2013). A lifestyle with poorly regulated glucose and insulin levels can alter neurochemical pathways and disrupt endocrine function. Insulin resistance and visceral obesity lower testosterone levels and increase the risk of ED (Knoblovits et al., 2010; Russo et al., 2014).

HORMONAL CONDITIONS OF ADOLESCENCE

Adolescence is a time of substantial hormonal, mental, and emotional transformations. Hormone imbalances caused by dietary and lifestyle patterns can lead to significant disruptions in meeting normal developmental milestones. Diets high in processed foods and low in fruits, vegetables, and high-quality protein can significantly disrupt hormone levels in developing teens, contributing to an increased risk of developing a psychiatric disorder.

Precocious puberty, defined as the onset of secondary sexual characteristics before the age of eight in girls such as breast development and pubic hair growth, and nine in boys such as facial hair and vocal changes, represents a significant endocrine disorder with implications beyond physical development, including notable effects on mental health. The early and abrupt transition into puberty can lead to psychosocial challenges for affected children, stemming from both biological and social factors. Biologically, the premature activation of the hypothalamic-pituitary-gonadal axis (HPG) may disrupt the neurological processes underlying emotional regulation and cognitive development, potentially predisposing individuals to mood disorders (Viner, 2015). Additionally, the psychosocial implications of precocious puberty are profound, as affected children may struggle to navigate social interactions and establish a sense of identity amidst peers who have not yet reached puberty (Çoban et al., 2021). This discrepancy in physical maturation can lead to feelings of social isolation, low self-esteem, and body image dissatisfaction, which may persist into adolescence and adulthood.

CLINICAL IMPLICATIONS AND TREATMENT APPROACHES

Hormones rise and fall throughout our lifespan both from the natural progression of aging, as well as in response to changes in our life, both exciting changes as well as difficult changes. Understanding our hormone levels can be very helpful to make lifestyle adjustments that will bring them into an optimal range. Unfortunately, hormone testing is often not covered under our current health insurance and is often not considered in early treatment plans in conventional medical practices. As an informed health consumer, if you have concerns about your hormone levels and would like to do some lab testing, you may have to seek out a more holistic style of medical practitioner, such as a Functional Medicine, Integrative Medicine, or Naturopathic doctor.

Pharmacological interventions that target hormone imbalances are often prescribed for conditions like hypothyroidism and diabetes. Unfortunately, these medications have numerous potential side effects. For example, women with severe menopausal symptoms are often prescribed hormone therapies to elevate their estrogen or improve the balance between their progesterone and estrogen levels. Estradiol, the most potent form of estrogen medication, is commonly prescribed for hormone replacement therapy in menopausal women. Estradiol can help decrease menopausal symptoms such as insomnia and hot flashes but comes with the risk of side effects including pain, heart palpitations (racing heartbeat), headache, and depression. Irritability and anger outbursts are also reported side effects, often linked to hormonal fluctuations.

Lifestyle factors such as diet, exercise, stress management, and sleep hygiene can also influence hormone levels. Integrative approaches that include a variety of treatment components to address hormonal imbalances are likely to yield the best results.

NUTRITION TO STABILIZE HORMONES

Disclaimer: The following section provides generalized nutritional information. Please consult a nutritionist, dietitian, or other qualified healthcare provider before changing your diet, especially if you are on any medications.

A low glycemic, low-processed whole food diet is crucial for balancing hormones. Foods with a low glycemic load (GL) are digested and absorbed more slowly, resulting in gradual increases in blood sugar. This helps maintain stable insulin and cortisol levels, reducing the risk of insulin resistance and its associated hormonal imbalances. Processed foods, on the other hand, often contain high levels of refined sugars which can cause rapid spikes and crashes in blood sugar levels. These fluctuations can disrupt the delicate balance of hormones such as insulin and cortisol, leading to increased stress responses and mood swings. Individuals can support more stable blood sugar levels and hormonal balance by choosing low glycemic, minimally processed foods. Foods high in omega-3 fatty acids, like salmon, flaxseeds, and walnuts, can help reduce inflammation and support the endocrine system. Increasing antioxidants from foods such as berries, citrus fruits, and green tea can protect the body's cells from oxidative stress, how it may be necessary to eat these in large quantities or add nutritional supplements to make a significant difference if your body is very depleted.

Moreover, a diet rich in whole, unprocessed foods provides essential nutrients vital for synthesizing and utilizing hormones effectively. For example, nutrition is pivotal in supporting estrogen balance, which is essential for maintaining various physiological functions and overall health. *Phytoestrogens* are plant-based compounds that mimic estrogen in the body and can help increase estrogen levels in those who may be deficient. Flaxseeds, soy products, and legumes are all excellent sources of phytoestrogens. Additionally, incorporating cruciferous vegetables like broccoli, cauliflower, and Brussels sprouts can aid estrogen clearance for those with excess estrogen. These vegetables contain compounds like indole-3-carbinol, which support healthy detoxification of excess estrogen. In addition, adequate fiber balances hormones and supports the microbiome. Women need 30–35 grams of fiber, and men need 25–30 grams daily.

Treatment for estrogen dominance also focuses on increasing progesterone levels. Certain foods support the body's natural progesterone production by providing essential nutrient building blocks and promoting optimal hormonal function. Vitamin B6, found in chickpeas and bananas, is vital in progesterone synthesis. Foods high in beta-carotene, such as red, yellow, and orange fruits, vegetables, and leafy greens, provide the necessary cofactors for healthy progesterone production. Additionally, zinc, abundant in pumpkin seeds, can help increase progesterone levels. Magnesium-rich foods like spinach, almonds, and dark chocolate support adrenal health and hormone production, including progesterone.

Testosterone production benefits from consuming lean proteins like eggs, chicken, turkey, and grass-fed beef, which provide the necessary amino acids for muscle repair and testosterone production. Fatty fish, including salmon, mackerel, and sardines, are abundant in necessary omega-3 fatty acids, which reduce inflammation and support healthy testosterone production. Nuts and seeds like almonds, walnuts, and pumpkin seeds deliver healthy fats, zinc, and magnesium, all essential for robust testosterone production.

Foods that generally support overall hormone health include cruciferous vegetables which help to regulate estrogen levels, and leafy greens, including spinach, kale, and Swiss chard, which are rich in magnesium which helps lower cortisol levels. Ginger has been shown to boost hormones and improve gastrointestinal function. Other beneficial foods include pomegranates, which are rich in antioxidants that enhance blood flow and reduce oxidative stress, oysters which are famously high in zinc, and avocados which provide healthy monounsaturated fats and vitamin E.

NUTRITION TO SUPPORT THYROID FUNCTION

Nutrition plays a critical role in supporting thyroid hormone balance. For individuals with thyroid disorders, especially those with autoimmune conditions like Hashimoto's thyroiditis, removing gluten from the diet can be beneficial, as gluten can trigger an immune response that exacerbates thyroid dysfunction. A diet rich in essential nutrients is crucial for thyroid health. Iodine, found in seaweed, fish, and dairy products, is a key component of thyroid hormones and is better when supplied through food sources rather than iodized salt which lacks many other minerals needed for proper balance. Selenium, present in Brazil nuts, sunflower seeds, and fish, helps to convert the storage form of the thyroid hormone, thyroxine (T4), to the active form, triiodothyronine (T3) and offers antioxidant protection to the thyroid gland. Zinc, abundant in meat, shellfish, legumes, and seeds, supports thyroid hormone production and metabolism. Iron, essential for thyroid function, can be sourced from animal products including red meat, poultry, and seafood, as well as in plant foods such as legumes, although it is more bio-available (easily digested and absorbed) through the consumption of animal sources.

Additionally, vitamin D, found in fatty fish and fortified foods and synthesized through sunlight exposure, is vital for immune function and may support thyroid health. A well-rounded gluten-free diet rich in these essential nutrients can help maintain thyroid hormone balance and health.

SUPPORT TO IMPROVE OXYTOCIN LEVELS

Options to increase oxytocin levels to improve physical and mental health have been gaining attention. Since 2005, there has been growing interest in pharmaceutical approaches to raising oxytocin, especially in administering exogenous (manufactured) oxytocin as a nasal spray as a treatment option for mood improvement, substance addiction, and weight loss. Another pharmaceutical approach is the therapeutic use of MDMA (3,4-methylenedioxymethamphetamine commonly known as ecstasy) to raise oxytocin levels (Carson et al., 2013; Skinner et al., 2018). Evidence for non-pharmaceutical approaches to increase endogenous (internally produced) oxytocin have also appeared in the literature.

Physical touch is one of the most powerful ways to increase oxytocin levels. There are many types of touch that show a positive benefit including holding hands, hugging, snuggling, making love, and giving or receiving a massage. Massage is associated with increased oxytocin levels, decreased pain, and increased feelings of wellbeing (Morhenn et al., 2012). Yet not all touch is the same. Context matters. The social intent and connection involved with touch is an important part of the equation. Gentle human touch paired with a friendly human face provides higher oxytocin levels than touch with a neutral or angry face (Ellingsen et al., 2014).

Physical touch with animals has also been proven to increase oxytocin levels. For example, petting a dog has been found to increase oxytocin and decrease blood pressure and cortisol levels (Uvnas-Moberg et al., 2015). A significant increase in oxytocin and a decrease in psychological stress can be seen after just 5–24 minutes of petting, with a stronger reaction when one is petting their own dog compared to an unfamiliar dog. The closer the human-animal relationship, the more oxytocin is released through the physical contact (Beetz et al., 2012).

Exercise is another avenue to increase oxytocin levels. Even moderate exercise makes a difference. For example, in a study of runners, oxytocin levels increased after just 10 minutes of moderate running, and further increased after 20, 30, and 60 minutes of running (Wirobski et al., 2024). Exercising with other people may offer additional benefits in both increased oxytocin levels and improved mood (Shima et al., 2024).

FOOD FOR THOUGHT: UNDERSTANDING AND NURTURING SENSITIVITY

Highly sensitive people (HSPs) represent a significant portion of the population, characterized by a heightened response to external stimuli and a deeper cognitive processing of sensory information. The development of acute sensitivity may be a result of trauma experienced during the formative years of life when the young human desires to experience safety, security, love, and belonging. Those whose childhoods lacked these fundamental needs are more likely to present in a continuous state of hypervigilance and increased sensitivity and awareness of their surroundings (Bunce et al., 1995). This sensitivity can manifest in various aspects of life, from emotional reactions to adverse response to environmental influences. Understanding HSPs, identifying their traits, and promoting their mental and emotional resilience through stable blood sugar levels are crucial for their overall wellbeing to prevent psychological burnout.

Highly sensitive people, a term popularized by psychologist Elaine Aron, are individuals with an increased sensitivity to sensory input. This trait, known as sensory processing sensitivity (SPS), is not a disorder but a normal variation in human temperament. HSPs tend to process sensory data more deeply, leading to heightened awareness of subtleties in their environment and a more intense experience of emotions, both positive and negative. According to Dr. Aron, HSP is a form of neuro-divergence and can often be mistaken for other personality types like empaths, as well as introversion, narcissism, and shyness (Acevedo et al., 2018; Aron, n.d.).

Critical characteristics of HSPs include deep processing, overstimulation, emotional reactivity, and sensitivity to subtleties. HSPs often reflect on and analyze information more deeply than others. This trait can lead to profound insights and creative thinking but can also cause overthinking and rumination. Due to their heightened sensitivity, HSPs can become easily overwhelmed by loud noises, bright lights, strong smells, or chaotic environments. They require more downtime to recover from sensory overload. HSPs experience emotions more intensely and may react strongly to positive and negative stimuli, making them more empathetic and compassionate and more susceptible to emotional exhaustion. They also notice details that others might miss, such as subtle changes in facial expressions or slight variations in their surroundings. This heightened perception can be advantageous in various situations but leads to overstimulation in others (Boterberg & Warreyn, 2016).

Many of the signs of being an HSP mirror the symptoms of post-traumatic stress disorder (PTSD). The symptoms of PTSD include being easily startled, feeling tense or a heightened awareness of surroundings, difficulty concentrating, difficulty falling or staying asleep, strong emotional response, and an increased experience of fight or flight. It is unclear if PTSD may be the start of HSP behavior or if being an HSP predisposes an individual to develop a PTSD disorder. A key difference between an HSP and a person with PTSD is the level of distress and dysfunction they experience due to their sensitivities and/or symptoms.

Maintaining stable blood sugar levels is crucial for everyone but is especially important for HSPs. Blood sugar fluctuations can significantly impact mood, energy levels, and overall mental and emotional resilience. Blood sugar fluctuations can lead to mood swings, irritability, and anxiety. For HSPs, who are already prone to emotional intensity, stable blood sugar levels can help maintain a more balanced and calm emotional state. Consistent blood sugar levels provide sustained energy throughout the day. HSPs often feel drained by sensory and emotional stimuli, so having a steady energy supply can help them manage their sensitivities better. Stable blood sugar supports cognitive function, helping HSPs avoid brain fog and maintain mental clarity. This is crucial for their deep processing abilities and can keep overthinking from becoming overwhelm and rumination. Blood sugar stability can enhance the body's ability to handle stress. For HSPs, who may experience higher stress levels due to their heightened sensitivity, this can help to prevent burnout and promote resilience.

To stabilize blood sugar, emphasize a diet rich in lean proteins, complex carbohydrates, healthy fats, and fiber. This combination helps slow sugar absorption into the bloodstream, preventing rapid spikes and crashes. Regular eating patterns, including balanced meals and healthy snacks, can help stabilize blood sugar. Avoiding long periods without food can prevent drops in blood sugar that lead to irritability and fatigue. Focus on foods with a lower glycemic index, such as vegetables, protein, nuts, and seeds. These foods release glucose more slowly, promoting stable blood sugar levels. In addition, staying hydrated is essential for overall health and can help maintain stable blood sugar levels. Regular physical activity helps regulate blood sugar levels and reduces stress. Activities and types of enjoyable movement help to avoid feeling overwhelmed, such as walking, yoga, swimming, and weight training, are best suited for HSPs. Incorporate stress reduction techniques such as mindfulness, meditation, deep breathing exercises, and strong social support. These practices can help HSPs manage emotional responses and prevent stress-induced blood sugar fluctuations. Finally, ensure that HSPs get enough restful sleep, as poor or insufficient sleep disrupts blood sugar regulation and increases sensitivity to stress.

HSPs have unique needs and strengths that require careful attention and nurturing. By understanding what it means to be highly sensitive, identifying these traits, and promoting stable blood sugar levels, HSPs can be supported in maintaining their mental and emotional resilience. Stable blood sugar is a cornerstone of their wellbeing, helping them avoid psychological burnout and thrive in an overwhelming world. Through balanced nutrition, regular meals, physical activity, stress reduction, and adequate sleep, HSPs can achieve a harmonious balance that allows them to leverage their sensitivity as a strength rather than a burden.

REFERENCES

Acevedo, B., Aron, E., Pospos, S., & Jessen, D. (2018). The functional highly sensitive brain: A review of the brain circuits underlying sensory processing sensitivity and seemingly related disorders. *Philosophical Transactions of the Royal Society B: Biological Sciences, 373*(1744), 20170161.

Aron, E. (n.d.). *The highly sensitive person.* https://hsperson.com/

Ayuso-Álvarez, A., Simón, L., Nuñez, O., Rodriguez-Blazquez, C., Martín-Méndez, I., Bel-Lán, A., Lopez-Abente, G., Merlo, J., Fernandez-Navarro, P., & Galan, I. (2019). Association between heavy metals and metalloids in topsoil and mental health in the adult population of Spain. *Environmental Research, 179*, 108784.

Bauermeister, S. D., Ben Yehuda, M., Reid, G., Howgego, G., Ritchie, K., Watermeyer, T., Gregory, S., Terrera, G. M., & Koychev, I. (2023). Insulin resistance, age and depression's impact on cognition in middle-aged adults from the PREVENT cohort. *BMJ Mental Health, 26*(1), e300665. https://doi.org/10.1136/bmjment-2023-300665

Baumgartner, A., Pietzcker, A., & Gaebel, W. (2000). The hypothalamic–pituitary–thyroid axis in patients with schizophrenia. *Schizophrenia Research, 44*(3), 233–243.

Beetz, A., Uvnäs-Moberg, K., Julius, H., & Kotrschal, K. (2012). Psychosocial and psychophysiological effects of human-animal interactions: The possible role of oxytocin. *Frontiers in Psychology, 3.* https://doi.org/10.3389/fpsyg.2012.00234

Boterberg, S., & Warreyn, P. (2016). Making sense of it all: The impact of sensory processing sensitivity on daily functioning of children. *Personality and Individual Differences, 92*, 80–86.

Bunce, S. C., Larson, R. J., & Peterson, C. (1995). Life after trauma: Personality and daily life experiences of traumatized people. *Journal of Personality, 63*(2), 165–188.

Caccappolo-van Vliet, E., Kelly-McNeil, K., Natelson, B., Kipen, H., & Fiedler, N. (2002). Anxiety sensitivity and depression in multiple chemical sensitivities and asthma. *Journal of Occupational and Environmental Medicine, 44*(10), 890–901.

Calkin, C. V., Ruzickova, M., Uher, R., Hajek, T., Slaney, C. M., Garnham, J. S., O'Donovan, M. C., & Alda, M. (2015). Insulin resistance and outcome in bipolar disorder. *British Journal of Psychiatry, 206*(1), 52–57. https://doi.org/10.1192/bjp.bp.114.152850

Carson, D., Guastella, A., Taylor, E., & McGregor, I. (2013). A brief history of oxytocin and its role in modulating psychostimulant effects. *Journal of Psychopharmacology, 27*(3), 231–247. https://doi.org/10.1177/0269881112473788

Chakrabarti, S. (2011). Thyroid functions and bipolar affective disorder. *Journal of Thyroid Research, 2011*, 1–13. https://doi.org/10.4061/2011/306367

Çoban, Ö. G., Bedel, A., Önder, A., Adanır, A. S., Tuhan, H., & Parlak, M. (2021). Psychiatric disorders, peer-victimization, and quality of life in girls with central precocious puberty. *Journal of Psychosomatic Research, 143*, 110401.

Corona, G., Ricca, V., Bandini, E., Mannucci, E., Petrone, L., Fisher, A. D., Lotti, F., Balercia, G., Faravelli, C., & Forti, G. (2008). Association between psychiatric symptoms and erectile dysfunction. *The Journal of Sexual Medicine*, *5*(2), 458–468.

Damone, A. L., Joham, A. E., Loxton, D., Earnest, A., Teede, H. J., & Moran, L. J. (2019). Depression, anxiety and perceived stress in women with and without PCOS: A community-based study. *Psychological Medicine*, *49*(9), 1510–1520.

Dayan, C. M., & Panicker, V. (2013). Hypothyroidism and depression. *European Thyroid Journal*, *2*(3), 168–179.

Ding, C., Leow, M. K. S., & Magkos, F. (2018). Oxytocin in metabolic homeostasis: Implications for obesity and diabetes management. *Obesity Reviews*, *20*(1), 22–40. https://doi.org/10.1111/obr.12757

Dokras, A. (2012). Mood and anxiety disorders in women with PCOS. *Steroids*, *77*(4), 338–341.

Ellingsen, D. M., Wessberg, J., Chelnokova, O., Olausson, H., Laeng, B., & Leknes, S. (2014). In touch with your emotions: Oxytocin and touch change social impressions while others' facial expressions can alter touch. *Psychoneuroendocrinology*, *39*, 11–20. https://doi.org/10.1016/j.psyneuen.2013.09.017

Fernandes, B. S., Salagre, E., Enduru, N., Grande, I., Vieta, E., & Zhao, Z. (2022). Insulin resistance in depression: A large meta-analysis of metabolic parameters and variation. *Neuroscience & Biobehavioral Reviews*, *139*, 104758. https://doi.org/10.1016/j.neubiorev.2022.104758

Freire, C., & Koifman, S. (2013). Pesticides, depression and suicide: A systematic review of the epidemiological evidence. *International Journal of Hygiene and Environmental Health*, *216*(4), 445–460.

Freuer, D., & Meisinger, C. (2023). Causal link between thyroid function and schizophrenia: A two-sample Mendelian randomization study. *European Journal of Epidemiology*, *38*(10), 1081–1088.

Fryar, C. D., Carroll, M. D., & Ogden, C. L. (2018). *Prevalence of overweight, obesity, and severe obesity among adults aged 20 and over: United States, 1960–1962 through 2015–2016*. Health E-Stats: National Center for Health Statistics. https://stacks.cdc.gov/view/cdc/58670

Gau, C. S., Chang, C. J., Tsai, F. J., Chao, P. F., & Gau, S. S. F. (2010). Association between mood stabilizers and hypothyroidism in patients with bipolar disorders: A nested, matched case-control study. *Bipolar Disorders*, *12*(3), 253–263.

Hendrick, V., Altshuler, L. L., & Suri, R. (1998). Hormonal changes in the postpartum and implications for postpartum depression. *Psychosomatics*, *39*(2), 93–101.

Herpertz-Dahlmann, B., Bühren, K., & Remschmidt, H. (2013). Growing up is hard: Mental disorders in adolescence. *Deutsches Ärzteblatt International*, *110*(25), 432.

Holt, R. I., De Groot, M., & Golden, S. H. (2014). Diabetes and depression. *Current Diabetes Reports*, *14*, 1–9.

Knoblovits, P., Costanzo, P. R., Valzacchi, G. J. R., Gueglio, G., Layus, A. O., Kozak, A. E., Balzaretti, M. I., & Litwak, L. E. (2010). Erectile dysfunction, obesity, insulin resistance, and their relationship with testosterone levels in Eugonadal patients in an andrology clinic setting. *Journal of Andrology*, *31*(3), 263–270. https://doi.org/10.2164/jandrol.109.007757

Kolhe, J. V., Chhipa, A. S., Butani, S., Chavda, V., & Patel, S. S. (2022). PCOS and depression: Common links and potential targets. *Reproductive Sciences*, 1–18.

Lefevre, A., Richard, N., Jazayeri, M., Beuriat, P. A., Fieux, S., Zimmer, L., Duhamel, J. R., & Sirigu, A. (2017). Oxytocin and serotonin brain mechanisms in the nonhuman primate. *Journal of Neuroscience*, *37*(28), 6741–6750. https://doi.org/10.1523/JNEUROSCI.0659-17.2017

Lipman, K., Betterly, H., & Botros, M. (2024). Improvement in selective serotonin reuptake inhibitor-associated sexual dysfunction with buspirone: Examining the evidence. *Cureus*, *16*(4).

Lodha, P., & Karia, S. (2019). Testosterone and schizophrenia: A clinical review. *Annals of Indian Psychiatry*, *3*(2), 92–96.

McCormack, S., Blevins, J., & Lawson, E. (2020). Metabolic effects of oxytocin. *Endocrine Reviews*, *41*(2), 121–145. https://doi.org/10.1210/endrev/bnz012

Misztak, P., Opoka, W., & Topór-Mądry, R. (2015). The serum concentration of magnesium as a potential state marker in patients with diagnosis of bipolar disorder. *Psychiatria Polska*, *49*(6), 1277–1287.

Moerkerke, M., Peeters, M., de Vries, L., Daniels, N., Steyaert, J., Alaerts, K., & Boets, B. (2021). Endogenous oxytocin levels in autism—a meta-analysis. *Brain Sciences*, *11*(11), 1545. https://doi.org/10.3390/brainsci11111545

Morhenn, V., Beavin, L. E., & Zak, P. J. (2012). Massage increases oxytocin and reduces adrenocorticotropin hormone in humans. *Alternative Therapies in Health and Medicine*, *18*(6), 11.

Nechifor, M. (2011). Magnesium in psychoses (schizophrenia and bipolar disorders). In R. Vink & M. Nechifor (Eds.), *Magnesium in the central nervous system* (pp. 303–312). University of Adelaide Press. https://www.ncbi.nlm.nih.gov/books/NBK507255

Pilver, C. E., Levy, B. R., Libby, D. J., & Desai, R. A. (2011). Posttraumatic stress disorder and trauma characteristics are correlates of premenstrual dysphoric disorder. *Archives of Women's Mental Health, 14,* 383–393.

Quang, N., Van Truong, L., Chung, E., Van Quang, B., Long, L. Q., Ngoc, N. T., Minh, N. A., Anh, D. M., Thanh, N. D., & Nam, N. T. (2024). Predicting anxiety and depression among erectile dysfunction patients: A cross-sectional study. *American Journal of Men's Health, 18*(1), 15579883231223502.

Russo, G. I., Cimino, S., Fragalà, E., Privitera, S., La Vignera, S., Condorelli, R., Calogero, A. E., Castelli, T., Favilla, V., & Morgia, G. (2014). Insulin resistance is an independent predictor of severe lower urinary tract symptoms and of erectile dysfunction: Results from a cross-sectional study. *The Journal of Sexual Medicine, 11*(8), 2074–2082. https://doi.org/10.1111/jsm.12587

Saito, J., Kumano, H., Ghazizadeh, M., Shimokawa, C., & Tanemura, H. (2024). Differences in psychological inflexibility among men with erectile dysfunction younger and older than 40 years: Web-based cross-sectional study. *JMIR Formative Research, 8,* e45998.

Sakuragi, Y., Takada, H., Sato, H., Kubota, A., Terasaki, M., Takeuchi, S., Ikeda-Araki, A., Watanabe, Y., Kitamura, S., & Kojima, H. (2021). An analytical survey of benzotriazole UV stabilizers in plastic products and their endocrine-disrupting potential via human estrogen and androgen receptors. *Science of the Total Environment, 800,* 149374.

Scott, E. M., Carpenter, J. S., Iorfino, F., Cross, S. P. M., Hermens, D. F., Gehue, J., Wilson, C., White, D., Naismith, S. L., Guastella, A. J., & Hickie, I. B. (2019). What is the prevalence, and what are the clinical correlates, of insulin resistance in young people presenting for mental health care? A cross-sectional study. *BMJ Open, 9*(5), e025674. https://doi.org/10.1136/bmjopen-2018-025674

Shima, T., Iijima, J., Sutoh, H., Terashima, C., & Matsuura, Y. (2024). Augmented-reality-based multi-person exercise has more beneficial effects on mood state and oxytocin secretion than standard solitary exercise. *Physiology & Behavior, 283,* 114623. https://doi.org/10.1016/j.physbeh.2024.114623

Skinner, J., Garg, M., Dayas, C., Fenton, S., & Burrows, T. (2018). Relationship between dietary intake and behaviors with oxytocin: A systematic review of studies in adults. *Nutrition Reviews, 76*(5), 303–331. https://doi.org/10.1093/nutrit/nux078

Tyagi, V., Scordo, M., Yoon, R. S., Liporace, F. A., & Greene, L. W. (2017). Revisiting the role of testosterone: Are we missing something? *Reviews in Urology, 19*(1), 16.

Uvnas-Moberg, K., Handlin, L., & Petersson, M. (2015). Self-soothing behaviors with particular reference to oxytocin release induced by non-noxious sensory stimulation. *Frontiers in Psychology, 5.* https://doi.org/10.3389/fpsyg.2014.01529

Van Bussel, J. C., Spitz, B., & Demyttenaere, K. (2006). Women's mental health before, during, and after pregnancy: A population-based controlled cohort study. *Birth, 33*(4), 297–302.

Vigil, P., Orellana, R. F., Cortés, M. E., Molina, C. T., Switzer, B. E., & Klaus, H. (2011). Endocrine modulation of the adolescent brain: A review. *Journal of Pediatric and Adolescent Gynecology, 24*(6), 330–337.

Viner, R. (2015). Puberty, the brain and mental health in adolescence. In J.-P. Bourguignon, J.-C. Carel, & Y. Christen (Eds.), *Brain crosstalk in puberty and adolescence* (pp. 75–83). Springer Nature.

Vivian-Taylor, J., & Hickey, M. (2014). Menopause and depression: Is there a link? *Maturitas, 79*(2), 142–146.

Wirobski, G., Crockford, C., Deschner, T., & Neumann, I. (2024). Oxytocin and cortisol concentrations in urine and saliva in response to physical exercise in humans. *Psychoneuroendocrinology, 168,* 107144. https://doi.org/10.1016/j.psyneuen.2024.107144

Yao, F., Liu, L., Zhang, Y., Huang, Y., Liu, D., Lin, H., Liu, Y., Fan, R., Li, C., & Deng, C. (2013). Erectile dysfunction may be the first clinical sign of insulin resistance and endothelial dysfunction in young men. *Clinical Research in Cardiology, 102*(9), 645–651. https://doi.org/10.1007/s00392-013-0577-y

Section III

The Emergence of
Nutritional Psychology

7 Evidence for Integrating Nutrition to Treat Mental Illness

The evidence is mounting to show that our current mental health treatment methods are not effective for a large portion of the population. The prevalence of mood and anxiety disorders remains high, despite substantial increases in access to treatment, particularly in the form of prescriptions for antidepressants (Jorm et al., 2017). Chronic mental illness is debilitating many members of our communities while presenting a substantial social, economic, and health burden for all of us (Marx et al., 2017). According to the 2017 Global Burden of Disease study, which included 195 countries, major depressive disorder is recognized as one of the top five leading causes of long-term disability worldwide, a list which also includes substance use disorders, anxiety, and Alzheimer's disease as leading causes of disability (Vos et al., 2017).

MENTAL HEALTH TREATMENT

It is of great concern that despite increased access to psychiatric treatment, so many people remain mentally unwell. For example, the rates of depression continue to rise in the face of substantial increases in antidepressant prescriptions, with the rate of long-term antidepressant use (at least five years) estimated to have tripled from 2000 to 2014 (Carey & Gebeloff, 2018). Antidepressants are currently one of the three most commonly prescribed medications in the U.S. (Pratt et al., 2017), yet our rates of depression continue to rise. It is clear we need to make changes in our mental healthcare system that focus on prevention and providing a broader range of viable treatment options.

THE NEED FOR A NEW TREATMENT PARADIGM

Treatment for mental health disorders is predominantly focused on psychopharmacology (e.g., antidepressants, antipsychotics) and psychotherapy (e.g., psychodynamic and cognitive-behavior therapies). Yet even with increased access to these treatments, the number of people struggling with debilitating mental health issues continues to rise. Clearly, we need to embrace other strategies that expand treatment options for people who are mentally ill. Toward that end, there is now compelling evidence that nutrition is a crucial factor in the high prevalence and incidence of mental disorders, which suggests that diet is as important to mental illness as it is to physical illnesses such as heart disease and diabetes (Sarris et al., 2015).

Systematic reviews and meta-analyses of the existing research have demonstrated significant associations between diet and mental health (Itsiopoulos et al., 2015; Lai et al., 2014; O'neil et al., 2014; Psaltopoulou et al., 2013). We now have a clearer understanding of the potential biological pathways such as inflammation (see more on inflammation later in this chapter) and an imbalanced gut microbiome (as discussed in Chapter 5) that can be acted upon through dietary changes to improve a person's mental health (Marx et al., 2017). Diets characterized by a high intake of vegetables, fruit, whole grains, nuts, seeds, and fish, with limited processed foods that are high in fat and sugar, show clear benefits in children and adults for reducing the risk of mental illness.

A recent article by the American Psychologic Association concurred there is considerable evidence that diets high in ultra-processed foods with little nutritional variety or micronutrients exacerbate depression and other mental health problems (DeAngelis, 2023). Sadly, over the last two decades, consumption of ultra-processed foods has continually increased in the majority of the population so that 57 percent of adult diets and 67 percent of youth diets (ages 2–19) are made up of ultra-processed foods, especially ready-to-eat or ready-to-heat foods such as pizza, fast food, and frozen foods (Juul et al., 2022; Wang et al., 2021).

Serious Mental Illness, Diet, and Weight Gain

To make matters worse, mental illness negatively impacts eating behavior. Research shows that a person with a serious mental illness (SMI) is more likely to have a poor diet with low intakes of fruit and vegetables and high intakes of fast food, convenience foods, and sweetened beverages (Teasdale et al., 2019). There is a dose response in that those with a very high consumption of ultra-processed foods are likely to suffer from elevated psychological distress (Lane et al., 2023). Not only does this contribute to the inflammation and dysbiosis that exacerbate psychiatric symptoms, but it also is a known driver of weight gain and obesity. This is a big issue for those living with SMI. In a qualitative study regarding diet and eating behavior, 28 participants with SMI reported one of their primary concerns was about their body weight and their strong inner conflict regarding their dietary behavior (Mueller-Stierlin et al., 2022).

Weight gain due to the combination of a poor diet and psychotropic medication is a big problem for people with SMI. We have known for decades that patients who take psychotropic medication are at high risk of weight gain and its associated negative physical and emotional consequences (Sachs & Guille, 1999). Many report dramatic weight gain when they begin taking psychotropic medication, which is consistent with the known common side effects of these medications, especially antipsychotics, mood stabilizers, and antidepressants, which are used to treat disorders such as schizophrenia, bipolar disorder, and depression (Alonso-Pedrero et al., 2019; Burin et al., 2022; Cuerda et al., 2014; Gafoor et al., 2018).

Apart from the effects of the medication, people with a trauma history are also more likely to gain weight. Trauma often impacts eating behavior when people use food as a coping strategy to distract from overwhelming emotions. When treatment for trauma includes psychotropic medication, patients are even more vulnerable to weight gain and its associated physical and psychological consequences that can exacerbate mental illness.

The situation is worsened by the lack of discussion about nutrition in the mental health treatment world. People are shamed and humiliated by the disparaging comments, bullying, weight-related discrimination, and micro-aggressions they endure from family, in social settings, while at work, and at the hands of mental health and health professionals, all of which make it harder to ask for help and to stay in treatment. It becomes a vicious cycle, where their poor eating behavior and weight gain make them feel worse both physically and psychologically, while also leading them feeling more trapped and ashamed. It is difficult to tease apart the cause and effect of poor diet quality, medication side effects, and weight gain since they are often highly correlated, and each contributes to perpetuating the unhealthy spiral.

Lack of Nutrition Education

As you may have noticed in Chapter 3, nutrition has not been a part of treatment as usual for mental health disorders. Sadly, much of the resistance to including nutrition in treatment comes from the absence of training in nutrition in most medical and mental health graduate school programs even though there is substantial evidence that nutrition is a leading risk factor to poor health. A 2013 report on the state of U.S. health from 1990 to 2010 found dietary factors to be the single most significant risk factor for disability and premature death (U.S. Burden of Disease Collaborators, 2013). Yet our medical practitioners receive almost no training in nutrition and many feel inadequately trained to provide nutritional counseling, even though patients expect them to be credible sources of nutrition information (Devries et al., 2014). The situation is the same in the field of mental health. In a study that surveyed 1056 mental health professionals (including psychiatrists, psychologists, and psychotherapists) in 52 countries, the majority reported having no training in nutrition, recognized that people with SMI tend to have worse diets compared to the general population, and almost all said they would like to expand their knowledge of "nutritional psychiatry" (Mörkl et al., 2021).

CASE STUDY: PANIC ATTACKS AND GLUTEN

Dr. Cook provided psychotherapy for a client who had previously been diagnosed with generalized anxiety disorder and panic disorder, for which the patient had been prescribed antidepressant and antianxiety medications but discontinued because she felt they were not improving her mental health. Panic disorder includes persistent worry about having a panic attack and feeling mental pressure to change your lifestyle to avoid or alleviate fear of having panic attacks. Panic attacks are defined in the DSM-5 as "an abrupt surge of intense fear or intense discomfort that reaches a peak within minutes," and include four or more of the following symptoms: pounding heart, sweating, trembling, shortness of breath, choking, chest pain, nausea, dizziness, chills or heat, tingling, feeling detached, fear of losing control, and fear of dying (American Psychiatric Association, 2013).

The client was a female college student in her 20s who was completing the last three months of her undergraduate degree program. She was struggling with nearly daily panic attacks that often presented with abdominal discomfort and diarrhea. The symptoms were severe enough for her family to drive her to a hospital emergency room on two occasions. She avoided seeing her doctor or her dentist, had stopped going on walks with her mother, and was generally becoming afraid to leave her home for fear of having a panic attack while away from home. The panic attacks and fear of reoccurrence had truly become debilitating and were impeding her ability to move on after graduation to begin her career.

The emergency room medical providers ruled out any major medical issues that would account for her anxiety and frequent panic attacks, so the cause seemed to be purely psychological. During the initial assessment, Dr. Cook asked the client to discuss different aspects of her family history, current potentially triggering events (such as graduating from college), as well as self-care habits including sleep, exercise, stress management, and nutrition. Psychotherapy focused on examining her worries about what to do after graduating college and some of her challenging family dynamics, with an identified goal to travel out of the area when she was feeling better. She had enjoyed travel in the past and yearned to feel free enough to travel again in the future.

Since abdominal discomfort and diarrhea were key aspects of the panic attacks, Dr. Cook asked the client if she was also open to experimenting with dietary changes that might help identify if there was a food or foods that her body was not handling well. The client was interested in exploring this adjunctive treatment. The client reported she had been staying away from alcohol, cannabis, and caffeine for the past year due to concerns that they would trigger a panic attack. She also avoided dairy because it upset her stomach. After discussing foods that tend to be included in an elimination diet to explore food sensitivities (e.g., gluten, dairy, sugar), the client chose to abstain from gluten to see if she noticed any difference in her symptoms. The results were startling. Within three weeks, the client reported that eating no gluten was helping and that she was, "feeling normal for the first time in a long time." The diarrhea had stopped, and the panic attacks had greatly subsided both in frequency and intensity.

In addition to abstaining from gluten, the client was able to connect through therapy that her panic attacks started when she stopped expressing anger with her family about her childhood abuse. In therapy, she worked to find her voice, to express her emotions, and to set better limits with her family and at work. She also worked to create better self-care coping strategies, including taking breaks at work, eating more whole foods and less processed foods, and regularly practicing self-compassion and self-soothing behaviors.

After six weeks of being gluten-free plus weekly psychotherapy sessions, the client felt ready to start traveling for short weekend excursions. She still had mild panic attacks associated with social triggers (e.g., midterm exams, family fights), but they were no longer exacerbated by stomach aches or diarrhea. At 12 weeks, she graduated from college and started job hunting. She eventually found employment in her field in preparation for graduate school. The client continued to expand her travel. She started with a few weekend vacations to nearby destinations, then, over the course of the next year, expanded to taking short airplane flights, and eventually took a longer flight to vacation in Hawaii.

NEW MENTAL HEALTH FIELDS

The idea of using food as a means of treating disease has been around for a long time. Hippocrates (460–370 BC), the ancient Greek physician considered the father of Western medicine, is credited with the axiom, "Let food be thy medicine and medicine be thy food." The medical use of vitamins began in the 18th century. In the early 20th century, some doctors hypothesized that vitamins could cure disease. Megadose nutritional supplements were prescribed by the 1930s, however their effects on health were disappointing. By the 1950s and 1960s, nutrition was downplayed in standard medical curricula (Menolascino et al., 1988). While there has been recognition of the importance of good nutrition for physical health, there has been less discussion about its importance for mental health. However, that is changing.

EARLY EVIDENCE OF THE IMPACT OF FOOD ON MENTAL HEALTH

Beginning in the 1950s, an early voice for a nutritional approach to psychiatric illness was Canadian biochemist, physician, and psychiatrist Abram Hoffer, MD, PhD. Both a clinician and a researcher, in his 60-year career from 1949 until he died in 2009, Dr. Hoffer took a unique approach to treatment where he would carefully assess each client to determine if there was a root cause behind their psychotic symptoms, such as nutritional deficiencies, infections, and disorders of metabolism (Sealey et al., 2019). Dr. Hoffer discovered that for a subset of patients with schizophrenia, their symptoms could be successfully treated with high doses of niacin, a B vitamin. He was joined by Dr. Humphry Osmond, a British psychiatrist, who brought his work with Dr. John Smythies to develop additional theories about biochemical underpinnings that cause psychotic symptoms. Their work became the basis of orthomolecular psychiatry and the use of megavitamin treatment for mental illness (Carter, 2019).

Two-time Nobel Prize winner Linus Pauling, PhD (1901–1994), a U.S. chemist, biochemist, chemical engineer, and peace activist, coined the term *Orthomolecular Psychiatry* in his 1968 article in the journal *Science* (Pauling, 1968) to describe a popular but controversial megavitamin therapy movement. Ortho is the Greek word for "correct" or "right" and molecular refers to studying the behavior of molecules, so orthomolecular means "right molecule." Orthomolecular psychiatry aims to vary the concentrations of substances (e.g., vitamins and minerals) that are normally present in the human body to prevent and treat psychiatric illness by providing the body with the necessary resources for optimal functioning (Orthomolecular.org, n.d.). In recognition of the growing body of research that there is a genetic component to mental illness (which is why we see them cluster in families), Pauling believed that it is the genes that regulate how the brain metabolizes essential nutrients that have the greatest influence on mental health rather than the genetic influence on other functions of the body (Kaplan & Rucklidge, 2021).

The *Journal of Orthomolecular Medicine* has continued to publish research and commentary on orthomolecular psychiatry since its inception in 1967. Unfortunately, while some of the initial research showed promising results, follow-up studies were not able to replicate the effects (possibly due to using lower doses) and the results were disappointing. At the same time, psychotropic medications were becoming more popular while orthomolecular psychiatry became less popular (Menolascino et al., 1988), largely due to the increasing influence of the pharmaceutical industry over medical and psychiatric education (Brody, 2009; Frances, 2013). However, now the tides are turning again with the growing wave of disillusionment about the effectiveness of psychotropic medicine, and attention is returning to the impact of dietary interventions for mental illness.

Until recently, nutrition research has only focused on the impact of nutrition on physical illness, especially chronic diseases like cardiovascular disease and diabetes. It is only in recent decades that the research lens has expanded and examining nutrition's impact on mental health has gained interest and growing support. Clinical nutrition research now includes studies focused on using structured dietary changes and/or nutrient-based supplements (generally a pill or powder made of food components such as vitamins, minerals, dietary fiber, and probiotics) to treat a range of mental health disorders.

One important early work was published in the 1990s when the respected journal *The Lancet* compared prevalent dietary practices in different countries and found a correlation between eating a lot of fish and lower rates of major depressive disorder (DeAngelis, 2023; Hibbeln, 1998). This research was followed by an impressive array of studies that demonstrated mental health can be improved by dietary changes. Articles in well-respected, peer-reviewed journals began reporting on various avenues of research on nutrition and mental health. For example, in 2006, an article in the *American Journal of Psychiatry* concluded there was sufficient evidence to support continuing exploration of treating unipolar and bipolar depressive disorders with omega-3 fatty acid supplementation (Parker et al., 2006). This finding was supported by the Committee on Research on Psychiatric Treatments of the American Psychiatric Association (APA) in the featured report of their meta-analyses of randomized controlled trials published in the *Journal of Clinical Psychiatry* confirming a protective effect of omega-3 fatty acids (Freeman et al., 2006). This led to the APA recommendation that all adults should eat fish at least two times a week, and patients with mood, impulse control, or psychotic disorders should also consider a fish oil supplement to ensure adequate consumption of omega-3 fatty acids (Richardson, 2008).

In 2001, Bonnie Kaplan, PhD, research psychologist and professor at the Cumming School of Medicine at the University of Calgary, began publishing data showing that micronutrient supplementation could resolve psychiatric symptoms for some patients. For example, in a small trial of 11 patients taking medication for bipolar disorder, after six months of taking a high-dose broad-based vitamin and mineral supplement, clients reported a 55 percent to 66 percent symptom reduction and a 50 percent decrease in their need for psychotropic medication with minimal side effects (Kaplan et al., 2001). Kaplan later partnered with Julia Rucklidge, PhD, Professor of Clinical Psychology at the University of Canterbury, to run clinical trials investigating the role of broad-spectrum micronutrients in treating mental illness. Their research journey is documented in their book *The Better Brain* (Kaplan & Rucklidge, 2021) where they discuss their rigorous study of the impact of nutrition on mental health.

An important aspect of Kaplan and Rucklidge's work is the focus on using high-quality broad-spectrum multinutrient formulas which they used consistently throughout their research and with which they have no financial ties that might influence their work. They argued that much of the research examining nutritional supplementation to treat mental illness focuses on identifying a single nutrient (e.g., vitamin D). This approach is likely too narrow because many nutrients work synergistically in the body, combining and acting on each other in different quantities and chemical reactions to satisfy the body's needs. Often, if you are deficient in one nutrient, you are likely to be deficient in other nutrients as well. Therefore, providing a spectrum of nutrients is more beneficial than offering just one or two nutrients in a treatment protocol (Rucklidge et al., 2023).

According to Kaplan and Rucklidge, over the last 20 years, there has been greater recognition that "the 'single ingredient solution' is no solution at all. Giving your brain *all* the nutrients it needs is what optimizes its health." Their research demonstrated that approximately 80 percent of people with psychiatric symptoms experience some benefit from taking a broad-spectrum multinutrient formula, with about 50 percent being "much to very much improved." A meta-analysis of studies using multinutrients for the treatment of psychiatric symptoms confirmed that participants who took broad-spectrum formulas showed more robust improvement than those given formulas with fewer ingredients (Johnstone et al., 2020). From this breadth of research, they made a bold statement,

> We now know that there are many people with underlying risk factors, often genetic, that may make them more vulnerable to emotional distress when their diet is poor. Improve and fix their nutritional needs, and many of them can and will get better. (Kaplan & Rucklidge, 2021, pp. 15–22).

THE FIELD OF NUTRITIONAL PSYCHOLOGY

Establishing a new field of study is not an easy task and is the accumulation of the hard work of many bright minds seeing the same evidence and moving in the same direction. In 2008, California-based wellness consultant Ephimia Morphew-Lu proposed, developed, and taught the first university-based nutritional psychology course, *Introduction to Nutritional Psychology*, at John F. Kennedy University as a continuing education course for psychologists, mental health professionals, and nurses. This popular course was followed by the development of a second course, *Advanced Nutritional Psychology*. In response to continued demand for this area of study, in 2011 Morphew-Lu collaborated with Australian psychologist Amanda Hull, PhD, to develop a seven-course certificate program in Nutritional Psychology for psychologists which includes methodology for how to appropriately provide nutrition education to their clients. The course was approved for continuing education credits by the American Psychological Association (APA) which represents 146,000 researchers, educators, clinicians, consultants, and students as its members (American Psychological Association, 2022).

In 2015, Morphew-Lu and Dr. Hull founded the non-profit Center for Nutritional Psychology (CNP), an online organization recognizing and supporting the field of nutritional psychology. CNP continues to consolidate nutritional psychology research and develop common language for use within the field to define, develop, and promote the interdisciplinary field of nutritional psychology. Their mission is to formalize education and training programs to facilitate the inclusion of nutritional psychology interventions in mental healthcare. The Nutritional Psychology certificate course was retired from JFK University in 2020, revamped, and offered through CNP. CNP went on to develop a nutritional psychology research library with links to nearly 3000 articles, an *Encyclopedia of Nutritional Psychology*, and now offers five Nutritional Psychology courses plus a 100-hour *Introductory Certificate in Nutritional Psychology* course in English and Greek languages (CNP, 2020). The current CNP courses are approved for continuing education by the APA, the Commission on Dietetic Registration (CDR), and the California Board of Behavioral Sciences (BBS).

According to CNP, the field of nutritional psychology is interdisciplinary and utilizes information from the disciplines of "psychology, behavioral and social sciences, nutrition science, neuroscience, biochemistry, physiology, and psychiatry." CNP focuses on the "diet-mental health relationship (DMHR)" which is an umbrella term used to describe a theoretical model that pulls from the different fields of study to understand how diet influences all aspects of "psychological functioning, processes, experience, and outcomes to shape how we think, feel, act, sense, and experience the world around us" (CNP, n.d.). CNP breaks down DMHR into six elements:

- Psychological, e.g., mood and emotions
- Behavioral, e.g., craving and conditioning
- Cognitive, e.g., learning and attention
- Sensory-perceptual, e.g., sight, smell, and taste
- Interoceptive, e.g., hunger and sensation
- Psychosocial, e.g., environment and social norms

The mental health field continues to embrace the importance of nutritional psychology. In addition to approving the CNP continuing education courses, the APA, one of the largest mental health professional organizations in the U.S., offers other nutritional psychology courses. In collaboration with the American Nutrition Association (ANA), the APA now offers a three-part continuing education course on nutrition and mental health for clinical psychologists (American Psychological Association, 2024). These courses explore the relationship between nutrition and mental health by examining eating behavior, the impact of nutrition on anxiety, and the bidirectional relationship of the gut–brain connection.

THE FIELD OF NUTRITIONAL PSYCHIATRY

In parallel with nutritional psychology, the new field of nutritional psychiatry has been gaining momentum as well. As discussed in Chapter 1, the difference between the field of Psychology and the field of Psychiatry is largely based on how the practitioners are trained. Psychologists complete a doctoral degree program to earn a degree as a Doctor of Philosophy (PhD) in a university or professional school where the training is focused on talk therapy and/or research. A psychiatrist completes medical school for training in general medicine during which they specialize in psychiatry and graduate with a degree as a Medical Doctor (MD). While these two fields have different training backgrounds and approaches to care, the fields of nutritional psychology and nutritional psychiatry are both solidly rooted in an understanding that there is an impact and importance in nutrition when it comes to preventing and treating psychiatric illness.

As the field of nutritional psychiatry evolves, there is a growing understanding that clinical interventions can be bolstered through an integrative approach that recognizes body systems, including the importance of nutrition and lifestyle choices. In 2014, an article written by Alan Logan and Felice Jacka acknowledged the growing body of research on the relationship between diet, brain function, and the risk of developing a mental disorder, including emerging studies demonstrating the importance of quality nutrition for developing brains during pregnancy and throughout the early childhood years (Logan & Jacka, 2014). This was followed by an article in 2015 in *The Lancet Psychiatry* (a top international journal in psychiatry) which took the position that, "Psychiatry is at an important juncture" where there is recognition that psychotropic medication only provides "modest benefits in addressing the burden of poor mental health worldwide" and that there is now "compelling evidence for nutrition as a crucial factor in the high prevalence and incidence of mental disorders" (Sarris et al., 2015).

The Lancet article authors are from an international collaboration of academics who are members of the International Society for Nutritional Psychiatry Research (ISNPR). The ISNPR supports the emerging field of research in nutritional psychiatry and advocates for "nutritional approaches to the prevention and treatment of mental disorders" (ISNPR, n.d.). In 2019, Professor Felice Jacka, Director of the Food & Mood Centre at Deakin University in Australia, and founder and president of the ISNPR, published the book *Brain Changer: How Diet Can Save Your Mental Health – Cutting-Edge Science from an Expert*, which documented current research in nutritional psychiatry, especially links between a whole-foods diet, gut health, and mental health (Jacka, 2019). The book discussed the goal of developing new, evidence-based mental health prevention and treatment strategies that include dietary changes. This is important because, while many factors contribute to poor mental health, such as early childhood trauma, a person's current diet is a modifiable risk factor that can frequently offer immediate benefits.

Jacka's work includes the SMILES Study (Supporting the Modification of Lifestyles in Lowered Emotional States). This was one of the first studies to test the hypothesis that clients diagnosed with clinical depression could improve their mood by making modifications to their diet (Jacka et al., 2017). This three-month study randomly assigned clients to either a dietary support group or a social support group and found depression scores demonstrating remission of depressive symptoms improved far more (over 30 percent) for participants in the dietary support group compared to the control group (8 percent). This research was validated in follow-up studies such as the HELFIMED Study (Healthy Eating for LiFe with a MEDiterranean-style diet) (Parletta et al., 2019), and the AMMEND Study (A Mediterranean Diet in MEN with Depression) (Bayes et al., 2022), which also demonstrated mental health improvement in response to changes in eating habits.

In addition to demonstrating that dietary modification can improve mood, the SMILES study also reported on the cost-effectiveness of healthy eating. In this study, 67 participants with major depressive disorder and a poor diet were randomly assigned to dietary support or social support as an adjunct to their current treatment. The dietary support group was coached to follow the Mediterranean diet with a focus on increasing whole foods consumption – vegetables, fruit, legumes, nuts, whole grains, fish, olive oil, and small servings of red meat – and a reduction in "extra" foods like chips, cakes, pastries, fast food, and packaged food. Not only was there a large effect size for decreasing symptoms of depression, but there was also a cost savings found in fewer health professional visits, fewer missed days of work, and more energy for unpaid roles such as household chores, volunteering, and child care (Jacka, 2019).

THE FIELD OF METABOLIC PSYCHIATRY

A similar area of study is the emerging field of *Metabolic Psychiatry*. This term was coined by Shebani Sethi, MD, ABOM, the founding director of the world's first academic Metabolic Psychiatry clinic and research program established in 2015 at Stanford University School of Medicine's Department of Psychiatry and Behavioral Sciences. The research at this clinic examines the intersection between metabolic health and mental health and how poor metabolic functioning, such as chronic inflammation, oxidative stress, and insulin resistance, may be at the root of some brain disorders and psychiatric illnesses. Their metabolic interventions emphasize reducing sugar, ultra-processed foods, and refined carbohydrates to improve overall wellbeing (Sethi, 2024).

TREATMENT APPROACHES

THE KETOGENIC DIET

The ketogenic diet (described in more detail in Chapter 8) has increasingly been the focus of research on dietary changes to improve mental health, especially in metabolic psychiatry (Chrysafi et al., 2024; Danan et al., 2022; Tillery et al., 2021). Many of the current clinical trials run through the Stanford Metabolic Psychiatry program focus on the benefits of a ketogenic diet to improve symptoms of psychiatric disorders including depression, bipolar disorder, Alzheimer's disease, anorexia nervosa, and schizophrenia. The *Frontiers in Psychiatry* journal has a research topic titled *Dietary and Metabolic Approaches for Mental Health Conditions* which lists articles about ketogenic and low carbohydrate diets to help address mental health issues (Frontiers in Psychiatry, 2024). To help organize the influx of research on this topic, the CNP recently added a *Keto Diet and Mental Health* research category to their nutritional psychology library to help readers follow this new research trend.

NUTRACEUTICALS AND PHYTOCEUTICALS

Nutritional psychology research has demonstrated substantial benefits of diet modification for specific psychiatric disorders. The research has included adding fresh fruits and vegetables, decreasing the intake of sugar and ultra-processed foods, and adding nutritional supplements to the overall food plan. Nutrient-based and plant-based supplements given for the treatment of health disorders (referred to as *nutraceuticals* and *phytoceuticals*, respectively) are often the treatment protocol for clinical studies since they allow a study to have a placebo control group and are less expensive studies to run compared to tracking people to make whole food dietary changes.

In an effort to consolidate the research on mental health nutraceuticals and phytoceuticals, the World Federation of Societies of Biological Psychiatry (WFSBP) and the Canadian Network for Mood and Anxiety Disorders (CANMAT) created an international taskforce that developed clinical guidelines for administering supplements in the course of a psychiatric treatment plan. These guidelines ranked the recommended use of different supplements based on the strength of the research evidence supporting their use for different psychiatric diagnoses, and identified the top 15 nutraceuticals (e.g., vitamin D and omega-3 fatty acids) and ten phytoceuticals (e.g., St. John's wort and Ginkgo) for mood disorders, anxiety disorders, psychotic disorders, and ADHD (Sarris et al., 2022). It was noted in the guidelines that adding a nutritional supplement to a treatment plan that already included a psychotropic medication could change the function of that medication and could increase its side effects, so consultation with a healthcare provide may be necessary before making any treatment changes.

SCREENING FOR RISK

While there is sufficient evidence of the benefits of nutritional support to prevent or treat mental health disorders, it can be difficult to clarify which clients are more likely to benefit from this approach. Since making dietary changes can be challenging and expensive, it is important to understand which clients are most likely to derive the maximum benefit from any nutritional changes. Development is underway for a nutrition and eating behavior screening tool to help clinicians decide how best to use their resources to achieve optimal results. Information about the NutriMental Screener was first published in 2021 as a tool for use in clinical practice to determine which clients living with SMI are at risk for common nutrition issues (Teasdale et al., 2021). The goal once development is complete is to encourage mental health clinicians to use the NutriMental Screener as part of their routine assessments in mental health services, which would facilitate including nutritional and eating behavior support in client treatment plans.

BRAIN INFLAMMATION MODEL OF DEPRESSION

Brain inflammation as an underlying cause or contributor to mental illness was briefly discussed in Chapter 3. An in-depth analysis of this topic can be found in the book *The Inflamed Mind* (Bullmore, 2019), which examines how the immune system interacts with the mind and mental health. In the 20th century, we thought the brain was separated from the immune system by the blood–brain barrier (BBB) (see Chapter 5 for more on the BBB). Scientists believed that this physical membrane did not allow inflammatory proteins associated with the immune system, such as cytokines, to make contact with the brain. The current field of neuro-immunology shows that cytokines (a protein that produces inflammatory effects in the body) also affect the brain by sending signals across the BBB from the body to the brain. Thus, the brain becomes inflamed.

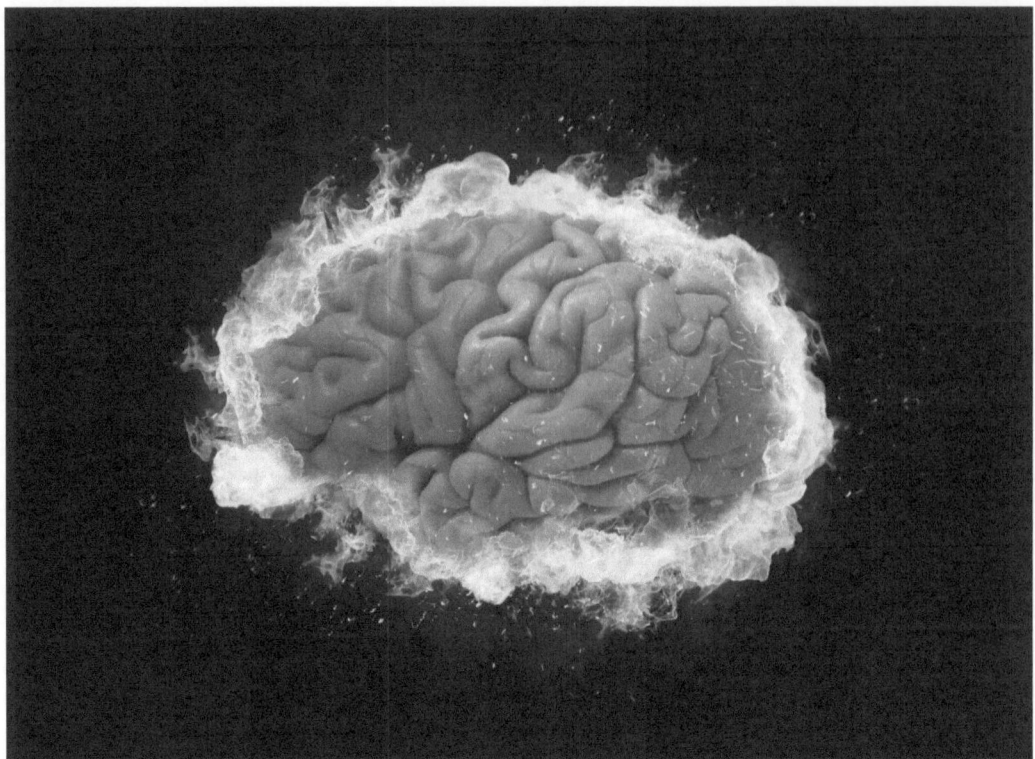

FIGURE 7.1 Brain inflammation. Credit: Alones (Shutterstock).

You may be thinking, "Okay, so the brain is inflamed. What does that have to do with mental health?" Here's the deal. We know there is a correlation between higher levels of inflammatory markers (such as cytokines and C-reactive protein [CRP]) and symptoms of mental illness, especially depression. A meta-analysis of 24 studies found that depressed people have higher blood concentrations of cytokines compared to healthy controls, which supports the idea that there is a connection between depression and the inflammatory response system (Dowlati et al., 2010). A landmark study that looked at 73,131 men and women aged 20–100 years found elevated levels of CRP in participants with higher levels of psychological distress and depression (Wium-Andersen et al., 2013).

The word inflammation continues to make the news, especially when associated with the benefits of anti-inflammatory medication, foods, and nutritional supplements. Inflammation can be understood as the body's protective response to a perceived threat such as an infection or damaged cells. It is an activation of the immune system to restore homeostasis in the body. Inflammation is protective when it clears away pathogens (like harmful viruses) and damaged tissue (such as from an injury) to support the body to repair any damage. Ideally, the inflammation does its job and tissues return to baseline in days or weeks. Inflammation can be harmful when it fails to resolve and becomes chronic, either because it was unable to remove the agent causing the inflammation or because it accelerated and spread where it is doing damage to tissues and organs without a pathogen, as in the case of an autoimmune disease. Chronic inflammation is associated with many medical conditions including inflammatory bowel disease, cancer, type 2 diabetes, heart disease, and autoimmune disorders such as rheumatoid arthritis, multiple sclerosis, and lupus (Oronsky et al., 2022).

Beyond correlation, there is growing evidence that systemic inflammation not only increases when someone is depressed but that the inflammation itself may be at least partly causing the depression. When inflammation activates the immune system, it triggers *sickness behavior* in mammals (Dantzer et al., 2008). Think about the last time you were sick with a cold or flu. Sickness behavior includes social withdrawal, pain and discomfort, lethargy, changes in sleep and appetite, and anhedonia. We often become sad and irritable when we are sick and have a hard time concentrating or remembering things. When these same symptoms do not abate, they match the diagnostic criteria for depression.

Many factors can cause an inflammatory response in the body. Traumatic life events, disease, poison, and nutritional deficiencies have all been associated with elevated levels of inflammatory biomarkers in the blood (Raison et al., 2006; Raison & Miller, 2013). Chronic irritants can cause long-term low-level inflammation in the body, such as dental issues like periodontitis (a form of gum disease) (Hashioka et al., 2018). Adverse childhood experiences (see Chapter 9) increase the risk of adult inflammation, as does having a higher BMI (see Chapter 11 for more information about BMI) (Danese et al., 2009; Das, 2001).

Dietary factors that increase or decrease inflammation have remained a popular concept. Many marketing strategies promote the benefits of anti-inflammatory foods such as berries, fatty fish, leafy greens, turmeric, and walnuts, as well as food supplement products that contain one of these or similar ingredients. Other foods are pro-inflammatory in that they tend to increase inflammation, such as ultra-processed foods (e.g., chips and candy), some processed meats and cheeses, fried foods, and sugary beverages (Wang et al., 2023). Of particular concern are pro-inflammatory foods with trans fatty acids (trans fats) in which vegetable oils are partially hydrogenated for use in margarine, food manufacturing, and commercial cooking and frying (Mozaffarian, 2006).

In addition to depression, there is some evidence that systemic inflammation also contributes to bipolar disorder, anxiety, and schizophrenia, but there is much less research on these other disorders compared to the large body of research about inflammation and depression (Ye et al., 2021). However, there is consistent evidence that individuals with SMI consume more pro-inflammatory foods and fewer anti-inflammatory foods than the general population, with the highest dietary risks among people with schizophrenia. Also, while much of the focus for this understanding has been on brain inflammation, there is also evidence that inflammation impacts mental health through other pathways including gut microbiome disruption and alterations in gut–brain communication (Firth et al., 2019).

The inflammatory model of mental illness provides a scientific approach to understanding some of the underlying mechanisms for how nutrition can impact mental health. It also supports mental health treatment that prioritizes anti-inflammatory foods or supplements as an important part of the treatment protocol for individuals with biomarkers for high inflammation. While there is no agreement on which is the best diet to lower inflammation, there are common factors across the studies of effective dietary treatment protocols to reduce depressive symptoms, such as reduced refined and ultra-processed foods while increasing intake of nutrient-dense and fiber-rich whole foods.

FOOD FOR THOUGHT: EIGHT SYSTEMS APPROACH TO MENTAL HEALTH

As discussed in the chapters thus far in the book, nutrition impacts the entire body. For a big-picture view, we can look at the body as having eight major systems to see how nutrition impacts each of these systems. The following infographic (Figure 7.2) provides a visual display of this full-body approach to mental health.

BIDIRECTIONAL INTERPLAY OF THE 8 SYSTEMS OF THE BODY ON MENTAL HEALTH

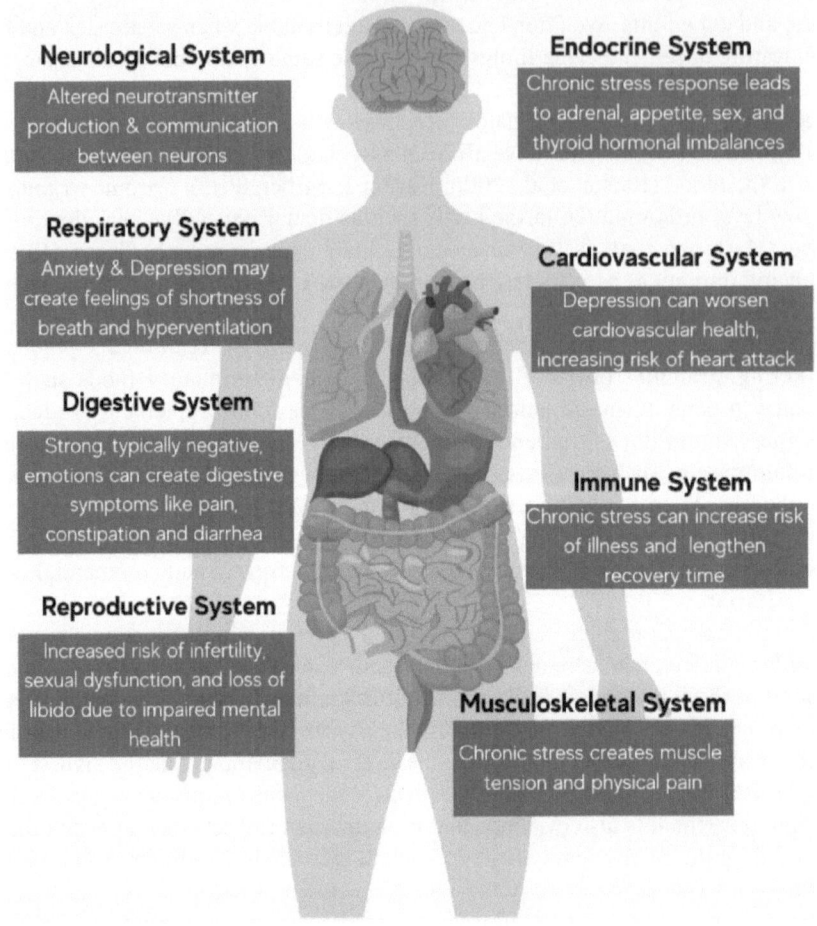

Neurological System
Altered neurotransmitter production & communication between neurons

Respiratory System
Anxiety & Depression may create feelings of shortness of breath and hyperventilation

Digestive System
Strong, typically negative, emotions can create digestive symptoms like pain, constipation and diarrhea

Reproductive System
Increased risk of infertility, sexual dysfunction, and loss of libido due to impaired mental health

Endocrine System
Chronic stress response leads to adrenal, appetite, sex, and thyroid hormonal imbalances

Cardiovascular System
Depression can worsen cardiovascular health, increasing risk of heart attack

Immune System
Chronic stress can increase risk of illness and lengthen recovery time

Musculoskeletal System
Chronic stress creates muscle tension and physical pain

FIGURE 7.2   Bidirectional interplay of the eight systems of the body on mental health. (Artwork by Jennifer Champion, 2024.)

REFERENCES

Alonso-Pedrero, L., Bes-Rastrollo, M., & Marti, A. (2019). Effects of antidepressant and antipsychotic use on weight gain: A systematic review. *Obesity Reviews*, *20*(12), 1680–1690.

American Psychiatric Association. (2013). *Diagnostic and statistical manual of mental disorders: DSM-5* (5th ed.). American Psychiatric Association. http://dsm.psychiatryonline.org/doi/book/10.1176/appi. books.9780890425596

American Psychological Association. (2022). *About APA*. https://www.apa.org/about

American Psychological Association. (2024). *Understanding nutrition and mental health*. https://on.apa. org/3zww71A

Bayes, J., Schloss, J., & Sibbritt, D. (2022). The effect of A Mediterranean diet on the symptoms of depression in young males (the "AMMEND: A Mediterranean Diet in MEN with depression" study): A randomized controlled trial. *The American Journal of Clinical Nutrition*, *116*(2), 572–580. https://doi. org/10.1093/ajcn/nqac106

Brody, H. (2009). Pharmaceutical industry financial support for medical education: Benefit, or undue influence? *Journal of Law, Medicine & Ethics, 37*(3), 451–460. https://doi.org/10.1111/j.1748-720X.2009.00406.x

Bullmore, E. T. (2019). *The inflamed mind: A radical new approach to depression* (1st U.S. ed.). Picador.

Burin, L. M., Hahn, M. K., da Rocha, N. S., van Amelsvoort, T., Bartels-Velthuis, A. A., Bruggeman, R., de Haan, L., Schirmbeck, F., Simons, C. J. P., van Os, J., & Cahn, W. (2022). Long-term treatment of antipsychotics and combined therapy with other psychotropic medications inducing weight gain in patients with non-affective psychotic disorder: Evidence from GROUP, a longitudinal study. *Psychiatry Research, 314*, 114680. https://doi.org/10.1016/j.psychres.2022.114680

Carey, B., & Gebeloff, R. (2018). Many people taking antidepressants discover they cannot quit. *New York Times.* https://www.nytimes.com/2018/04/07/health/antidepressants-withdrawal-prozac-cymbalta.html

Carter, S. (2019). Origins of orthomolecular medicine. *Integrative Medicine (Encinitas), 18*(3), 76–77.

Chrysafi, M., Jacovides, C., Papadopoulou, S. K., Psara, E., Vorvolakos, T., Antonopoulou, M., Dakanalis, A., Martin, M., Voulgaridou, G., Pritsa, A., Mentzelou, M., & Giaginis, C. (2024). The potential effects of the ketogenic diet in the prevention and co-treatment of stress, anxiety, depression, schizophrenia, and bipolar disorder: From the basic research to the clinical practice. *Nutrients, 16*(11), 1546.

CNP. (n.d.). *What is nutritional psychology?* The Center for Nutritional Psychology. Retrieved February 21, 2024, from https://www.nutritional-psychology.org/what-is-nutritional-psychology/

CNP. (2020). *The history of nutritional psychology: A new field of study to support a new model of mental healthcare.* The Center for Nutritional Psychology. https://www.nutritional-psychology.org/the-history-of-nutritional-psychology-a-new-field-of-study-to-support-a-new-model-of-mental-healthcare/

Cuerda, C., Velasco, C., Merchán-Naranjo, J., García-Peris, P., & Arango, C. (2014). The effects of second-generation antipsychotics on food intake, resting energy expenditure and physical activity. *European Journal of Clinical Nutrition, 68*(2), 146–152. https://doi.org/10.1038/ejcn.2013.253

Danan, A., Westman, E. C., Saslow, L. R., & Ede, G. (2022). The ketogenic diet for refractory mental illness: A retrospective analysis of 31 inpatients [Original research]. *Frontiers in Psychiatry, 13.* https://doi.org/10.3389/fpsyt.2022.951376

Danese, A., Moffitt, T. E., Harrington, H., Milne, B. J., Polanczyk, G., Pariante, C. M., Poulton, R., & Caspi, A. (2009). Adverse childhood experiences and adult risk factors for age-related disease: Depression, inflammation, and clustering of metabolic risk markers. *Archives of Pediatrics & Adolescent Medicine, 163*(12), 1135–1143. https://doi.org/10.1001/archpediatrics.2009.214

Dantzer, R., O'Connor, J. C., Freund, G. G., Johnson, R. W., & Kelley, K. W. (2008). From inflammation to sickness and depression: When the immune system subjugates the brain. *Nature Reviews Neuroscience, 9*(1), 46–56. https://doi.org/10.1038/nrn2297

Das, U. (2001). Is obesity an inflammatory condition? *Nutrition, 17*(11-12), 953–966.

DeAngelis, T. (2023). That salad isn't just good for your nutrition – It may help stave off depression. *Monitor on Psychology, 54*(4). https://www.apa.org/monitor/2023/06/nutrition-for-mental-health-depression

Devries, S., Dalen, J. E., Eisenberg, D. M., Maizes, V., Ornish, D., Prasad, A., Sierpina, V., Weil, A. T., & Willett, W. (2014). A deficiency of nutrition education in medical training. *The American Journal of Medicine, 127*(9), 804–806.

Dowlati, Y., Herrmann, N., Swardfager, W., Liu, H., Sham, L., Reim, E. K., & Lanctôt, K. L. (2010). A meta-analysis of cytokines in major depression. *Biological Psychiatry, 67*(5), 446–457.

Firth, J., Veronese, N., Cotter, J., Shivappa, N., Hebert, J. R., Ee, C., Smith, L., Stubbs, B., & Sarris, J. (2019). What is the role of dietary inflammation in severe mental illness? A review of observational and experimental findings. *Frontiers in Psychiatry, 10*, 443755.

Frances, A. (2013). *Saving normal: an insider's revolt against out-of-control psychiatric diagnosis, DSM-5, Big Pharma, and the medicalization of ordinary life* (1st ed.). William Morrow.

Freeman, M. P., Hibbeln, J. R., Wisner, K. L., Davis, J. M., Mischoulon, D., Peet, M., Keck, P. E. Jr, Marangell, L. B., Richardson, A. J., & Lake, J. (2006). Omega-3 fatty acids: Evidence basis for treatment and future research in psychiatry. *Journal of Clinical Psychiatry, 67*(12), 1954.

Frontiers in Psychiatry. (2024). *Dietary and metabolic approaches for mental health conditions.* https://www.frontiersin.org/research-topics/34945/dietary-and-metabolic-approaches-for-mental-health-conditions/magazine

Gafoor, R., Booth, H. P., & Gulliford, M. C. (2018). Antidepressant utilisation and incidence of weight gain during 10 years' follow-up: Population based cohort study. *BMJ, 361*, k1951.

Hashioka, S., Inoue, K., Hayashida, M., Wake, R., Oh-Nishi, A., & Miyaoka, T. (2018). Implications of systemic inflammation and periodontitis for major depression. *Frontiers in Neuroscience, 12*, 483.

Hibbeln, J. R. (1998). Fish consumption and major depression. *The Lancet, 351*(9110), 1213.

ISNPR. (n.d.). *International Society for Nutritional Psychiatry Research.* http://www.isnpr.org/

Itsiopoulos, C., Jacka, F. N., Opie, R. S., & O'Neil, A. (2015). The impact of whole-of-diet interventions on depression and anxiety: A systematic review of randomised controlled trials. *Public Health Nutrition, 18*(11), 2074–2093. https://doi.org/10.1017/S1368980014002614

Jacka, F. (2019). *Brain changer: How diet can save your mental health–cutting-edge science from an expert.* Yellow Kite, Hatchette.

Jacka, F. N., O'Neil, A., Opie, R., Itsiopoulos, C., Cotton, S., Mohebbi, M., Castle, D., Dash, S., Mihalopoulos, C., Chatterton, M. L., Brazionis, L., Dean, O. M., Hodge, A. M., & Berk, M. (2017). A randomised controlled trial of dietary improvement for adults with major depression (the 'SMILES' trial). *BMC Medicine, 15*(1), 23. https://doi.org/10.1186/s12916-017-0791-y

Johnstone, J. M., Hughes, A., Goldenberg, J. Z., Romijn, A. R., & Rucklidge, J. J. (2020). Multinutrients for the treatment of psychiatric symptoms in clinical samples: A systematic review and meta-analysis of randomized controlled trials. *Nutrients, 12*(11). https://doi.org/10.3390/nu12113394

Jorm, A. F., Patten, S. B., Brugha, T. S., & Mojtabai, R. (2017). Has increased provision of treatment reduced the prevalence of common mental disorders? Review of the evidence from four countries. *World Psychiatry, 16*(1), 90–99. https://doi.org/10.1002/wps.20388

Juul, F., Parekh, N., Martinez-Steele, E., Monteiro, C. A., & Chang, V. W. (2022). Ultra-processed food consumption among US adults from 2001 to 2018. *The American Journal of Clinical Nutrition, 115*(1), 211–221. https://doi.org/10.1093/ajcn/nqab305

Kaplan, B. J., & Rucklidge, J. J. (2021). *The better brain: Overcome anxiety, combat depression, and reduce ADHD and stress with nutrition.* Houghton Mifflin Harcourt Publishing Company.

Kaplan, B. J., Simpson, J. S., Ferre, R. C., Gorman, C. P., McMullen, D. M., & Crawford, S. G. (2001). Effective mood stabilization with a chelated mineral supplement: An open-label trial in bipolar disorder. *Journal of Clinical Psychiatry, 62*(12), 936–944. https://doi.org/10.4088/jcp.v62n1204

Lai, J. S., Hiles, S., Bisquera, A., Hure, A. J., McEvoy, M., & Attia, J. (2014). A systematic review and meta-analysis of dietary patterns and depression in community-dwelling adults. *The American Journal of Clinical Nutrition, 99*(1), 181–197.

Lane, M. M., Lotfaliany, M., Hodge, A. M., O'Neil, A., Travica, N., Jacka, F. N., Rocks, T., Machado, P., Forbes, M., Ashtree, D. N., & Marx, W. (2023). High ultra-processed food consumption is associated with elevated psychological distress as an indicator of depression in adults from the Melbourne Collaborative Cohort Study. *Journal of Affective Disorders, 335*, 57–66, https://doi.org/10.1016/j.jad.2023.04.124

Logan, A. C., & Jacka, F. N. (2014). Nutritional psychiatry research: An emerging discipline and its intersection with global urbanization, environmental challenges and the evolutionary mismatch. *Journal of Physiological Anthropology, 33*(1), 22. https://doi.org/10.1186/1880-6805-33-22

Marx, W., Moseley, G., Berk, M., & Jacka, F. (2017). Nutritional psychiatry: The present state of the evidence. *Proceedings of the Nutrition Society, 76*(4), 427–436. https://doi.org/10.1017/S0029665117002026

Menolascino, F. J., Donaldson, J. Y., Gallagher, T. F., Golden, C. J., & Wilson, J. E. (1988). Orthomolecular therapy: Its history and applicability to psychiatric disorders. *Child Psychiatry and Human Development, 18*, 133–150. https://link.springer.com/article/10.1007/BF00709727

Mörkl, S., Stell, L., Buhai, D. V., Schweinzer, M., Wagner-Skacel, J., Vajda, C., Lackner, S., Bengesser, S. A., Lahousen, T., Painold, A., Oberascher, A., Tatschl, J. M., Fellinger, M., Müller-Stierlin, A., Serban, A. C., Ben-Sheetrit, J., Vejnovic, A. M., Butler, M. I., Balanzá-Martínez, V.,…Holasek, S. J. (2021). 'An Apple a Day'?: Psychiatrists, psychologists and psychotherapists report poor literacy for nutritional medicine: International Survey Spanning 52 countries. *Nutrients, 13*(3). https://doi.org/10.3390/nu13030822

Mozaffarian, D. (2006). Trans fatty acids – Effects on systemic inflammation and endothelial function. *Atherosclerosis Supplements, 7*(2), 29–32. https://doi.org/10.1016/j.atherosclerosissup.2006.04.007

Mueller-Stierlin, A. S., Cornet, S., Peisser, A., Jaeckle, S., Lehle, J., Moerkl, S., & Teasdale, S. B. (2022). Implications of dietary intake and eating behaviors for people with serious mental illness: A qualitative study. *Nutrients, 14*(13). https://doi.org/10.3390/nu14132616

O'Neil, A., Quirk, S. E., Housden, S., Brennan, S. L., Williams, L. J., Pasco, J. A., Berk, M., & Jacka, F. N. (2014). Relationship between diet and mental health in children and adolescents: A systematic review. *American Journal of Public Health, 104*(10), e31–e42.

Oronsky, B., Caroen, S., & Reid, T. (2022). What exactly is inflammation (and what is it not?). *International Journal of Molecular Sciences, 23*(23), 14905. https://www.mdpi.com/1422-0067/23/23/14905

Orthomolecular.org. (n.d.). *Welcome to Orthomolecular.org.* http://orthomolecular.org/

Parker, G., Gibson, N. A., Brotchie, H., Heruc, G., Rees, A. M., & Hadzi-Pavlovic, D. (2006). Omega-3 fatty acids and mood disorders. *American Journal of Psychiatry, 163*(6), 969–978. https://doi.org/10.1176/ajp.2006.163.6.969

Parletta, N., Zarnowiecki, D., Cho, J., Wilson, A., Bogomolova, S., Villani, A., Itsiopoulos, C., Niyonsenga, T., Blunden, S., & Meyer, B. (2019). A Mediterranean-style dietary intervention supplemented with fish oil improves diet quality and mental health in people with depression: A randomized controlled trial (HELFIMED). *Nutritional Neuroscience*, *22*(7), 474–487.

Pauling, L. (1968). Orthomolecular psychiatry. *Science*, *160*(3825), 265–271. https://doi.org/doi:10.1126/science.160.3825.265

Pratt, L. A., Brody, D. J., & Gu, Q. (2017). Antidepressant use among persons aged 12 and over: United States, 2011-2014. *NCHS Data*, *Brief* (283), 1–8. https://www.cdc.gov/nchs/data/databriefs/db283.pdf

Psaltopoulou, T., Sergentanis, T. N., Panagiotakos, D. B., Sergentanis, I. N., Kosti, R., & Scarmeas, N. (2013). Mediterranean diet, stroke, cognitive impairment, and depression: A meta-analysis. *Annals of Neurology*, *74*(4), 580–591.

Raison, C. L., Capuron, L., & Miller, A. H. (2006). Cytokines sing the blues: Inflammation and the pathogenesis of depression. *Trends in Immunology*, *27*(1), 24–31.

Raison, C. L., & Miller, A. H. (2013). Do cytokines really sing the blues? *Cerebrum*, *2013*, 10.

Richardson, A. J. (2008). n-3 fatty acids and mood: The devil is in the detail. *British Journal of Nutrition*, *99*(2), 221–223. https://doi.org/10.1017/S0007114507824123

Rucklidge, J. J., Johnstone, J. M., Villagomez, A., Ranjbar, N., & Kaplan, B. J. (2023). Broad-spectrum micronutrients and mental health. In T. Dinan (Ed.), *Nutritional psychiatry: A primer for clinicians* (pp. 152–171). Cambridge University Press. https://doi.org/DOI:10.1017/9781009299862.010

Sachs, G. S., & Guille, C. (1999). Weight gain associated with use of psychotropic medications. *Journal of Clinical Psychiatry*, *60*, 16–19.

Sarris, J., Logan, A. C., Akbaraly, T. N., Amminger, G. P., Balanzá-Martínez, V., Freeman, M. P., Hibbeln, J., Matsuoka, Y., Mischoulon, D., & Mizoue, T. (2015). Nutritional medicine as mainstream in psychiatry. *The Lancet Psychiatry*, *2*(3), 271–274.

Sarris, J., Ravindran, A., Yatham, L. N., Marx, W., Rucklidge, J. J., McIntyre, R. S., Akhondzadeh, S., Benedetti, F., Caneo, C., Cramer, H., Cribb, L., de Manincor, M., Dean, O., Deslandes, A. C., Freeman, M. P., Gangadhar, B., Harvey, B. H., Kasper, S., Lake, J., & …Berk, M. (2022). Clinician guidelines for the treatment of psychiatric disorders with nutraceuticals and phytoceuticals: The World Federation of Societies of Biological Psychiatry (WFSBP) and Canadian Network for Mood and Anxiety Treatments (CANMAT) Taskforce. *The World Journal of Biological Psychiatry*, *23*(6), 424–455. https://doi.org/10.1080/15622975.2021.2013041

Sealey, R., Smith, R. G., & Saul, A. W. (2019). Abram Hoffer's 60 years of research and discovery of the orthomolecular approach to psychiatry. *Orthomolecular Medicine News Service*. http://www.orthomolecular.org/resources/omns/v15n03.shtml

Sethi, S. (2024). *Metabolic psychiatry*. Stanford Medicine. https://www.metabolicpsychiatry.com/what-is-metabolic-psychiatry

Teasdale, S. B., Moerkl, S., Moetteli, S., & Mueller-Stierlin, A. (2021). The development of a nutrition screening tool for mental health settings prone to obesity and cardiometabolic complications: Study protocol for the NutriMental screener. *International Journal of Environmental Research and Public Health*, *18*(21), 11269. https://www.mdpi.com/1660-4601/18/21/11269

Teasdale, S. B., Ward, P. B., Samaras, K., Firth, J., Stubbs, B., Tripodi, E., & Burrows, T. L. (2019). Dietary intake of people with severe mental illness: Systematic review and meta-analysis. *The British Journal of Psychiatry*, *214*(5), 251–259.

Tillery, E. E., Ellis, K. D., Threatt, T. B., Reyes, H. A., Plummer, C. S., & Barney, L. R. (2021). The use of the ketogenic diet in the treatment of psychiatric disorders. *Mental Health Clinician*, *11*(3), 211–219. https://doi.org/10.9740/mhc.2021.05.211

U.S. Burden of Disease Collaborators (2013). The State of US health, 1990-2010: Burden of diseases, injuries, and risk factors. *The Journal of the American Medical Association*, *310*(6), 591–606. https://doi.org/10.1001/jama.2013.13805

Vos, T., Abajobir, A. A., Abate, K. H., Abbafati, C., Abbas, K. M., Abd-Allah, F., Abdulkader, R. S., Abdulle, A. M., Abebo, T. A., & Abera, S. F. (2017). Global, regional, and national incidence, prevalence, and years lived with disability for 328 diseases and injuries for 195 countries, 1990–2016: A systematic analysis for the Global Burden of Disease Study 2016. *The Lancet*, *390*(10100), 1211–1259.

Wang, A., Wan, X., Zhuang, P., Jia, W., Ao, Y., Liu, X., Tian, Y., Zhu, L., Huang, Y., & Yao, J. (2023). High fried food consumption impacts anxiety and depression due to lipid metabolism disturbance and neuro-inflammation. *Proceedings of the National Academy of Sciences*, *120*(18), e2221097120.

Wang, L., Martínez Steele, E., Du, M., Pomeranz, J. L., O'Connor, L. E., Herrick, K. A., Luo, H., Zhang, X., Mozaffarian, D., & Zhang, F. F. (2021). Trends in consumption of ultraprocessed foods among US youths aged 2-19 years, 1999-2018. *The Journal of the American Medical Association*, *326*(6), 519–530. https://doi.org/10.1001/jama.2021.10238

Wium-Andersen, M. K., Ørsted, D. D., Nielsen, S. F., & Nordestgaard, B. G. (2013). Elevated C-reactive protein levels, psychological distress, and depression in 73 131 individuals. *JAMA Psychiatry*, *70*(2), 176–184. https://doi.org/10.1001/2013.jamapsychiatry.102

Ye, Z., Kappelmann, N., Moser, S., Davey Smith, G., Burgess, S., Jones, P. B., & Khandaker, G. M. (2021). Role of inflammation in depression and anxiety: Tests for disorder specificity, linearity and potential causality of association in the UK Biobank. *eClinicalMedicine*, *38*. https://doi.org/10.1016/j.eclinm.2021.100992

8 Using a Nutritional Approach to Treat Disease

Using nutrition to treat disease adds another layer of consideration to the already complicated decision-making process of making dietary changes. Different benefits and concerns must be considered when examining what each diet has to offer. There are many pros and cons of popular dietary trends, with individual responses to how they impact mental health. Keep in mind that no single diet is going to be perfect for every human being. We are all biochemically unique. Therefore, it is important to explore different dietary options when working to treat a mental health condition.

CHOOSING THE RIGHT DIET

It is important to keep in mind the previous discussion about calories and the incorrect vilification of fat that continues to influence dietary decisions. Some healthcare providers still believe that "eat less and exercise more" is a sufficient guide to good health. Does eat less mean eat fewer calories? Which type of calories? The research reminds us that the quality of the calories counts as much as the number of calories (Booth & Gibson, 2022; Ludwig et al., 2020). Most people find they require more accurate information to clarify what works best for their body.

Macro-based Diets

As anyone in the fitness industry can attest, macronutrients are often a focal point for those trying to get healthier or lose weight. As mentioned in Chapter 4, macronutrients include protein, fat, and carbohydrates. A macro-based diet focuses on calculating a percentage goal for each macronutrient to help reach a specific intake goal. After calculating the caloric need for the person, the calories are divided into proteins, fats, and carbohydrates, regardless of micronutrient density, meaning there is little differentiation between carbohydrates from vegetables and those from ultra-processed foods. Some use this style of eating as a way of being able to lose weight or build muscle mass. Others find it overly restrictive and less intuitive. Ideally, macronutrients *and* micronutrients should be balanced to help provide the mind and body with all the necessary building blocks (Muscaritoli, 2021). Focusing solely on the macronutrient ranges can also lead to an excessive intake of chemicals and "fake food" products just to hit the numbers. For example, high protein diets often promote the use of protein supplements to reach macronutrient goals, which can be high in sugar and preservatives. There is substantial literature demonstrating how important it is to balance meals for blood sugar stability, weight, muscle, and mental health, which are not necessarily mutually exclusive (Dye et al., 2000). Therefore, caution should be used with a macro-based diet to be sure there are healthy whole-food representatives of all three macros included in the daily diet.

Popular Diets

Many diets come and go, gaining and losing popularity. Each diet listed below has been popular at one point or another and could be beneficial if used by the right person at the right time in their life. When we look at the entire person and not just their symptoms, we recognize the need for bio-individuality in our eating.

The nutrition industry once assumed that everyone could and should eat the same things. We have now learned that not everyone tolerates the same foods or has the same nutrient needs. We also have different abilities to tolerate and adapt to some of the new challenges in our foods, such as

DOI: 10.1201/9781032647647-11

the addition of chemical additives, preservatives, stabilizers, and dyes. Therefore, it is important to consider different options to decide which is our highest priority need to which we are tailoring our food. Below are descriptions of six popular diets followed by a chart of mental health considerations associated with each diet plan.

The *ketogenic diet*, often called keto, is a high-fat, low-carbohydrate diet designed to induce a metabolic state known as ketosis, where the body primarily utilizes fat for fuel instead of carbohydrates. This diet significantly reduces the intake of carbohydrates, typically in a range of 20–50 grams per day. This is a drastic reduction compared to the average consumption of 200–350 grams of carbohydrates per day eaten in the Standard American Diet (SAD). Fats are increased to approximately 70 percent of the daily caloric intake to compensate for the reduction in carbohydrates, which are down to about 10 percent of the daily calories. Many people report needing fewer calories daily because the increase in fat keeps them feeling satiated longer with fewer cravings for snack foods. Protein is still consumed but in moderate amounts, usually accounting for approximately 20 percent of the dietary intake. When carbohydrate intake is low, the liver converts fatty acids into ketones, which the body can use for energy in place of glucose. This creates the state of ketosis.

The *paleo diet*, also referred to as the caveman diet or paleolithic diet, is based on the idea of eating in a way that mimics the diet of our prehistoric ancestors during the paleolithic era, before the agricultural revolution. This diet emphasizes whole, unprocessed foods that would have been available to early humans, believing that modern processed foods contribute to many of today's chronic health problems. Foods are avoided that are heavily processed, contain artificial ingredients, or are high in refined sugars. The diet typically includes many animal-based proteins (such as meat, fish, and eggs) alongside healthy fats from sources like nuts, seeds, and avocados. While not as carbohydrate restrictive as the ketogenic diet, the Paleo diet tends to have fewer carbohydrates because it excludes grains, legumes, and dairy.

The *carnivore diet* is an extreme form of a low-carbohydrate diet that involves eating only animal-based foods, such as meat, fish, eggs, and certain dairy products. It eliminates all plants, including fruits, vegetables, grains, legumes, nuts, and seeds. The diet is based on the ideology that some humans thrive best on a diet composed solely of animal products, similar to what some believe our ancestors consumed, because they do not digest carbohydrates very well which disrupts the digestive system and creates inflammation. The carnivore diet advocates that animal products, especially organ meats, are the most nutrient-dense non-inflammatory foods available and provide all essential nutrients.

On the complete opposite end of the spectrum lie the *vegetarian and vegan diets*, in which meat, poultry, fish, and, for some, eggs and dairy are removed from the diet in favor of eating only plant-based foods. The diet is often adopted for health reasons, ethical concerns, environmental considerations, or a combination of these factors. Vegetarian diets include the lacto-ovo vegetarian, who eats plant-based but also adds in dairy (lacto) and eggs (ovo) while excluding meat, poultry, and fish. The vegan diet is a more restrictive form of vegetarianism by excluding all animal products, including dairy, eggs, and honey, in addition to meat, poultry and fish. Some individuals will also avoid wearing animal products (e.g., leather) or using any personal products containing animal ingredients or tested on animals.

The *Mediterranean diet* is a dietary pattern inspired by the traditional eating habits of people living in countries bordering the Mediterranean Sea, such as Greece, Italy, and Spain. It emphasizes whole, minimally processed foods, a high intake of fruits, vegetables, and healthy fats, and moderate consumption of fish, poultry, and dairy. The diet is rich in fruits, vegetables, whole grains, legumes, nuts, and seeds, which form the basis of daily meals. Olive oil is the primary source of fat. Other sources of fats include nuts, seeds, and cold-water fatty fish. Fish and seafood are the preferred sources of animal protein, consumed between two and four times weekly. Poultry, eggs, and dairy are consumed in moderation, while red meat is limited. Like the keto and paleo diets, the Mediterranean diet limits processed foods, especially added sugars and refined grains. Herbs and spices are used in abundance to enhance the foods and naturally intensify the flavor palettes.

Finally, the *MIND diet (Mediterranean-DASH Intervention for Neurodegenerative Delay)* is a hybrid of the Mediterranean diet and the DASH diet. The DASH diet (Dietary Approaches to Stop Hypertension) focuses on foods that are rich in calcium, potassium, protein, fiber, and magnesium, and which are low in sodium, added sugars, and saturated fat. The MIND diet is specifically designed to enhance brain health while reducing the risk of Alzheimer's disease and other forms of dementia. This diet emphasizes foods that support cognitive function, such as leafy greens, berries, nuts, and fish, and limits those that might contribute to cognitive decline, such as red meat, butter, cheese, sweets, and fried/fast foods. Of the six popular dietary plans, the MIND diet is the least restrictive and encourages moderation and gradual incorporation of its principles into daily eating habits.

DIETS AND MENTAL HEALTH

The following chart lists the benefits and concerns about these six diet plans viewed through the lens of mental health and socioeconomic equality.

Ketogenic	Paleo	Carnivore
Pros:	Pros:	Pros:
• Healthy, quality fats that are brain-supportive and may help with anxiety (Platero et al., 2020) • Increased satiety which helps people feel calmer • Improved glucose management which increases insulin sensitivity and decreases reactive hypoglycemia • High potential for weight loss • Decreases cravings for processed foods which supports a diet that lowers inflammation	• There are many anti-inflammatory benefits from the phytonutrients, polyphenols, and antioxidants which can help with mental health • Increased iron consumption (red meat) • Increased protein intake often improves satiety • Weight loss is possible since simple carbs and sugar are eliminated • Eliminates reliance on refined carbohydrates which may be reducing mental health	• Provides sufficient protein which increases muscle building, wound healing, and provides the structure for many enzymes and hormones, all of which impacts mental health • Weight loss potential • Suitable for those who have severe food allergies; most people are not allergic to meat so those who tend to react to plant-based foods can worry less about reactions • Can be helpful as a short-term gut resent
Cons:	Cons:	Cons:
• Difficult to learn a new style of eating that accommodate high levels of healthy fats • Confusing advertising for keto that promotes processed foods that use almond or cassava flour in place of wheat flour, which pulls some people out of ketosis and encourages them to eat more sugar and sweeteners • Increased risk of kidney stones (Acharya et al., 2021) • A tendency to focus on fats and not pay enough attention to maintain a healthy assortment of vegetables in the diet	• Difficult for vegetarians and vegans since it doesn't include legumes • Without the cost-cutting carbohydrates and starches, this diet can be expensive • May increase the risk of kidney stones in some individuals due to high protein intake	• Difficult to follow through – the options are limited and may be boring after a while • Low in fiber and other key nutrients like vitamin C, polyphenols, and antioxidants that help with overall health • High in sodium for those who are using processed meats like bacon and deli meats to fill in the gaps • Socially restrictive – very few people eat this way and this can leave a person feeling isolated • Too much protein can be taxing to the kidneys and liver • Insufficient research to identify benefits

Plant-Based/Vegan	Mediterranean	MIND Diet
Pros: • May help with anxiety and depression due to increased phytonutrient intake (Agarwal et al., 2015) • May reduce inflammation that is exacerbating mental health conditions (Lucas et al., 2014) • Increased affordability without consumption of animal products	Pros: • Most widely studied diet regarding mental health with over 215,000 studies • Can help with blood sugar regulation (Da Porto et al., 2021) • Positive impact on the gut–brain axis by modulating the microbiome (Merra et al., 2020) • Anti-inflammatory, including reducing brain inflammation (Hornedo-Ortega et al., 2018) • High nutrient profile improves mental health (Ventriglio et al., 2021)	Pros: • Combines the best of the Mediterranean and DASH diets • Provides the brain with essential nutrients for cognitive function • Can help protect the brain, increase the ability to learn, focus, and make decisions. (Dhana et al., 2021) • May help prevent cognitive decline (Morris et al., 2015)
Cons: • Multiple nutrient deficiencies such as B12, iron, choline, taurine, omega-3, zinc, vitamin D, calcium, iodine, and protein (Sakkas et al., 2020) • The increased consumption of grains can lead to gas and bloating • Decreased ability to detoxify due to a lack of protein to support phase I and phase II of detoxification. • Insufficient consumption of fat • Potential increase in blood glucose levels if carbohydrates are the primary nutrient source • Potential increase in homocysteine levels due to insufficient B12 and B6 consumption (Ueno et al., 2022)	Cons: • Contains wheat and dairy products, which may not be suitable for all • Is not very specific and may require more guidance from a nutritionist • Recommends daily wine consumption, which may not be suitable for all	Cons: • Limited consumption of processed and prepared foods can be a difficult lifestyle adjustment • Eliminates dairy and red meat, which may be sources of calcium and iron for some

All of these diets have in common that they recommend eating only whole foods, minimizing processed and packaged foods, and reducing consumption of sodium, sugar, trans fats, and alcohol. The SAD diet is often deficient in whole foods, opting more for processed and packaged foods, which are convenient and require little preparation or cooking skills, but can be inflammatory and do not provide the necessary nutrients for mental health.

Of Note . . . THE HEALING PROPERTIES OF MUSHROOMS

Mushrooms have been a part of the human diet and healthcare practices for thousands of years due to their amazing array of nutritional and therapeutic benefits. Traditionally, mushrooms have been added to meals for both flavor and as an environmentally friendly, relatively inexpensive protein source. *Culinary mushrooms* are those species of mushrooms primarily used for cooking, whereas *medicinal mushrooms* have been focused on for their therapeutic benefits, however, there is no true differentiation because many mushrooms are often used for both. Culinary mushrooms have been valued not only for their taste and texture, but also for their plethora of nutritional benefits. Mushrooms are high in dietary fiber and protein, as well as vitamins B1, B2, B12, C, D, and E, and trace minerals such as zinc and selenium. Taking care when cooking mushrooms helps maintain their nutritional value, with grilling and microwaving being preferable to boiling and frying in order to preserve their antioxidant activity and nutritional profile (Roncero-Ramos et al., 2016).

While medicinal mushrooms such as Reishi and Turkey Tail have an established history of therapeutic use in ancient traditional therapies, it is only recently that contemporary research has validated and documented these benefits. We now have evidence that medicinal mushrooms can: decrease cancer tumor growth; reduce viral, bacterial, parasitic, and fungal overgrowths in the body; improve the body's ability to detoxify; and improve blood glucose levels (Wasser, 2011). The exponential increase in medicinal mushroom research has been exploring both consumption of whole mushrooms as well as the therapeutic use of mushroom extracts and supplements (Venturella et al., 2021).

In addition to physical health, there are now numerous studies demonstrating the ability of mushrooms to improve mental health. A systematic review of epidemiological and intervention studies concluded that a higher mushroom intake, especially of the Lion's Mane mushroom species, reduces depressive symptoms and decreases dementia (Cha et al., 2024). For example, in an analysis of data from the National Health and Nutrition Examination Survey (NHANES) that analyzed survey results and PHQ-9 scores for over 24,000 participants, researchers found evidence that regular mushroom consumption is associated with a decreased risk of depressive symptoms (Ba et al., 2021). Similarly, another study of NHANES respondents compared mushroom consumption by a nationally representative sample of over 2800 U.S. older adults over age 60 to results on cognitive function tests. The results of the study provide evidence that mushrooms may have neuroprotective properties and that regular mushroom consumption may reduce the risk of cognitive decline (Ba et al., 2022). While other species of mushrooms have demonstrated cognitive benefits, white button and oyster mushrooms, which are some of the most common species of culinary mushrooms in the U.S., do not appear to offer the same types of cognitive support (Uffelman et al., 2024).

Another avenue where mushrooms can be used for treatment of mental illness is in the realm of psychedelic mushrooms (Stamets, n.d.). The mental health field is beginning to recognize the potential value of psychedelic-supported psychotherapy, especially for PTSD and treatment-resistant depression, and psilocybin mushrooms are included in that expansion. *Psilocybin* is a psychedelic mushroom (known colloquially as "magic mushrooms") that has recently gained a lot of attention for its psychiatric therapeutic benefits (Pollan, n.d.). A systematic review published by the American Psychological Association in 2020 concluded that psilocybin "demonstrates wide ranging potential for treating anxiety, depression, OCD, and substance use disorders associated with alcohol and nicotine" and promotes connection, acceptance, and processing of emotions (Wheeler & Dyer, 2020, p. 26). We are just beginning to explore the promising uses for psilocybin in the psychiatric clinical setting.

BENEFITS OF TESTING

Part of the challenge of working with mental health conditions is obtaining the proper testing to get to the root of what is happening. As mentioned in Chapter 3, mainstream medicine has long focused on the chemical imbalance theory of mental illness and the serotonin theory of depression, even though recent research has challenged these concepts and argued for a more nuanced approach to understanding mental illness. Still, as a community, we continue to accept the idea that anyone with symptoms of depression, anxiety, or any other mental health condition must have a chemical imbalance since that theory endures and is promoted within the healthcare system.

Analyte	Result	Unit per Creatinine	L	WRI	H	Reference Interval
Serotonin	63.6	µg/g				60–125
Dopamine	120	µg/g				125–250
Norepinephrine	16.6	µg/g				22–50
Epinephrine	1.5	µg/g				1.6–8.3

FIGURE 8.1   Sample neurotransmitter level lab report. (Courtesy of Doctor's Data Inc. https://www.doctors data.com/NeuroBasic-Profile-urine.)

Fortunately, modern laboratory tests give us more insight and allow us to test this theory on an individual basis. We can consider neurotransmitter levels through a laboratory test such as an *organic acids test (OAT)*, which allows practitioners to assess the levels of an individual's neurotransmitters and make decisions about how to address any imbalances if the values are out of range. Figure 8.1 demonstrates a sample report which shows low serotonin, dopamine, norepinephrine, and epinephrine levels (Result) compared to population average levels of these neurotransmitters (Reference Interval). The green column in the center identifies results that are Within Reference Interval (WRI), which are considered optimal neurotransmitter levels. In this report, the serotonin levels are in the low WRI range, which is not optimal, and the other neurotransmitters are in the Low (L) range which is significantly below the WRI and may be associated with anxiety, depression, and other mood-related symptoms.

As discussed in Chapter 5, it is important to remember that the gut health of the individual can have a significant impact on their mental health. The gut–brain axis conveys messages between the intestinal tract and the brain. Many neurotransmitters (such as dopamine and serotonin) are produced in the intestinal tract, with additional production in various body areas, such as the central nervous system (Berger et al., 2009; Terry & Margolis, 2017). The OAT looks at neurotransmitter levels via a urine sample and, when combined with a stool sample that also measures overall gut health and neurotransmitters, can be a powerful indicator of an underlying root-cause imbalance to why a person feels the way they do.

The field of Functional Medicine (FM) is driven by a healthcare approach that works to address the root causes of disease rather than just manage the visible symptoms (IFM, n.d.). An FM practitioner is likely to use sophisticated lab testing to elucidate imbalances, such as neurotransmitter, hormone, and gut microbiome levels, in order to guide the treatment recommendation. FM treatment includes consideration of the impact of a person's diet on their health issues and works with patients to make dietary changes to improve their health. While there are many testing options in the FM approach, in mainstream medicine, this type of testing is generally limited, and prescriptions for psychotropic medications for mental illness are written based on symptoms alone with no lab testing.

In conventional or mainstream medicine, many patients with chronic conditions such as a mental health issue seek answers, help, and understanding from their primary care practitioner but feel disappointed in the care they receive. Since most appointments last only 15–20 minutes, there is little time to evaluate and comprehend the symptoms and lifestyle choices with the patient to explore potential underlying factors. In conventional medicine, after hearing a brief description of symptoms from the patient, a prescription is often written, and the patient heads to the pharmacy. While these medications may help in the short term, many people feel only partial relief of their symptoms and have concerns about their long-term side effects.

When we use lab testing, we get data from the body that we need to help the client make the right changes in diet and lifestyle, changes that are individualized. Testing is an essential tool to guide people to make effective changes that will help them feel better. When we give the body what it needs, especially natural foods in their whole state, and avoid processed and packaged foods with a list of ingredients we cannot pronounce, it allows our body to thrive. These changes through individualized care plans empower the body to do the healing work it was designed to do.

CASE STUDY: MOOD, ENERGY, AND CANDIDA

On a typically gloomy Pacific Northwest (PNW) day, Dr. Champion met with a new client, Michelle, age 48, who was coming for help with recent changes in mood and energy levels. While a common complaint of those living in the PNW associated with many days of overcast and rainy weather, Dr. Champion also noticed a paleness to Michelle's skin as she sat timidly on the couch. Michelle's eyes were sunken in, with dark circles around them. She wore no makeup, and her fingernails were bitten so low that they showed signs of previous bleeding. Michelle's chin quivered and tears welled in her eyes as she said she was desperate to find answers to what was wrong with her.

For years, Michelle had faithfully taken her daily antidepressant, which no longer worked as it once did. After careful probing, Dr. Champion discovered that Michelle's symptoms often worsened during wintertime but seemed year-round to some extent. Her mother's health history included major depression and generalized anxiety that worsened into agoraphobia around the same age that Michelle was now.

A review of Michelle's dietary history described periods when she consumed almost no food, skipping meals to "get work done" because if she did not, she had to work later or on weekends to ensure she completed her work. She reported working for a boss who has "no compassion or care for work-life balance." When Michelle made the time to eat, she did not want to cook and opted to swing through a drive-thru or grab takeout on her way home, which left very little space for variety and fresh produce in her diet. On the days when she cooked, she felt as though her family did not appreciate the food she made and would often go to the kitchen to find something else. The lack of appreciation made it difficult for her to find the motivation to cook, even though she used to love cooking.

Michelle reported having no outside activities that brought her joy. She could not remember the last time she did anything for herself. She said her recent 30-pound weight gain greatly hindered her physical activity. She felt ashamed to be outside and often opted for staying inside where she could hide from the judgment she felt.

Dr. Champion ordered an OAT to see if any micronutrients (e.g., vitamin B) or microorganisms (e.g., bacteria or fungi) were out of balance. Michelle's OAT results (see Figure 8.2) showed a *Candida albicans* overgrowth was present, with a result of 8.04e2 (8.04e2 is equivalent to 8.04×10^2) on a reference scale where less than 5.00e2 is optimal, indicating very high levels of *Candida*. *Candida* is a type of yeast (which is a type of fungus) that can create symptoms of fatigue, yeast infections, oral thrush, skin redness, itching, pain or discomfort, and vaginal discharge. It may also interfere with sleep and mood and create emotional fluctuations with big highs and lows. Multiple factors can encourage *Candida* overgrowth, including: increased stress; poorly managed diabetes; decreased immune system function; consuming a diet with excess refined carbohydrates, yeast, and sugar; and taking antibiotics, steroids,

FUNGI/YEAST			
FUNGI/YEAST	Result		Reference
Candida spp.	9.51e2		<5.00e3
Candida albicans	8.04e2	High ↑	<5.00e2
Geotrichum spp.	<dl		<3.00e2
Microsporidium spp.	<dl		<5.00e3
Rhodotorula spp.	<dl		<1.00e3

FIGURE 8.2 Sample lab report showing *Candida* overgrowth. (Courtesy of Jennifer Champion, DCN.)

hormones, or oral contraceptives. The other fungi shown in the report are normal since the *Candida* spp. result of 9.51e2 is well below the reference range of 5.00e3, as e2 (10^2) is 10 times smaller than e3 (10^3), and the other fungi levels are so low they are not detectable (<dl represents results below the detectable limit).

To facilitate remediation of her yeast overgrowth, Dr. Champion recommended adding coconut oil, quality fats, oregano, and thyme to her diet, while at the same time reducing foods higher in sugar, such as dairy, grains, and sweets. At the 6-week check-in, the client reported a 40 percent improvement in symptoms. At the 12-week check-in, the client reported improved sleep, digestion, and mood, and was satisfied with the course and success of the treatment.

GASTROINTESTINAL HEALTH

Another critical consideration when working with mental health clients is overall gastrointestinal health. Previously, we discussed the impact of nutrient deficiencies on overall health, including mental health. Maintaining healthy micronutrient levels depends on all systems functioning well to break down and utilize all the nutrients we consume. While many tests are available that provide data on gut health, choosing the right one for the client is essential. Making these tests affordable and accessible is critical to the healing journey, including reporting which tests are covered by insurance companies. This can be frustrating because often the tests that are covered by insurance lack many important components for understanding gut health, especially testing for intestinal permeability and beneficial and opportunistic bacteria levels, the importance of which is discussed in Chapter 5. As a practitioner, lab tests which provide information regarding the client's digestion and absorption rates can be essential to developing an appropriate treatment plan.

When working with a client struggling with mental health challenges, it can be helpful to start with an examination of overall gastrointestinal health. If the nutrients are not absorbed properly in the gut, anything changed downstream (e.g., hormones or neurotransmitters) will not hold for long. The body cannot maintain hormone and neurotransmitter levels without the proper building blocks made up of micronutrients from our food.

For simplicity's sake, let us assume that you, as the practitioner, did the root work of helping the client get their digestion on track. After working together, the client is no longer experiencing constipation or diarrhea, is having at least one bowel movement daily, and is not noticing food particles in their stool any more (Ma et al., 2023; McCormick, 2019). This can be taken as evidence that their digestive tract is now functioning more optimally and that nutrients are likely being absorbed sufficiently.

Once the gut has been repaired, it is important to begin looking into the health of both the neurological and endocrine systems that maintain neurotransmitter and hormone levels in the body. This assessment can be done through a variety of tests as well. It is often helpful to combine urine, blood, stool, and genetic testing to get the full picture to best identify and address the root cause of any potential imbalances through diet and lifestyle changes.

Medication can be a temporary bandage to help stabilize the system and support the necessary energy and focus to make diet and lifestyle changes, but their long-term use can be problematic. When we experience specific nutrient, sleep, hydration, and movement deficiencies, they cannot be remediated long-term by medication. You cannot medicate your way out of an unhealthy lifestyle. This is not to say that the temporary use of medications has no place in our healthcare system. Sometimes we need something to help us get over a hump. However, that hump does not usually last five or more years, while sometimes the prescriptions do.

FOOD ALLERGIES AND SENSITIVITIES

Once an individual is eating a whole-food-based diet, it may be necessary to refine which whole foods are appropriate for that person based on whether or not they have a food allergy or sensitivity to that food. Approximately 11 percent of U.S. adults have one or more food allergies and up to 20 percent have food sensitivities (sometimes referred to as food intolerances) (IFM, 2024). Food allergies are generally defined as having an immunoglobulin E (IgE) immune system response after ingesting the food, whereas food sensitivities do not trigger an IgE response but do contribute to discomfort and dysfunction. Therefore, assessing food allergies and sensitivities may be a helpful part of developing a nutrition plan to treat mental health.

Skin-prick Test

One of the most common methods of testing for food allergies is the *skin-prick test*. The first skin-prick or skin-scratch test to assessfor food allergies was created in 1912 by pediatrician Oscar Menderson Schloss, MD. This type of testing remains popular today and is often completed during an office visit. The skin is poked or "scratched" with a sterile needle containing a small amount of the food in question. This type of testing often yields a 50 percent accuracy rate for food allergies and does not provide indicators of any food sensitivities. Since food sensitivities do not trigger the release of IgE antibodies, nor will they lead to major allergic reactions like anaphylaxis, they are often disregarded despite uncomfortable symptoms when consuming these foods. For this reason, very early on there was concern that we should not rely solely on IgE testing but should also include food challenge testing (removing and carefully reintroducing suspected foods) to assess if a person has food allergies and/or sensitivities (Bahna, 2024).

The Elimination Diet

The *elimination diet* origin is credited to Albert Rowe, M.D., a California-based physician who began using the elimination diet in 1926 to help identify suspected food sensitivities (Wuthrich, 2014). The elimination diet removes the most common food allergens and sensitivities, many of which are not identified in a food allergy test. The length of elimination varies, as does the number of foods that need to be removed. However, the standard rule of thumb is eliminating higher-risk foods such as gluten and dairy for three weeks. This allows the inflammation to subside and the gut mucosa to begin the healing process. After three weeks, foods are reintroduced one at a time, and any symptoms that occur are noted. Symptoms can be physical, like gas, bloating, constipation or diarrhea, as well mental or emotional, such as an inability to think clearly (brain fog), fatigue, or irritability.

With the elimination diet, the client does not have to invest in costly food allergy testing, which often has a high rate of false positives and can be frustrating to someone already challenged by food choices. False positives can result in misdiagnosis of a food allergy and lead to overly restrictive dietary avoidance (Bird et al., 2015). The client's principal investment in the elimination diet is food, which must already be purchased to live. The elimination diet is not suitable for all patients such as patients who are struggling with an acute medical illness, those with a history of or an active eating disorder, and pregnant women (IFM, 2024).

REACTIVE HYPOGLYCEMIA

An area of clear connection between nutrition and mood is *reactive hypoglycemia*, where blood sugar (glucose) rapidly drops in response to eating foods high in simple carbohydrates. The body responds to a sudden drop in glucose by increasing cortisol and adrenaline. This is often associated with feeling uncomfortable, edgy, shaky, lightheaded, and irritable.

Highly processed or ultra-processed foods have been through a manufacturing process where the ingredients have been broken down into tiny food particles, and no longer have much resemblance to their original form in nature. These foods are generally low in fiber and high in starches and added sugars. The process of heating, grinding, squeezing, filtering, and chemically breaking down the ingredients (e.g., grinding wheat, juicing oranges) makes the food particles very small and thereby more quickly digested in the stomach and absorbed in the small intestine so that they rapidly enter the bloodstream and raise our glucose levels (see Chapter 5 for more details about digestion).

When we eat ultra-processed food, our glucose quickly increases and signals the body to produce insulin to bring our blood sugar back into a healthy range. As a result, our body goes through a glucose roller-coaster ride. Our glucose spikes right after we eat the ultra-processed food and then quickly drops when the body releases insulin and the glucose is shuttled from the bloodstream to the fat cells, sometimes resulting in glucose levels in the body quickly dropping to a level below the standard range, generally 70 milligrams per deciliter (mg/dl) known as hypoglycemia. Stress, poor sleep, caffeine consumption, irregular eating patterns, and a diet high in sugar and low in healthy fats and protein can exacerbate the symptoms of hypoglycemia.

With hypoglycemia, the body senses that glucose (often the body's primary energy source) is low and releases cortisol and adrenaline to motivate us to find more fuel (i.e., food). Cortisol and adrenaline can create sensations of shakiness, sweating, headache, hunger or nausea, fatigue, irritability, anxiety, difficulty concentrating, lightheadedness, confusion, panic, and nightmares. Feeling "hangry" is a common experience for many people who have not eaten for a while, are experiencing hypoglycemia, and feel grouchy and unfocused. This drives them to quickly grab whatever food is at hand that will give them another boost of glucose, which can then start the rollercoaster ride all over again.

A diet high in processed foods can maintain this cycle of reactive hypoglycemia throughout the day and perpetuate a sense of urgency and panic around food that often leads to impulsive food choices of whatever is accessible to help them feel better quickly. The rapid blood sugar spike and subsequent drop an hour or two later increases anxiety and fatigue, adding more drive for a "quick fix" to feel better as quickly as possible. Over time, these constant highs and lows can take a toll on a person's mental health and contribute to symptoms of anxiety, depression, and panic attacks. In contrast, foods high in water, fiber, protein, and fat all slow down the digestive process and decrease this glucose-insulin rollercoaster ride, increasing feelings of calm and the ability to consistently make healthier food choices.

COLLABORATION

Being part of a care team for a client is a privilege. As a practitioner, we work for the client, not vice versa. It is essential that we, as practitioners, collaborate with other skilled practitioners for the overall betterment of the client. Collaboration also helps keep us in our professional scope of practice. Getting pulled into another scope by the client's questions or concerns is easy. Collaborating puts the client at the forefront of their healing and helps to build a strong care team. When someone is concerned about mental health, making sure that we are addressing the entire person (e.g., nutrition, trauma, lifestyle, hormones) needs to be practiced by every person on the care team.

Using a combination protocol to address the physical and psychological impact of life stressors is beneficial for clients. Many people with mental health disorders see a therapist and a primary care provider, but they rarely consider seeing a nutritionist to help them focus on the necessary nutrients to help them combat chronic emotional, mental, and physical stress. Both nutrition and psychological support can help increase resilience to better manage stressful and traumatic situations.

MEDICALLY TAILORED MEALS

There is abundant evidence that eating more whole foods and less processed foods leads to improved mental health. Therefore, the healthcare system is an obvious place where assistance with obtaining, cooking, and storing foods should be available. Unfortunately, that is generally not the case. Medical providers usually receive little training in nutrition and face many barriers to helping patients navigate the confusing food system to establish a healthy diet (Mozaffarian et al., 2018).

One interesting model that is gaining momentum to address this issue is the provision of *Medically Tailored Meals (MTMs)*. MTMs are nutritionally tailored to best match a person's medical needs. They are fully prepared and home-delivered meals for individuals with advanced and costly diet-sensitive conditions like diabetes, heart failure, end-stage kidney disease, and cancer. A standard program provides ten weekly meals (lunch and dinner for five days per week) designed by a registered dietitian based on the patient's disease diagnosis and nutritional assessment.

These programs are designed to provide quality dietary access to lower-income and homebound patients at higher risk for food insecurity, especially those with physical or mental limitations that make it hard to perform activities like shopping or cooking due to their disease. To evaluate if MTMs are a financially viable option for the healthcare system, a 2022 article in the Journal of the American Medical Association (JAMA) performed an economic evaluation of MTMs to examine if helping patients with diet-sensitive conditions improve the quality of their diet decreases their hospital visits and overall use of the healthcare system. The result was a resounding Yes! The study authors reported an estimated net savings (after paying for MTM program costs, including clinical screenings and meals) of $13.6 billion by decreasing the number of hospitalizations and other healthcare costs (Hager et al., 2022).

FOOD FOR THOUGHT: COMORBID DIABETES, NAFLD, DEPRESSION, AND ANXIETY

Diabetes (also known as diabetes mellitus) is, by definition, a disease of the inability to process and regulate insulin, contributing to an inability to process carbohydrates and glucose effectively. There are two types of diabetes, *type 1 diabetes (T1D)* and *type 2 diabetes (T2D)*. T1D is an autoimmune condition that shows up early in life and is thought to be more genetically based, whereas T2D is generally diagnosed later in life (but not always) and occurs in response to a lifestyle where glucose and insulin levels remain chronically high.

According to the CDC an estimated 38.4 million U.S. adults have diabetes (11.6 percent of the population) and 97.6 million (38.0 percent) have pre-diabetes (defined as a higher-than-normal blood sugar level that is not high enough to be diagnosed with T2D). Higher rates of diabetes are found in ethnic minorities including American Indian, Puerto Rican, Black, Filipino, Pacific Islander, and Mexican (CDC, 2024). The disparity of diabetes diagnoses aligns with the food deserts that many of these individuals live in, which we will discuss more in Chapter 14. It is clear that those who live in a lower socioeconomic group are more likely to receive unfavorable health diagnoses such as diabetes.

A diabetes diagnosis nearly doubles the risk of developing depression (Holt et al., 2014). Managing diabetes can be a stressful task, which can cause people to feel discouraged and seek out more comfort foods, which are often sugar-based and exacerbate diabetes symptoms. This is made worse by the fact that when someone is depressed, they often do not feel like they are worth the time and energy to eat healthy foods or move the body in ways that build health. Both conditions – diabetes and depression – tend to have similar causal factors: *hypothalamus-pituitary-adrenal (HPA)* axis over-activation due to stress, inflammation, erratic sleep patterns, poor dietary and lifestyle choices, and an environmental toxic burden (such as mold or poor air quality) (Holt et al., 2014). The HPA axis is the tightly connected system of communication between the hypothalamus, the pituitary gland, and the adrenal glands and is the body's primary way of responding to stress (discussed in more detail in Chapter 9).

Depression is not the only mental health comorbidity that presents with diabetes. Those diagnosed with schizophrenia are two to five times more likely to be diagnosed with T2D, likely due to the common risk factors of obesity, sedentary lifestyle, and lower socioeconomic status shared by these two disorders. In addition, antipsychotic medications often prescribed for schizophrenia and other psychotic disorders increase the risk of a T2D diagnosis by directly affecting insulin processing and weight gain (Suvisaari et al., 2016).

Anxiety risk also increases with the development of diabetes (Smith et al., 2013). As blood sugar levels spike and fall, it becomes more challenging to control moods. Our minds become less resilient and more sensitive to the daily onslaught of negativity that can be found in every area of life – from home and career to social media and our social lives. We become more sensitive to the fears of life and feel like we need to control every aspect or everything will crumble. Anxiety can be an unrelenting intruder in our thoughts. At first, it may feel as if an uneasiness has taken over our minds, and then we feel the racing heart, sinking feeling in the pit of our stomach, the sweaty skin, and potentially the room spinning, which are symptoms associated with both anxiety and rapid drops in blood sugar.

In addition to the brain, another organ heavily affected by glucose levels is the liver. The liver plays a significant role in glucose processing and regulation by acting as a storage unit to keep the circulating blood sugar levels steady and constant. When there is chronically too much glucose in the bloodstream, the liver develops increased fat deposits, which can interfere with its ability to regulate glucose. *Non-Alcoholic Fatty Liver Disease (NAFLD)* is a common comorbidity with diabetes and the most common liver disorder worldwide (Shea et al., 2021).

Research around the association between NAFLD and mental health is becoming more robust. Researchers have drawn connections between the increased oxidative stress load caused by NAFLD and mental health disorders (Soto-Angona, 2020). Growing evidence supports the connection between NAFLD and mental health conditions such as schizophrenia, bipolar disorder, and depression (Acharya et al., 2021). One study found an especially high prevalence of NAFLD among patients with schizophrenia in a psychiatric hospital setting (Li et al., 2023). This common comorbidity between metabolic diseases like T2D and NAFLD and mental disorders like depression, anxiety, and schizophrenia speaks to the importance of addressing the potential causal underlying factors for all of these disorders, namely poorly managed glucose and insulin levels due to a diet high in processed foods and low in nutrient-dense whole foods.

REFERENCES

Acharya, P., Acharya, C., Thongprayoon, C., Hansrivijit, P., Kanduri, S. R., Kovvuru, K., Medaura, J., Vaitla, P., Garcia Anton, D. F., Mekraksakit, P., Pattharanitima, P., Bathini, T., & Cheungpasitporn, W. (2021). Incidence and characteristics of kidney stones in patients on ketogenic diet: A systematic review and meta-analysis. *Diseases*, 9(2). https://doi.org/10.3390/diseases9020039

Agarwal, U., Mishra, S., Xu, J., Levin, S., Gonzales, J., & Barnard, N. D. (2015). A multicenter randomized controlled trial of a nutrition intervention program in a multiethnic adult population in the corporate setting reduces depression and anxiety and improves quality of life: The GEICO study. *American Journal of Health Promotition*, 29(4), 245–254. https://doi.org/10.4278/ajhp.130218-QUAN-72

Ba, D., Gao, X., Al-Shaar, L., Muscat, J., Chinchilli, V., Beelman, R., & Richie, J. (2021). Mushroom intake and depression: A population-based study using data from the US National Health and Nutrition Examination Survey (NHANES), 2005–2016. *Journal of Affective Disorders*, 294, 686–692. https://doi.org/10.1016/j.jad.2021.07.080

Ba, D., Gao, X., Al-Shaar, L., Muscat, J., Chinchilli, V., Ssentongo, P., Beelman, R., & Richie, J. (2022). Mushroom intake and cognitive performance among US older adults: The National Health and Nutrition Examination Survey, 2011–2014. *British Journal of Nutrition*, 128(11), 2241–2248. https://doi.org/10.1017/S0007114521005195

Bahna, S. L. (2024). History of food allergy and where we are today. *World Allergy Organization Journal*, *17*(5), 100912. https://doi.org/10.1016/j.waojou.2024.100912

Berger, M., Gray, J. A., & Roth, B. L. (2009). The expanded biology of serotonin. *Annual Review of Medicine*, *60*, 355–366. https://doi.org/10.1146/annurev.med.60.042307.110802

Bird, J. A., Crain, M., & Varshney, P. (2015). Food allergen panel testing often results in misdiagnosis of food allergy. *The Journal of Pediatrics*, *166*(1), 97–100.e101. https://doi.org/10.1016/j.jpeds.2014.07.062

Booth, D. A., & Gibson, E. L. (2022). Physics and physiology of obesity: Higher rate of energy input than output. Comment on "The carbohydrate-insulin model: A physiological perspective on the obesity pandemic. *American Journal of Clinical Nutrition*, *115*(2), 590–591. https://doi.org/10.1093/ajcn/nqab382

CDC. (2024). *National diabetes statistics report*. Retrieved August 12, 2024, from https://www.cdc.gov/diabetes/php/data-research/index.html

Cha, S., Bell, L., Shukitt-Hale, B., & Williams, C. (2024). A review of the effects of mushrooms on mood and neurocognitive health across the lifespan. *Neuroscience & Biobehavioral Reviews*, *158*, 105548. https://doi.org/10.1016/j.neubiorev.2024.105548

Da Porto, A., Brosolo, G., Casarsa, V., Bulfone, L., Scandolin, L., Catena, C., & Sechi, L. A. (2021). The pivotal role of oleuropein in the anti-diabetic action of the Mediterranean diet: A concise review. *Pharmaceutics*, *14*(1). https://doi.org/10.3390/pharmaceutics14010040

Dhana, K., James, B. D., Agarwal, P., Aggarwal, N. T., Cherian, L. J., Leurgans, S. E., Barnes, L. L., Bennett, D. A., & Schneider, J. A. (2021). MIND diet, common brain pathologies, and cognition in community-dwelling older adults. *Journal of Alzheimer's Disease*, *83*(2), 683–692. https://doi.org/10.3233/JAD-210107

Dye, L., Lluch, A., & Blundell, J. E. (2000). Macronutrients and mental performance. *Nutrition*, *16*(10), 1021–1034. https://doi.org/10.1016/s0899-9007(00)00450-0

Hager, K., Cudhea, F. P., Wong, J. B., Berkowitz, S. A., Downer, S., Lauren, B. N., & Mozaffarian, D. (2022). Association of national expansion of insurance coverage of medically tailored meals with estimated hospitalizations and health care expenditures in the US. *JAMA Network Open*, *5*(10), e2236898.

Holt, R. I., de Groot, M., & Golden, S. H. (2014). Diabetes and depression. *Current Diabetes Reports*, *14*(6), 491. https://doi.org/10.1007/s11892-014-0491-3

Hornedo-Ortega, R., Cerezo, A. B., de Pablos, R. M., Krisa, S., Richard, T., Garcia-Parrilla, M. C., & Troncoso, A. M. (2018). Phenolic compounds characteristic of the Mediterranean diet in mitigating microglia-mediated neuroinflammation. *Frontiers in Cellular Neuroscience*, *12*, 373. https://doi.org/10.3389/fncel.2018.00373

IFM. (n.d.). *What is functional medicine?* Institute for Functional Medicine. Retrieved September 28, 2024, from https://www.ifm.org/

IFM. (2024). *IFM's elimination diet: Personalized optimized nutrition*. Institute for Functional Medicine. Retrieved August 12, 2024, from https://www.ifm.org/news-insights/heal-the-gut-with-the-ifm-elimination-diet/

Li, X., Gao, Y., Wang, Y., Wang, Y., & Wu, Q. (2023). Prevalence and influence factors for non-alcoholic fatty liver disease in long-term hospitalized patients with schizophrenia: A cross-sectional retrospective study. *Neuropsychiatric Disease and Treatment*, *19*, 379–389. https://doi.org/10.2147/NDT.S398385

Lucas, M., Chocano-Bedoya, P., Shulze, M. B., Mirzaei, F., O'Reilly, É. J., Okereke, O. I., Hu, F. B., Willett, W. C., & Ascherio, A. (2014). Inflammatory dietary pattern and risk of depression among women. *Brain, Behavior, and Immunity*, *36*, 46–53. https://doi.org/10.1016/j.bbi.2013.09.014

Ludwig, D. S., Greco, K. F., Ma, C., & Ebbeling, C. B. (2020). Testing The carbohydrate-insulin model of obesity in a 5-month feeding study: The perils of post-hoc participant exclusions. *European Journal of Clinical Nutrition*, *74*(7), 1109–1112. https://doi.org/10.1038/s41430-020-0658-8

Ma, C., Li, Y., Mei, Z., Yuan, C., Kang, J., Grodstein, F., Ascherio, A., Willett, W., Chan, A., Huttenhower, C., Stampfer, M., & Wang, D. (2023). Association between bowel movement pattern and cognitive function. *Neurology*, *101*(20). https://doi.org/10.1212/WNL.0000000000207849

McCormick, D. (2019). Managing costs and care for chronic idiopathic constipation. *American Journal of Managed Care*, *25*(4), S63–S69. https://www.ncbi.nlm.nih.gov/pubmed/31002490

Merra, G., Noce, A., Marrone, G., Cintoni, M., Tarsitano, M. G., Capacci, A., & De Lorenzo, A. (2020). Influence of Mediterranean diet on human gut microbiota. *Nutrients*, *13*(1). https://doi.org/10.3390/nu13010007

Morris, M. C., Tangney, C. C., Wang, Y., Sacks, F. M., Barnes, L. L., Bennett, D. A., & Aggarwal, N. T. (2015). MIND diet slows cognitive decline with aging. *Alzheimer's Dementia*, *11*(9), 1015–1022. https://doi.org/10.1016/j.jalz.2015.04.011

Mozaffarian, D., Angell, S. Y., Lang, T., & Rivera, J. A. (2018). Role of government policy in nutrition—Barriers to and opportunities for healthier eating. *BMJ, 361*.

Muscaritoli, M. (2021). The impact of nutrients on mental health and well-being: Insights from the literature. *Frontiers in Nutrition, 8*, 656290. https://doi.org/10.3389/fnut.2021.656290

Platero, J. L., Cuerda-Ballester, M., Ibanez, V., Sancho, D., Lopez-Rodriguez, M. M., Drehmer, E., & Orti, J. E. R. (2020). The impact of coconut oil and epigallocatechin gallate on the levels of IL-6, anxiety and disability in multiple sclerosis patients. *Nutrients, 12*(2). https://doi.org/10.3390/nu12020305

Pollan, M. (n.d.). *Psychedelics*. Michael Pollan. https://michaelpollan.com/psychedelics-resources/

Roncero-Ramos, I., Mendiola-Lanao, M., Pérez-Clavijo, M., & Delgado-Andrade, C. (2016). Effect of different cooking methods on nutritional value and antioxidant activity of cultivated mushrooms. *International Journal of Food Sciences and Nutrition, 68*(3), 287–297. https://doi.org/10.1080/0963 7486.2016.1244662

Sakkas, H., Bozidis, P., Touzios, C., Kolios, D., Athanasiou, G., Athanasopoulou, E., Gerou, I., & Gartzonika, C. (2020). Nutritional status and the influence of the vegan diet on the gut Microbiota and human health. *Medicina, 56*(2). https://doi.org/10.3390/medicina56020088

Shea, S., Lionis, C., Kite, C., Atkinson, L., Chaggar, S. S., Randeva, H. S., & Kyrou, I. (2021). Non-alcoholic fatty liver disease (NAFLD) and potential links to depression, anxiety, and chronic stress. *Biomedicines, 9*(11). https://doi.org/10.3390/biomedicines9111697

Smith, K. J., Beland, M., Clyde, M., Gariepy, G., Page, V., Badawi, G., Rabasa-Lhoret, R., & Schmitz, N. (2013). Association of diabetes with anxiety: A systematic review and meta-analysis. *Journal of Psychosomatic Research, 74*(2), 89–99. https://doi.org/10.1016/j.jpsychores.2012.11.013

Soto-Angona, Ó. (2020). Non-alcoholic fatty liver disease (NAFLD) as a neglected metabolic companion of psychiatric disorders: Common pathways and future approaches. *BMC Medicine*. https://doi.org/10.1186/s12916-020-01713-8

Stamets, P. (n.d.). *MushroomReferences.com*. Paul Stamets. https://mushroomreferences.com/

Suvisaari, J., Keinanen, J., Eskelinen, S., & Mantere, O. (2016). Diabetes and schizophrenia. *Current Diabetes Reports, 16*(2), 16. https://doi.org/10.1007/s11892-015-0704-4

Terry, N., & Margolis, K. G. (2017). Serotonergic mechanisms regulating the GI tract: Experimental evidence and therapeutic relevance. *Handbook of Experimental Pharmacology, 239*, 319–342. https://doi.org/10.1007/164_2016_103

Ueno, A., Hamano, T., Enomoto, S., Shirafuji, N., Nagata, M., Kimura, H., Ikawa, M., Yamamura, O., Yamanaka, D., Ito, T., Kimura, Y., Kuriyama, M., & Nakamoto, Y. (2022). Influences of vitamin B(12) supplementation on cognition and homocysteine in patients with vitamin B(12) deficiency and cognitive impairment. *Nutrients, 14*(7). https://doi.org/10.3390/nu14071494

Uffelman, C., Harold, R., Hodson, E., Chan, N., Foti, D., & Campbell, W. (2024). Effects of consuming white button and oyster mushrooms within a healthy Mediterranean-style dietary pattern on changes in subjective indexes of brain health or cognitive function in healthy middle-aged and older adults. *Foods, 13*(15), 2319. https://doi.org/10.3390/foods13152319

Ventriglio, A., Sancassiani, F., Contu, M. P., Latorre, M., Di Salvatore, M., Fornaro, M., & Bhugra, D. (2021). Erratum: Mediterranean diet and its benefits on health and mental health: A literature review. *Clinical Practice and Epidemiology in Mental Health, 17*, 9. https://doi.org/10.2174/1745017902117010009

Venturella, G., Ferraro, V., Cirlincione, F., & Gargano, M. (2021). Medicinal mushrooms: Bioactive compounds, use, and clinical trials. *International Journal of Molecular Sciences, 22*(2), 634. https://doi.org/10.3390/ijms22020634

Wasser, S. (2011). Current findings, future trends, and unsolved problems in studies of medicinal mushrooms. *Applied Microbiology and Biotechnology, 89*(5), 1323–1332. https://doi.org/10.1007/s00253-010-3067-4

Wheeler, S. W., & Dyer, N. L. (2020). A systematic review of psychedelic-assisted psychotherapy for mental health: An evaluation of the current wave of research and suggestions for the future. *Psychology of Consciousness: Theory, Research, and Practice, 7*(3), 279–315. https://doi.org/10.1037/cns0000237

Wuthrich, B. (2014). History of food allergy. *Chemical Immunology and Allergy, 100*, 109–119. https://doi.org/10.1159/000358616

Section IV

Nutrition and Mental Health Challenges

9 Risk Factors That Impact Mental Health

The previous chapters have focused on the interconnected relationship between nutrition and mental health. This chapter discusses other risk factors for mental illness to help you understand how complex and multi-faceted the connections can be between mental health, physical health, and our environment. The risk factors discussed here focus on some basic human challenges: housing, stress, trauma, sleep, and loneliness.

HOUSING AND PSYCHIATRIC CARE

Unfulfilled basic needs like food, clothing, shelter, and community are clear risks for physical and mental illness. For the seriously mentally ill, homelessness has increasingly become a problem. Our city streets are strewn with tent cities that bring conflict and confusion to city and public health managers who are struggling to find kind and ethical solutions to this complicated issue. Many question why the homeless population has been growing and are seeking fair and effective solutions. To better understand this issue, it is important to look at some of the history of mental healthcare.

In early 18th-century Europe, mental hospitals as public institutions became more common and the first hospital with psychiatric care opened in the U.S. (Scult, 2018). These evolved into mental *asylums* whose primary purpose was to care for people suffering from severe mental illness (Comer & Comer, 2024). Born of good intentions, these facilities quickly began to overflow and become overcrowded, leading to tragic living conditions and the inhumane treatment of patients. With little to no recognized medical treatment options, patient symptoms were not treated but managed by isolating this population from greater society. Asylums more closely resembled prisons than medical facilities.

In the U.S., asylum use transitioned to state-run public mental hospitals in the late 18th century. The initial goal of these hospitals was to provide ethical treatment for mentally ill patients. However, between the mid-19th to the mid-20th centuries, state hospitals once again faced overcrowding and understaffing to properly care for patients. Rather than function as a place of treatment and support, institutions became a method to "warehouse" patients keeping them out of the public eye. They maintained a large patient population with a relatively small staff by suppressing mental health physical symptoms and associated behaviors using sedating medication (such as Thorazine), physical restraints, and isolation rooms, resulting in a very poor quality of life for the patients.

Increased public awareness about the often-inhumane treatment in the public mental health hospitals combined with increased access to safer antipsychotic medications started the movement to get patients out of the large state hospitals and into small community facilities (Torrey, 2015). Initially, the effort was focused on placing them in small residential group homes with the goal of eventually integrating them back into their communities rather than separating them from society.

THE EFFECTS OF DEINSTITUTIONALIZATION

U.S. state hospital populations swelled to almost 559,000 patients in 1955, and then fell to 47,000 by 2003 due to changes in mental health treatment funding generally referred to as *deinstitutionalization* (Davis et al., 2012). The federal Community Mental Health Centers Act of 1963 enacted by President John F. Kennedy was intended to transition 50 percent of patients from state hospitals to community-based mental health services including residential programs, nursing

DOI: 10.1201/9781032647647-13

homes, and general hospital psychiatric wards. When President Kennedy was assassinated, the Community Mental Health Centers Act was not fully funded and many patients had little to no mental health treatment services after they were released from the state hospitals (Cor Media, 2017). As a result of this legislation, by 2003 there was a startling 90 percent reduction in state hospital patients with minimal funding to create new treatment programs to provide support for these former state hospital patients.

Additionally, people with severe mental illness were unable to receive newly adopted health insurance options, such as Medicare. This challenge to receive funding to pay for mental health services was compounded by passage of the Omnibus Budget Reconciliation Act of 1981, which cut federal mental health spending by 30 percent and effectively ended federally funded community-based treatment by shifting treatment costs to individual states. These budget cuts removed major support structures designed to help people with serious mental illness transition into their communities and left them without adequate resources to manage their illness and function in society.

Changes in federal government funding meant that many of the planned residential group homes were never built. Forced discharges without continued care and resources overwhelmed patients and their families as increasing numbers of the mentally ill struggling to survive while their mental health symptoms intensified and their ability to cope diminished. This resulted in a rapid rise in incarceration, unemployment, and homelessness for people with mental illness (Gutwinski et al., 2021; Lamb & Weinberger, 2020; Lin et al., 2022; Torrey, 2015).

People diagnosed with schizophrenia and substance use disorders were particularly at risk. The veteran population has long been at high risk of suffering comorbid mental health and substance abuse disorders, which fosters a greater probability of experiencing incarceration, homelessness, and higher unemployment rates; this likelihood increases if the comorbidity is substance abuse and schizophrenia (Lin et al., 2022).

DEINSTITUTIONALIZATION AND INCARCERATION

Deinstitutionalization increases the likelihood of incarceration for people with severe mental health symptoms such as hallucinations and delusions. Authors Lamb and Weinberger (2020) cited deinstitutionalization as one of the leading causes of the recent spike of people with mental illness becoming involved in the criminal justice system. When people with serious mental illness are left without the ability to meet basic needs like food and housing, they become more anxious and distressed, and less able to care for themselves. In this state, with their symptoms highly activated, they are less able to make use of services (such as consistently taking medication and eating at soup kitchens) and often have poor insight into their illness and dysfunction. They are also at higher risk of abusing substances, which makes them more likely to become violent when stressed or confronted and thereby more likely to get arrested.

It is no surprise that our homeless population generally has a poor diet and suffers from nutritional deficiencies as a result. A systematic review of studies of the nutritional status of adults experiencing homelessness estimated that up to two-thirds of participants were overweight or obese and nearly one in five were underweight, with low blood levels of iron, folate, vitamins C, D, and B12 due to a diet higher in dietary fats and alcohol, and lower in fruits and vegetables compared to housed individuals (Huang et al., 2022). Recommendations to improve the nutritional status of this population include additional funding and resources for soup kitchens and other food sources, and the exclusion of certain products (such as sugar-sweetened beverages) from the SNAP national food assistance program (see more on this in Chapter 14) to encourage increased consumption of fruits and vegetables (Cuffey et al., 2016; Seale et al., 2016).

Our society as a whole and local communities in particular continued to be challenged with providing viable solutions to homelessness, especially in times of inflation and lack of affordable housing options. Our current situation where we are increasing our prison population by incarcerating our mental ill is expensive, ineffective, and cruel. Based on the evidence of the powerful impact improved nutrition has on mental health, homeless support programs that emphasize improved nutrition and access to healthier food could go a long way in decreasing psychiatric symptoms in the seriously mentally ill. Access to whole foods and education about the mental health benefits of a healthy diet would increase their ability to stabilize, utilize other resources such as housing and healthcare programs, and create an improved and more independent quality of life.

IMPACT OF STRESS

Stress is an important factor in any discussion of mental health because it affects human functioning in so many ways. Stress can be a response to an immediate threat, like swerving the car to avoid hitting a pedestrian, which is a type of acute stress. It can also be in the form of chronic stress with longer-term stressors that occur over months or years, such as when a child grows up with periods of hunger due to limited access to food or unsafe living conditions due to domestic violence in the household.

Stress can be defined as "conditions where an environmental demand exceeds the natural regulatory capacity of an organism, in particular situations that include unpredictability and uncontrollability" (Koolhaas et al., 2011, p. 1). It includes physical and psychological demands that put pressure on a person and test their current coping abilities. Stress is a natural part of life. We are designed to respond to challenging and stressful situations by maximizing our biochemical, mental, and emotional resources to overcome the challenge. Knowing how our body responds to stress provides important information for understanding the interconnections between stress, eating behavior, nutritional deficiencies, and mental health.

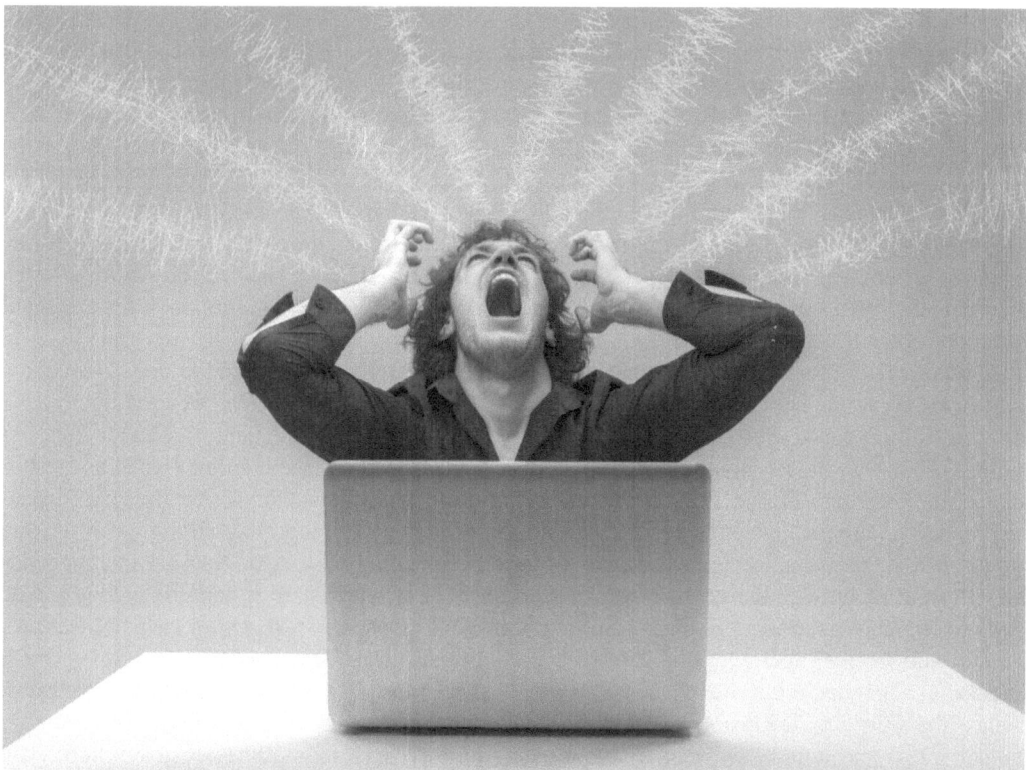

FIGURE 9.1   Stress response. Credit: Giulio_Fornasar (Shutterstock).

POLYVAGAL THEORY

"Fight-or-flight" is a well-known concept about how the body amps up to face a threat in either a physical battle or by running away. Our heart pounds in our ears, our muscles tense and our breath quickens, our senses are on full alert, and our mind is fully focused. All systems are on full alert and ready for action. The term fight-or-flight was coined by American physiologist Walter Cannon in 1915, and has since been expanded to "fight, flight, freeze, or fawn" (Raypole, 2021), which can be understood as:

- Fight: battling against a perceived threat
- Flight: fleeing from danger
- Freeze: becoming immobilized in response to a threat
- Fawn: trying to please an aggressor to avoid conflict or calm a tense situation

The *polyvagal theory* posited by Stephen Porges has added nuance to the concept of fight-flight-freeze-or-fawn to provide a more vivid acknowledgment of what is happening in our body and mind when we respond to stress (Dana, 2018; Porges, 2011). Polyvagal theory focuses on how the nervous system functions during stressful and non-stressful events. The focus is on the autonomic nervous system, which handles communication between your brain and your internal organs, and its two primary branches, the sympathetic and parasympathetic nervous systems (Cleveland Clinic, 2022).

The *sympathetic nervous system (SNS)* is part of the central nervous system (brain and spinal cord) and cues the body to act during a fight-or-flight response. This activation is counterbalanced by the *parasympathetic nervous system (PNS)*, which cues the body to be inactive and quiet through the vagus nerve. This inactive PNS state can occur both when we are feeling relaxed and happy (ventral vagal pathway) and when we are feeling overwhelmed and shut down (dorsal vagal pathway), such as in a freeze or fawn response.

The SNS classic *fight or flight response* is designed to equip us with the physical resources that will help us survive the next five minutes when responding to an immediate threat. Imagine you are walking peacefully in the woods and suddenly you come upon a sabretooth tiger. The alarm bells go off and the SNS is activated. The body prioritizes its resources to survive by either fighting the sabretooth tiger or running as fast as possible. Adrenaline, heart rate, and blood sugar surge to supply plenty of blood, oxygen, and fuel to the muscles and tendons. At the same time the body slows down the core resources designed for long-term survival that are not necessary in a crisis. Digestion, immune system, reproduction, and memory are all inhibited and put on the back burner to be saved for later when you survived this sabretooth tiger encounter and want to sit around a feast and tell your kids about it.

When we shift into the PNS, the ventral vagal nerve cues the body and mind to slow down; muscles relax, breathing slows, and we feel connected, safe, and happy. You survived the tiger attack and are ready to party! Pretty soon your stomach growls and you become interested in food or your groin flushes with blood and you become interested in sex. This phase is often known as "rest & digest" or "feed & breed." In PNS, our core long-term survival systems are active: the gut is digesting food, the immune system is working on repairs to the body, the reproductive system is gearing up to make a baby, and the brain's memory center is reviewing and organizing our memory files so we can think through our next important decisions. The whole system is humming along nicely.

Now let's look at another scenario. If our first active response to a threat with the SNS is unsuccessful and we then feel overwhelmed by the continued threat, a secondary response through the dorsal vagal nerve initiates some alternate stress response behaviors. This is where we experience the freeze or fawn portion of the fight-flight-freeze-fawn stress response. Overwhelm, helplessness, and hopelessness have taken over. If we *freeze*, our body goes heavy and limp, emotions feel numb, facial expression is blank, and the mind checks out, so we are not fully aware of what is happening around us. In the case of your tiger attack, perhaps you ran and climbed a tree, but the tiger is still after you and starting to climb the tree as well. At this point you are exhausted and overwhelmed, consumed by feelings of hopelessness and helplessness. Your mind goes blank, you feel weak, numb, and unable to move, and are incapable of considering your options like shouting, throwing things at the tiger, and climbing higher in the tree. Truly frozen in terror.

Fawning happens when the response is an attempt to calm or distract the aggressor by moving into people-pleasing mode. Smiling, talking softly, encouraging, and soothing are all ways to accomplish the goal of lessening the threatening situation. You might coo at the tiger, "Nice tiger. You are such a nice tiger. You are *so* handsome. You don't *really* want to eat me. Let's be friends." Fawning is common in children struggling to withstand an attack from an abusive parent and can lead to feelings of confusion and shame afterward for behaving in a "weak" manner by being nice to someone who was being mean rather than being "strong" and fighting back.

Recognizing that you are in a state of SNS or PNS activation can be a helpful, more objective way of understanding uncomfortable reactions to stress. We can recognize our experience as a normal response to stressors, and then take steps to counteract our body's stress response with tools like *deep breathing* (Seppälä et al., 2020). Breathing is one of the few functions that is both automatic (happens without our intention) as well as something we can control (e.g., holding our breath). When we slow and deepen our breathing, it cues the body to shift from SNS to PNS, so that we feel calmer and can think more clearly.

Deep breathing is also a powerful tool to help your body to function properly. Remember that when you are in SNS, your body prioritizes essential resources for surviving the immediate crisis, and slows resources equipped for long-term survival, like reproduction, immune system function, and digestion. For example, during a crisis, digestion slows, and the body often experiences a desire to lighten the load and discard any undigested food through vomiting or diarrhea. Nature is not dainty. More of a dump-and-run strategy. This can be an effective short-term strategy to deal with a crisis, but in the long term can be a problem. Deep breathing helps deactivate the SNS cycle and return the body to PNS more quickly, enabling you to relax and repair.

HPA Axis

A secondary arousal process in the body after the SNS is the *hypothalamic-pituitary-adrenal (HPA) axis*. Whereas the SNS signals the body through nerve fibers in the autonomic nervous system, the HPA axis functions by releasing hormones that travel throughout the body in the bloodstream. During a stressful event, the hypothalamus in the brain (the H in HPA) signals the nearby pituitary gland (the P in HPA) to secrete a hormone that signals the adrenal glands that sit on top of the kidneys (the A in HPA) to release stress hormones including adrenaline and cortisol. These hormones travel to organs, skin, and muscles throughout the body and produce an arousal effect.

We all experience stress. It comes from many different sources, both external (e.g., work, finances, relationships) and internal (e.g., illness, inflammation, pain). When a stressor activates the HPA axis, at first, we feel energized and focused. However, frequent activation of the HPA during periods of chronic stress leads to over-stimulation of the adrenal glands as they pump out more and more stress hormones, which can leave us feeling tired and wired.

The HPA axis is designed to provide energy for a short burst of intense activity during acute stress followed by a period of recuperation. This era of chronic stress and frequent activation of the HPA axis can lead to HPA axis dysfunction where a person feels either constantly energized and tense (e.g., anxiety) or feels depleted and lacks energy (e.g., depression), or swings back and forth between these two states (Cleveland Clinic, 2024). Intense periods of HPA axis over-activation can develop into the frightening sensations of a panic attack that can include heart palpitations, shortness of breath, dizziness, nausea, sweating, and fear that you are dying. An over-used and depleted HPA axis system results in depressive symptoms like difficulty getting out of bed, focusing your attention, or staying motivated to accomplish simple tasks.

CHRONIC STRESS

Fight-or-flight is an effective mechanism for short-term, acute stress, but what about chronic stress? According to the Yale Stress Center, *chronic stress* can be defined as "a consistent sense of feeling pressured and overwhelmed over a long period of time" which "slowly drains a person's psychological resources and damages their brains and bodies" (Yale Medicine, 2023, p. 1). Chronic stress can come from many sources, including a dysfunctional relationship or family, poverty, a dissatisfying job, caring for a sick loved one, or moving to a new home. In response to chronic stress, people experience symptoms including aches and pains, insomnia, low energy, and brain fog.

American life currently provides an endless array of challenges and experiences that result in chronic stress. Survey results from *Stress in America* 2022 demonstrated high levels of chronic stress in American adults, where 27 percent of adults reported that "most days they are so stressed they can't function" and 56 percent of young adults ages 18–35 reported that "stress is completely overwhelming most days." Around a quarter of adults often felt their difficulties were piling up so high that they could not overcome them and that they were so stressed they felt numb (American Psychological Association, 2023).

In this era of chronic stress, we are continually in SNS activation, so the body sustains ongoing pressure to decrease function in our long-term survival activities (e.g., digestion, immune function), which can wreak havoc on our health over time. For example, when you are stressed, your body releases fewer digestive enzymes and less stomach acid, and the peristaltic movement slows in your stomach and intestines, so food does not break down as well and sits too long in your digestive tract, which can cause bloating and discomfort. In this case, your ability to digest food properly has decreased and you may have signs of indigestion.

Yet society conditions us to respond to chronic stress by eating to sooth ourselves. When our digestive system is getting signals to slow down while at the same time, we are eating more food, it can be like putting one foot on the gas pedal by eating food and the other foot on the brake pedal by eating when the body is in a state where it cannot properly digest food. Over time, this conflict can damage the digestive tract and lead to issues such as poor absorption of nutrients and chronic pain, both of which can contribute to symptoms of mental illness.

STRESS AND THE GUT

The gut does more than just process food. It also processes information! Recent research discovered the gut has more similarities to the brain than we thought. As discussed in Chapter 5, it turns out the gut has neurons just like the brain that communicate with each other using neurotransmitters like serotonin and dopamine. Therefore, the gut is capable of its own system of "thinking"(dubbed the "second brain") and is processing information about our body and the world. This information is transmitted to our consciousness as a "gut feeling" and is often interpreted as intuition (Foster, 2013). When our gut is impaired due to chronic stress, we lose access to some of that gut information. In addition, having an inflamed gut alters how the gut produces and utilizes neurotransmitters, which can contribute to mental illness (Clapp et al., 2017). New research is focusing on the links between gut health and mental health, and how to build new mental health treatment protocols that include repairing the gut for improved overall functioning.

CHILDHOOD TRAUMA

Some of the most challenging stressors are associated with childhood psychological abuse and trauma. Childhood trauma has lasting effects that ripple into adulthood and increase the risk of a wide range of chronic diseases, both physical and mental. One of the largest studies that demonstrates the negative impact of childhood trauma on lifelong health was the ACE Study.

ACE Study

In 1998, the landmark *Adverse Childhood Experiences Study (ACE Study)* clearly documented the connection between childhood abuse, neglect, and household dysfunction (discussed as childhood exposure) and adult health risk behavior and chronic disease (Felitti et al., 1998). The ACE study included physical exams, confidential surveys, and medical record reviews for over 17,000 patients. ACE survey categories of childhood exposure were divided into two main categories, *abuse* and *household dysfunction*, with seven subcategories. Abuse exposure included: psychological, physical, and sexual abuse. Household dysfunction included: household substance abuse, mental illness, mother treated violently, and criminal behavior.

The results showed a strong graded, dose-response relationship between the amount of exposure to childhood trauma and the number of risk factors for many of the leading causes of death in adults. The higher the number of ACEs or exposures, the higher the risk of lifelong health-risk behaviors and disease. For example, if a person grew up with a parent with mental illness and substance abuse issues who was physically violent in the family (three ACEs), they were at higher risk of developing health-risk behaviors such as alcoholism, drug use, and smoking. They were also at higher risk of suffering from chronic disease, disability, and social problems like cancer, stroke, and depression, as well as early death.

Data on ACEs have continued to be collected since the original research study, with variations to the survey questions and ACE categories, including expansion of the categories in some studies to include physical and emotional neglect and divorce. The Center for Disease Control (CDC) uses the Behavioral Risk Factor Surveillance System (BRFSS) to continue to gather data on ACEs in all 50 states. BRFSS data from 2011 to 2020 estimated that on average 63.9 percent of U.S. adults reported at least one ACE and 17.3 percent reported four or more ACEs. ACEs were highest among people aged 25–34, women, non-Hispanic American Indian or Alaska Native adults, non-Hispanic multiracial adults, adults with less than a high school education, and adults who were unemployed or unable to work (Swedo, 2023).

Armed with this information, the clinical world has been working to understand how to prevent ACEs in children. One important factor that has come to light is the tremendous impact of intergenerational trauma. A parent who struggled with multiple ACEs growing up is at greater risk of PTSD symptoms and of carrying forward some of those harmful practices in their own parenting style. ACE prevention work needs to address and provide support for parents as well as their children to promote resilience and thriving in families (Narayan et al., 2021). Rather than vilify parents for hurting their children, we need to recognize that they too were the victims of trauma and require support and the resources to change so they can interrupt the intergenerational cycle of abuse. When we help the parents, we help the children and thereby support the health and happiness of future adults.

Evidence is also mounting about the negative health impact of the chronic stress associated with childhood trauma. Children who are chronically stressed and worried show unhealthy changes to their neurological, immune, and endocrine system development and function (Boullier & Blair, 2018). Through epigenetic mechanisms, ACEs impact brain development in children by causing a chronic increase in the production of stress hormones like cortisol, which cause them to appraise situations as more dangerous and hopeless and decreases their ability to regulate (calm down) their stress response (Karatsoreos & McEwen, 2013). ACEs also impact gut development by making the gut more hypersensitive and hyper-responsive, which can have several effects including changes in gut motility and digestive juice production; disruptions to the gut microbiome, and thinning of the mucus that lines the walls of the colon (large intestine) which increases the risk of bacterial infection in the gut (IFM, n.d.; Labus et al., 2017). These physiological changes make a child less resilient when faced with new challenges which increases the likelihood they become overly emotional and less able to solve problems and make good decisions.

One way to help improve resilience to trauma and stress is with nutritional support. Research has shown that an improved diet and/or nutritional supplements such as probiotics, multivitamins, and B complex can help the body to heal from traumatic stressors (Kaplan et al., 2015; McKean et al., 2016; Rucklidge et al., 2011; Young et al., 2019). This can be especially helpful to mitigate the impact of ACEs on adult obesity, mental illness, and disease (Kim et al., 2019).

Multiple studies have shown clear connections to ACEs increased risk for both childhood and adult obesity (Felitti et al., 2019; Schroeder et al., 2021). A meta-analysis of ten cross-sectional studies identified a 46 percent increase in the odds of developing adult obesity following exposure to multiple ACEs, with the odds of becoming obese increasing as the number of ACEs increase (Wiss & Brewerton, 2020). The authors also explored possible mechanisms to explain the link between ACEs and obesity. They reported evidence that ACEs increase susceptibility to substance-related disorders and predispose a person to overeating. Increased cravings for hyper-palatable foods suggest food addiction (see more in Chapter 13) as a potential factor that increases the risk of obesity in people with multiple ACEs. Ultimately, there is clear evidence that ACEs can significantly harm the body and lead to long-term mental and physical health problems. Holistic healthcare needs to give greater consideration to the impact of trauma on intertwined physical and mental health conditions to provide more effective care that addresses the impact of trauma.

CASE STUDY: **TRAUMA AND MCAS**

Client Emily was a 32-year-old female who was unemployed due to her health problems. She began treatment with Dr. Champion looking for help with her diagnosis of Mast Cell Activation Syndrome (MCAS). MCAS is a condition with unexplained intense episodes of swelling, shortness of breath, numbness and tingling, trouble thinking (brain fog), hives, diarrhea, and vomiting, and in severe cases, may lead to life-threatening anaphylaxis (a reaction that can cause a person to suffocate). The episodes are due to mast cells (a part of the allergy immune system response) alerting your immune system that there is something harmful in your body, even if there is no clear trigger.

Emily presented with chronic anxiety and depressive episodes which she linked to past trauma, along with bouts of severe digestive issues, including frequent abdominal pain, bloating, alternating constipation, and diarrhea. Her digestive symptoms were initially managed with dietary adjustments and medications to stabilize mast cell activity. However, despite these interventions, Emily's symptoms persisted, severely affecting her quality of life.

Emily's symptoms began in her late 20s and progressively worsened. She underwent numerous medical evaluations, including blood tests, endoscopies, and allergen testing, which led to her diagnosis of MCAS. Conventional treatments provided limited relief, prompting her healthcare team to explore potential underlying causes, including psychological factors. A detailed psychological assessment revealed a history of childhood trauma. When she was young, Emily experienced emotional and physical abuse which she had not fully processed. Her healthcare team hypothesized that unresolved trauma might be exacerbating her MCAS symptoms.

Emily's treatment plan was expanded to include dialectical behavior therapy (DBT) and eye movement desensitization and reprocessing (EMDR) psychotherapies to address her trauma. DBT was chosen for its effectiveness in managing intense emotions and building distress tolerance, while EMDR was selected for its evidence-based success in processing traumatic memories. Over one year, Emily attended weekly DBT sessions, which helped her develop coping skills, emotion regulation, and mindfulness practices. Simultaneously, she underwent EMDR therapy, where she processed traumatic memories in a controlled, supportive environment.

Upon completion of the combined DBT and EMDR therapies, Emily reported a significant remission of her MCAS symptoms. Her abdominal pain, bloating, and irregular bowel movements reduced markedly. Furthermore, her anxiety and depressive symptoms also improved, contributing to an overall better quality of life.

This case illustrates the potential link between trauma and MCAS, suggesting that psychological factors may play a critical role in the manifestation and persistence of MCAS symptoms and other digestive disorders. For patients with MCAS, particularly those with a history of trauma, integrating psychological therapies such as DBT and EMDR may be crucial for symptom remission. Emily's case highlights the importance of an integrative approach that addresses both physiological and psychological aspects of health and encourages healthcare providers to consider comprehensive treatment plans that include mental health support for patients with chronic physical conditions like MCAS.

ACEs AND SLEEP

Exposure to trauma is clearly associated with sleep difficulties, especially interpersonal trauma (Lind et al., 2017). There is evidence of a graded effect of ACEs on sleep, where an increased number of ACE exposures increases the likelihood of trouble falling and staying asleep, and waking up tired after sleeping (Chapman et al., 2011). Sleep may be an important mediator of the relationship between ACEs and other serious health outcomes, such as immune dysfunction and depression, and metabolic syndrome (see the next section under Sleep Deprivation). There may also be a social mechanism to this connection, in that children exposed to ACEs grow up with increased family chaos and household disruption, with less support to learn proper sleep hygiene (Kajeepeta et al., 2015) (see more on sleep hygiene in Chapter 16). Sleep treatment for patients with exposure to ACEs may require more complex treatment strategies to address their trauma history.

SLEEP DEPRIVATION

Healthy sleep is essential for overall health and wellbeing. The amount of sleep required each night differs by individual. The American Academy of Sleep Medicine (AASM) recommends the following number of hours of sleep per night (AASM, 2024):

- 9–12 hours per night for children ages 6–12
- 8–10 hours per night for teens
- 7–9 hours per night for adults

Regularly sleeping more than 9 hours per night may be appropriate for young adults, especially if they are recovering from sleep losses or an illness (Paruthi et al., 2016; Watson et al., 2015).

Unfortunately, knowing how much sleep we need and actually getting that much sleep every night is not always easy. *Sleep deprivation* is defined as going a whole night without sleep (often dubbed by students as "pulling an all-nighter") or having very little sleep for multiple nights. Sleep deprivation includes sleep insufficiency and insomnia. *Sleep insufficiency* describes regularly sleeping for a shorter amount of time than the body requires to stay healthy or consistently maintaining only low-quality sleep due to sleep disruptions. *Insomnia* differs from sleep insufficiency. Both involve sleeping less than the recommended amount, but with sleep insufficiency a person is physically able to sleep but they sleep less because of a busy schedule where they prioritize other activities instead of sleep. With insomnia, time has been allotted to sleep, but they struggle to fall asleep, stay asleep, or both.

IMPACT OF SLEEP DEPRIVATION

In the U.S., chronic sleep deprivation is common. About 20 percent of U.S. adults sleep fewer than five hours each night, which, in the long term, can come with heavy consequences including increased risk of car crashes, workplace error, heart problems, reduced immune function, obesity, a lower quality of life, and an earlier death. "Sleep deprivation is a high interest loan with steep payments in the form of health consequences" (Summer & Singh, 2024). There is clear evidence that chronic sleep deprivation negatively impacts mood and cognitive function with symptoms that include anxiety, depression, irritability, trouble paying attention, impaired logical reasoning, and reduced sex drive.

College students are notorious for functioning under the weight of sleep deprivation. While many can overcome the challenges of chronic poor sleep, others become seriously affected. Many students are not aware of the impact of poor sleep on their struggles in school. Research tells us that sleep deprivation has an adverse effect on cognitive performance, including attention, memory, and decision making (Alhola & Polo-Kantola, 2007). There is a dose response to sleep deprivation in that more nights of insufficient sleep in college students was found to be associated with a greater likelihood of hopelessness, feeling overwhelmed, exhaustion, loneliness, depressed mood, anxiety, anger, a desire to self-harm, and suicidal ideation (Ramsey et al., 2019).

One of the factors that puts students at risk of sleep deprivation is an irregular sleep/wake cycle where they are going to bed and waking up at different times and sleeping for longer and shorter periods during the week. This can be a problem. As you read in the section on sleep hygiene in Chapter 16, working to maintain a regular sleep schedule is one of the tools to improve overall sleep quality if you are struggling with mental health symptoms. Going to bed and waking up around the same time each day, including weekends, has been shown to improve academic performance and to increase happiness and calmness in college students (Phillips et al., 2017; Sano et al., 2017).

MOOD AND SLEEP

In his landmark research on sleep deprivation, especially its impact on decreased REM (rapid eye movement) sleep associated with dreaming, William Dement noted psychological disturbances including anxiety, irritability, and difficulty concentrating, as well as a marked increase in appetite in response to sleep deprivation (Dement, 1960). Anxiety can be both the cause of poor sleep as well as the result of it. Insufficient sleep leads to increased feelings of anxiety, which can then turn into insomnia so that you cannot sleep even when you try (Pires et al., 2016). Similarly, chronically poor sleep increases symptoms of depression, and a diagnosis of a depressive disorder often includes insomnia as one of its key features (Riemann et al., 2020).

DIET AND SLEEP

Interestingly, there is evidence of an association between consumption of ultra-processed foods and insomnia. In a large sample of 38,570 adults, the NutriNet-Santé study found a significant association between greater consumption of ultra-processed foods (defined as Group 4 on the NOVA scale) and chronic insomnia, independent of sociodemographic and mental health status (Duquenne et al., 2024). One possible mechanism is that ultra-processed foods contribute to *nocturnal hypoglycemia*, which is when blood glucose levels fall to low levels while you sleep leading to sleep disturbance due to feeling restless, clammy, and shaky.

There is also mounting evidence that sleep can be improved with sufficient micronutrients. For example, foods high in the amino acid tryptophan, such as found in whole food diets rich in fruits, vegetables, and legumes, are associated with improved sleep. Tryptophan is an essential building block for the neurotransmitter serotonin and the hormone melatonin, both of which are part of the sleep mechanism in the body. So a diet rich in tryptophan, found in foods such as seeds and nuts (sunflower, pumpkin, chia, sesame, cashews, pistachios), eggs, spinach, and poultry helps maintain healthy levels of serotonin and melatonin in the body and improves your chances of getting a good night's rest (Zuraikat et al., 2021).

The timing of our meals also has an impact on the quality of our sleep as well as our blood glucose levels through its impact on the hormone melatonin (see Chapter 15 for more on late night eating.) *Melatonin* has long been connected with maintaining a steady circadian rhythm which heavily impacts our ability to fall and stay asleep. When properly functioning, melatonin peaks during the night and is low during the day. While there is conflicting data about the effect of melatonin on glucose control, there is some evidence that eating a meal late at night while our melatonin levels are high contributes to insulin resistance and hyperglycemia (high blood glucose), especially if you are taking a melatonin supplement at night (Garaulet et al., 2020).

Sleep and Obesity

Conversely, how we sleep has a big impact on our food choices. Sleep deprivation creates changes in our hunger and satiety cues due to hormonal changes, especially increases in ghrelin (our hunger hormone) and decreases in leptin (our satiety hormone) (Chaput et al., 2007). In a study that evaluated over 1000 participants for six days they examined ghrelin and leptin levels for people in the short sleep group (approximately five hours per night) compared to people in the sufficient sleep group (approximately eight hours per night). The short sleep group had a 14.9 percent increase in ghrelin and a 15.5 percent decrease in leptin compared to the sufficient sleep group (Taheri et al., 2004).

We are also more attracted to sweets and calorie dense foods when we have been struggling with chronically poor sleep, which puts us at higher risk for an increased caloric intake and its associated weight gain (see Figure 9.2) (Sejbuk et al., 2022). Sleep deprivation changes brain function associated with food decision making. When we are short on sleep, we have decreased activity in our prefrontal cortex which lowers our executive function and ability to fully recognize the consequences of our actions. We also have increased activity in the our amygdala, which makes us more impulsive and likely to make decisions based on our emotions (Greer et al., 2013; Taheri et al., 2004).

Sleep deprivation also impacts how the body lays down fat. A randomized controlled trial performed by Covassin et al. (2022) examined the impact of sleep loss on 12 healthy, non-obese

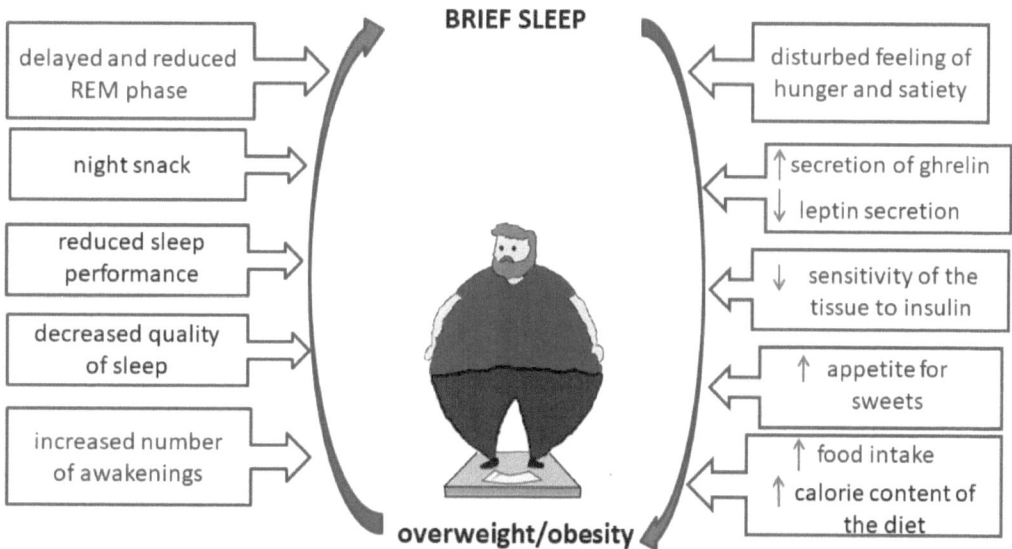

FIGURE 9.2   The relationship between inadequate sleep and calorie intake (Sejbuk et al., 2022).

participants age 19–39 years old. Participants were randomly divided into either the sleep restriction group (opportunity for 4 hours of sleep per night) or the control group (opportunity for 9 hours of sleep per night). Both groups spent 14 days in a research unit with unlimited food available. The results showed that the sleep restricted group consumed more calories and gained weight, particularly abdominal (visceral) fat, in that short period of time. The authors concluded that sleep loss predisposes people to "abdominal visceral obesity" where their BMI is in the obese range and they have excess belly fat, a body composition associated with poorer health and higher rates of inflammation than general adiposity where fatty deposits are more evenly distributed around the body, especially in the butt and thighs.

FOOD FOR THOUGHT: LONELINESS

Loneliness is a risk factor for poor mental health in children, adolescents and adults of all ages (Christiansen et al., 2021; Courtin & Knapp, 2017; Hards et al., 2022; Mann et al., 2022). In research, it is a predictor of depression, generalized anxiety, and suicidal ideation (Beutel et al., 2017). People with depression who perceive that they have a weak social support system tend to have worse outcomes in terms of symptoms, recovery, and social functioning (Wang et al., 2018). This is especially true for young people (ages 18–24) who reported that lack of in-person socializing with friends negatively impacts their mental health (Bala et al., 2024). A survey of over 400 undergraduate college students found that higher levels of loneliness predicted greater anxiety, stress, and depression over time. This study also found that students who reported concerns about loneliness were at greater risk of developing an eating disorder (Richardson et al., 2017).

Eating food when we are lonely is very common. This behavior generally falls under the heading of *Emotional Eating* which will be discussed in Chapter 10. For many, food helps ease the pain of loneliness, at least for a little while. In their book *Intuitive Eating: A Revolutionary Anti-Diet Approach*, authors Tribole and Resch discuss that many people are embarrassed to admit that food is their best friend, and yet that is a common feeling. "Food is love, food is comfort, food is reward, food is a reliable friend. And, sometimes, food becomes your only friend in moments of pain and loneliness" (Tribole & Resch, 2020, p. 179).

Loneliness can contribute to emotional dysregulation (trouble recognizing, understanding, and coping with your feelings) which can exacerbate disordered eating (Southward et al., 2014). A study that surveyed over 500 undergraduate college women found that loneliness increased binge eating. The authors reasoned that supportive connections help buffer difficult emotions, and the lack of that buffering may be associated with greater use of binge eating as a coping mechanism (Mason, 2024).

Loneliness impacts cravings. According to a study that used fMRI imaging, the same part of the brain that becomes active when we are hungry becomes active when we are lonely and can lead to cravings for both social interaction and for food. There is evidence that deprivation of one need (social connection) can lead to increased motivation to pursue other sources of pleasure, and that social isolation increases food consumption, susceptibility to addiction, and general reward-seeking behavior (Tomova et al., 2020). Loneliness is associated with lower fruit and vegetable intake, higher intake of energy-dense, nutrient-poor foods such as sugar-sweetened beverages, and lower overall diet quality (Doan et al., 2022; Hanna et al., 2023).

Eating alone is an important part of the equation. The study of *commensality*, which is the act of eating together, shows evidence that the preparation and sharing of food can improve people's social connections and feelings of overall wellbeing. Many cultures value mealtimes as essential for coming together and connecting with loved ones (Jönsson et al., 2021). Commensality is most beneficial when people feel they have the choice to gather or to eat alone and when it is a convivial gathering where people are friendly, agreeable, and welcoming while eating or feasting together (Bernardi & Visioli, 2024). Older adults can be particularly vulnerable to social isolation and are often better organized around eating regular meals when they eat in the company of others (Björnwall et al., 2024).

REFERENCES

AASM. (2024). *Healthy sleep*. American Academy of Sleep Medicine. https://sleepeducation.org/healthy-sleep/

Alhola, P., & Polo-Kantola, P. (2007). Sleep deprivation: Impact on cognitive performance. *Neuropsychiatric Disease and Treatment, 3*(5), 553–567. https://www.tandfonline.com/doi/full/10.2147/ndt.s12160203

American Psychological Association. (2023). *Stress in American 2022*. https://www.apa.org/news/press/releases/stress/2022/concerned-future-inflation

Bala, J., Newson, J. J., & Thiagarajan, T. C. (2024). Hierarchy of demographic and social determinants of mental health: analysis of cross-sectional survey data from the Global Mind Project. *BMJ Open, 14*(3), e075095.

Bernardi, E., & Visioli, F. (2024). Fostering wellbeing and healthy lifestyles through conviviality and commensality: Underappreciated benefits of the Mediterranean diet. *Nutrition Research, 126*, 46–57. https://doi.org/10.1016/j.nutres.2024.03.007

Beutel, M. E., Klein, E. M., Brähler, E., Reiner, I., Jünger, C., Michal, M., Wiltink, J., Wild, P. S., Münzel, T., & Lackner, K. J. (2017). Loneliness in the general population: Prevalence, determinants and relations to mental health. *BMC Psychiatry, 17*, 1–7.

Björnwall, A., Colombo, P. E., Sydner, Y. M., & Neuman, N. (2024). The impact of eating alone on food intake and everyday eating routines: A cross-sectional study of community-living 70- to 75-year-olds in Sweden. *BMC Public Health, 24*(1), 2214. https://doi.org/10.1186/s12889-024-19560-0

Boullier, M., & Blair, M. (2018). Adverse childhood experiences. *Paediatrics and Child Health, 28*(3), 132–137. https://doi.org/10.1016/j.paed.2017.12.008

Chapman, D. P., Wheaton, A. G., Anda, R. F., Croft, J. B., Edwards, V. J., Liu, Y., Sturgis, S. L., & Perry, G. S. (2011). Adverse childhood experiences and sleep disturbances in adults. *Sleep Medicine, 12*(8), 773–779. https://doi.org/10.1016/j.sleep.2011.03.013

Chaput, J. P., Després, J. P., Bouchard, C., & Tremblay, A. (2007). Short sleep duration is associated with reduced leptin levels and increased adiposity: Results from the Quebec family study. *Obesity, 15*(1), 253–261.

Christiansen, J., Qualter, P., Friis, K., Pedersen, S., Lund, R., Andersen, C., Bekker-Jeppesen, M., & Lasgaard, M. (2021). Associations of loneliness and social isolation with physical and mental health among adolescents and young adults. *Perspectives in Public Health, 141*(4), 226–236. https://doi.org/10.1177/17579139211016077

Clapp, M., Aurora, N., Herrera, L., Bhatia, M., Wilen, E., & Wakefield, S. (2017). Gut microbiota's effect on mental health: The gut–brain axis. *Clinics and Practice, 7*(4), 987. https://www.mdpi.com/2039-7283/7/4/987

Cleveland Clinic. (2022). *Autonomic nervous system*. https://my.clevelandclinic.org/health/body/23273-autonomic-nervous-system

Cleveland Clinic. (2024). *Hypothalamic-pituitary-adrenal (HPA) axis*. Body Systems & Organs. https://my.clevelandclinic.org/health/body/hypothalamic-pituitary-adrenal-hpa-axis

Comer, R. J., & Comer, J. S. (2024). *Psychopathology: Science and practice* (12th ed.). Worth Publishers.

Cor Media. (2017). *Deinstitutionalized*. https://www.youtube.com/watch?v=T3-1AYdfJ64

Courtin, E., & Knapp, M. (2017). Social isolation, loneliness and health in old age: A scoping review. *Health & Social Care in the Community, 25*(3), 799–812. https://doi.org/10.1111/hsc.12311

Covassin, N., Singh, P., McCrady-Spitzer, S. K. St. Louis E. K., Calvin, A. D., Levine, J. A., & Somers, V. K. (2022). Effects of experimental sleep restriction on energy intake, energy expenditure, and visceral obesity. *Journal of the American College of Cardiology, 79*(13), 1254–1265. https://doi.org/10.1016/j.jacc.2022.01.038

Cuffey, J., Beatty, T. K. M., & Harnack, L. (2016). The potential impact of supplemental nutrition assistance program (SNAP) restrictions on expenditures: A systematic review. *Public Health Nutrition, 19*(17), 3216–3231. https://doi.org/10.1017/S1368980015003511

Dana, D. (2018). *A beginner's guide to polyvagal theory*. University of Ottawa Faculty of Medicine.

Davis, L., Fulginiti, A., Kriegel, L., & Brekke, J. S. (2012). Deinstitutionalization? Where have all the people gone? *Current Psychiatry Reports, 14*(3), 259–269. https://doi.org/10.1007/s11920-012-0271-1

Dement, W. (1960). The effect of dream deprivation: The need for a certain amount of dreaming each night is suggested by recent experiments. *Science, 131*(3415), 1705–1707.

Doan, S. N., Xie, B., Zhou, Y., Lei, X., & Reynolds, K. D. (2022). Loneliness and cravings for sugar-sweetened beverages among adolescents. *Pediatric Obesity, 17*(1), e12834. https://doi.org/10.1111/ijpo.12834

Duquenne, P., Capperella, J., Fezeu, L. K., Srour, B., Benasi, G., Hercberg, S., Touvier, M., Andreeva, V. A., & St-Onge, M.-P. (2024). The association between ultra-processed food consumption and chronic insomnia in the NutriNet-Sante Study. *Journal of the Academy of Nutrition and Dietetics*. https://doi.org/10.1016/j.jand.2024.02.015

Felitti, V. J., Anda, R. F., Nordenberg, D., Williamson, D. F., Spitz, A. M., Edwards, V., Koss, M. P., & Marks, J. S. (2019). Reprint of: Relationship of childhood abuse and household dysfunction to many of the leading causes of death in adults: The Adverse Childhood Experiences (ACE) study. *American Journal of Preventive Medicine*, *56*(6), 774–786. https://doi.org/10.1016/j.amepre.2019.04.001

Felitti, V. J. Anda, R. F., Nordenberg, D., Williamson, D. F., Spitz, A. M., Edwards, V., Koss, M. P. P., Marks, J. S. (1998). Relationship of childhood abuse and household dysfunction to many of the leading causes of death in adults: The Adverse Childhood Experiences (ACE) Study. *American Journal of Preventive Medicine*, *14*(4), 245–258. https://doi.org/10.1016/S0749-3797(98)00017-8

Foster, J. A. (2013). Gut feelings: Bacteria and the brain. *Cerebrum*, *2013*, 9.

Garaulet, M., Qian, J., Florez, J. C., Arendt, J., Saxena, R., & Scheer, F. A. J. L. (2020). Melatonin effects on glucose metabolism: Time to unlock the controversy. *Trends in Endocrinology & Metabolism*, *31*(3), 192–204. https://doi.org/10.1016/j.tem.2019.11.011

Greer, S. M., Goldstein, A. N., & Walker, M. P. (2013). The impact of sleep deprivation on food desire in the human brain. *Nature Communications*, *4*(1), 2259. https://doi.org/10.1038/ncomms3259

Gutwinski, S., Schreiter, S., Deutscher, K., & Fazel, S. (2021). The prevalence of mental disorders among homeless people in high-income countries: An updated systematic review and meta-regression analysis. *PLoS Medicine*, *18*(8), e1003750.

Hanna, K., Cross, J., Nicholls, A., & Gallegos, D. (2023). The association between loneliness or social isolation and food and eating behaviours: A scoping review. *Appetite*, *191*, 107051. https://doi.org/10.1016/j.appet.2023.107051

Hards, E., Loades, M. E., Higson-Sweeney, N., Shafran, R., Serafimova, T., Brigden, A., Reynolds, S., Crawley, E., Chatburn, E., Linney, C., McManus, M., & Borwick, C. (2022). Loneliness and mental health in children and adolescents with pre-existing mental health problems: A rapid systematic review. *British Journal of Clinical Psychology*, *61*(2), 313–334. https://doi.org/10.1111/bjc.12331

Huang, C., Foster, H., Paudyal, V., Ward, M., & Lowrie, R. (2022). A systematic review of the nutritional status of adults experiencing homelessness. *Public Health*, *208*, 59–67. https://doi.org/10.1016/j.puhe.2022.04.013

IFM. (n.d.). *The microbiome, stress hormones, & gut function*. The Institute for Functional Medicine. https://www.ifm.org/news-insights/gut-stress-changes-gut-function/

Jönsson, H., Michaud, M., & Neuman, N. (2021). What is commensality? A critical discussion of an expanding research field. *International Journal of Environmental Research and Public Health*, *18*(12), 6235. https://www.mdpi.com/1660-4601/18/12/6235

Kajeepeta, S., Gelaye, B., Jackson, C. L., & Williams, M. A. (2015). Adverse childhood experiences are associated with adult sleep disorders: A systematic review. *Sleep Medicine*, *16*(3), 320–330.

Kaplan, B. J., Rucklidge, J. J., Romijn, A. R., & Dolph, M. (2015). A randomised trial of nutrient supplements to minimise psychological stress after a natural disaster. *Psychiatry Research*, *228*(3), 373–379. https://doi.org/10.1016/j.psychres.2015.05.080

Karatsoreos, I. N., & McEwen, B. S. (2013). Annual research review: The neurobiology and physiology of resilience and adaptation across the life course. *Journal of Child Psychology and Psychiatry*, *54*(4), 337–347. https://doi.org/10.1111/jcpp.12054

Kim, M., Basharat, A., Santosh, R., Mehdi, S. F., Razvi, Z., Yoo, S. K., Lowell, B., Kumar, A., Brima, W., Danoff, A., Dankner, R., Bergman, M., Pavlov, V. A., Yang, H., & Roth, J. (2019). Reuniting overnutrition and undernutrition, macronutrients, and micronutrients. *Diabetes/Metabolism Research and Reviews*, *35*(1), e3072. https://doi.org/10.1002/dmrr.3072

Koolhaas, J. M., Bartolomucci, A., Buwalda, B., de Boer, S. F., Flügge, G., Korte, S. M., Meerlo, P., Murison, R., Olivier, B., Palanza, P., Richter-Levin, G., Sgoifo, A., Steimer, T., Stiedl, O., van Dijk, G., Wöhr, M., & Fuchs, E. (2011). Stress revisited: A critical evaluation of the stress concept. *Neuroscience & Biobehavioral Reviews*, *35*(5), 1291–1301. https://doi.org/10.1016/j.neubiorev.2011.02.003

Labus, J. S., Hollister, E. B., Jacobs, J., Kirbach, K., Oezguen, N., Gupta, A., Acosta, J., Luna, R. A., Aagaard, K., Versalovic, J., Savidge, T., Hsiao, E., Tillisch, K., & Mayer, E. A. (2017). Differences in gut microbial composition correlate with regional brain volumes in irritable bowel syndrome. *Microbiome*, *5*(1), 49. https://doi.org/10.1186/s40168-017-0260-z

Lamb, H. R., & Weinberger, L. E. (2020). Deinstitutionalization and other factors in the criminalization of persons with serious mental illness and how it is being addressed. *CNS Spectrums*, *25*(2), 173–180.

Lin, D., Kim, H., Wada, K., Aboumrad, M., Powell, E., Zwain, G., Benson, C., & Near, A. M. (2022). Unemployment, homelessness, and other societal outcomes in patients with schizophrenia: A real-world retrospective cohort study of the United States Veterans Health Administration database: Societal burden of schizophrenia among US veterans. *BMC Psychiatry*, *22*(1), 458.

Lind, M. J., Baylor, A., Overstreet, C. M., Hawn, S. E., Rybarczyk, B. D., Kendler, K. S., Dick, D. M., & Amstadter, A. B. (2017). Relationships between potentially traumatic events, sleep disturbances, and symptoms of PTSD and alcohol use disorder in a young adult sample. *Sleep Medicine*, *34*, 141–147. https://doi.org/10.1016/j.sleep.2017.02.024

Mann, F., Wang, J., Pearce, E., Ma, R., Schlief, M., Lloyd-Evans, B., Ikhtabi, S., & Johnson, S. (2022). Loneliness and the onset of new mental health problems in the general population. *Social Psychiatry and Psychiatric Epidemiology*, *57*(11), 2161–2178. https://doi.org/10.1007/s00127-022-02261-7

Mason, T. B. (2024). Loneliness as a moderator of the association of affective symptoms and binge eating among college women. *Eating Behaviors*, *54*, 101903. https://doi.org/10.1016/j.eatbeh.2024.101903

McKean, J., Naug, H., Nikbakht, E., Amiet, B., & Colson, N. (2016). Probiotics and subclinical psychological symptoms in healthy participants: A systematic review and meta-analysis. *The Journal of Alternative and Complementary Medicine*, *23*(4), 249–258. https://doi.org/10.1089/acm.2016.0023

Narayan, A. J., Lieberman, A. F., & Masten, A. S. (2021). Intergenerational transmission and prevention of adverse childhood experiences (ACEs). *Clinical Psychology Review*, *85*, 101997. https://doi.org/10.1016/j.cpr.2021.101997

Paruthi, S., Brooks, L. J., D'Ambrosio, C., Hall, W. A., Kotagal, S., Lloyd, R. M., Malow, B. A., Maski, K., Nichols, C., Quan, S. F., Rosen, C. L., Troester, M. M., & Wise, M. S. (2016). Recommended amount of sleep for pediatric populations: A Consensus Statement of the American Academy of Sleep Medicine. *Journal of Clinical Sleep Medicine*, *12*(06), 785–786. https://doi.org/doi:10.5664/jcsm.5866

Phillips, A. J. K., Clerx, W. M., O'Brien, C. S., Sano, A., Barger, L. K., Picard, R. W., Lockley, S. W., Klerman, E. B., & Czeisler, C. A. (2017). Irregular sleep/wake patterns are associated with poorer academic performance and delayed circadian and sleep/wake timing. *Scientific Reports*, *7*(1), 3216. https://doi.org/10.1038/s41598-017-03171-4

Pires, G. N., Bezerra, A. G., Tufik, S., & Andersen, M. L. (2016). Effects of acute sleep deprivation on state anxiety levels: A systematic review and meta-analysis. *Sleep Medicine*, *24*, 109–118. https://doi.org/10.1016/j.sleep.2016.07.019

Porges, S. W. (2011). *The polyvagal theory: Neurophysiological foundations of emotions, attachment, communication, and self-regulation (Norton series on interpersonal neurobiology)*. WW Norton & Company.

Ramsey, T., Athey, A., Ellis, J., Tubbs, A., Turner, R., Killgore, W. D. S., Warlick, C., Alfonso-Miller, P., & Grandner, M. A. (2019). 0901 dose-response relationship between insufficient sleep and mental health symptoms in collegiate student athletes and non-athletes. *Sleep*, *42*(Supplement_1), A362–A362. https://doi.org/10.1093/sleep/zsz067.899

Raypole, C. (2021). *The Beginner's Guide to Trauma Responses*. Healthline. https://www.healthline.com/health/mental-health/fight-flight-freeze-fawn

Richardson, T., Elliott, P., & Roberts, R. (2017). Relationship between loneliness and mental health in students. *Journal of Public Mental Health*, *16*(2), 48–54. https://doi.org/10.1108/JPMH-03-2016-0013

Riemann, D., Krone, L. B., Wulff, K., & Nissen, C. (2020). Sleep, insomnia, and depression. *Neuropsychopharmacology*, *45*(1), 74–89. https://doi.org/10.1038/s41386-019-0411-y

Rucklidge, J., Johnstone, J., Harrison, R., & Boggis, A. (2011). Micronutrients reduce stress and anxiety in adults with attention-deficit/hyperactivity disorder following a 7.1 earthquake. *Psychiatry Research*, *189*(2), 281–287. https://doi.org/10.1016/j.psychres.2011.06.016

Sano, A., Phillips, A., McHill, A., Taylor, S., Barger, L., Czeisler, C., & Picard, R. (2017). 0182 influence of weekly sleep regularity on self-reported wellbeing. *Sleep*, *40*(suppl_1), A67–A68. https://doi.org/10.1093/sleepj/zsx050.181

Schroeder, K., Schuler, B. R., Koblusky, J. M., Sarwer, D. B. (2021). The association between adverse childhood experiences and childhood obesity: a systematic review. *Obesity Reviews*, *22*(7). https://doi.org/10.1111/obr.13204

Scult, M. (2018). How have mental disorders with hallucinations been treated in the past? A brief history of treating mental illnesses. *Massive Science*. https://massivesci.com/articles/drugs-excerpt-past-treatments/

Seale, J. V., Fallaize, R., & Lovegrove, J. A. (2016). Nutrition and the homeless: The underestimated challenge. *Nutrition Research Reviews*, *29*(2), 143–151. https://doi.org/10.1017/S0954422416000068

Sejbuk, M., Mirończuk-Chodakowska, I., & Witkowska, A. M. (2022). Sleep quality: A narrative review on nutrition, stimulants, and physical activity as important factors. *Nutrients*, *14*(9). https://doi.org/10.3390/nu14091912

Seppälä, E., Bradley, C., & Goldstein, M. R. (2020). *Research: Why Breathing Is So Effective at Reducing Stress*. https://hbr.org/2020/09/research-why-breathing-is-so-effective-at-reducing-stress

Southward, M. W., Christensen, K. A., Fettich, K. C., Weissman, J., Berona, J., & Chen, E. Y. (2014). Loneliness mediates the relationship between emotion dysregulation and bulimia nervosa/binge eating disorder psychopathology in a clinical sample. *Eating and Weight Disorders - Studies on Anorexia, Bulimia and Obesity, 19*(4), 509–513. https://doi.org/10.1007/s40519-013-0083-2

Summer, J., & Singh, A. (2024). *Sleep Deprivation: Symptoms, Treatment, & Effects*. Sleep Foundation. https://www.sleepfoundation.org/sleep-deprivation

Swedo, E. A. (2023). Prevalence of adverse childhood experiences among US adults—Behavioral risk factor surveillance system, 2011–2020. *MMWR. Morbidity and Mortality Weekly Report, 72*.

Taheri, S., Lin, L., Austin, D., Young, T., & Mignot, E. (2004). Short sleep duration is associated with reduced leptin, elevated ghrelin, and increased body mass index. *PLoS Medicine, 1*(3), e62.

Tomova, L., Wang, K. L., Thompson, T., Matthews, G. A., Takahashi, A., Tye, K. M., & Saxe, R. (2020). Acute social isolation evokes midbrain craving responses similar to hunger. *Nature Neuroscience, 23*(12), 1597–1605. https://doi.org/10.1038/s41593-020-00742-z

Torrey, E. F. (2015). Deinstitutionalization and the rise of violence. *CNS Spectrums, 20*(3), 207–214.

Tribole, E., & Resch, E. (2020). *Intuitive eating: A revolutionary anti-diet approach*. St. Martin's Essentials.

Wang, J., Mann, F., Lloyd-Evans, B., Ma, R., & Johnson, S. (2018). Associations between loneliness and perceived social support and outcomes of mental health problems: A systematic review. *BMC Psychiatry, 18*(1), 156. https://doi.org/10.1186/s12888-018-1736-5

Watson, N. F., Badr, M. S., Belenky, G., Bliwise, D. L., Buxton, O. M., Buysse, D., Dinges, D. F., Gangwisch, J., Grandner, M. A., Kushida, C., Malhotra, R. K., Martin, J. L., Patel, S. R., Quan, S. F., & Tasali, E. (2015). Recommended amount of sleep for a healthy adult: A joint consensus statement of the American Academy of Sleep Medicine and Sleep Research Society. *Journal of Clinical Sleep Medicine, 11*(06), 591–592. https://doi.org/doi:10.5664/jcsm.4758

Wiss, D. A., & Brewerton, T. D. (2020). Adverse childhood experiences and adult obesity: A systematic review of plausible mechanisms and meta-analysis of cross-sectional studies. *Physiology & Behavior, 223*, 112964.

Yale Medicine. (2023). *Chronic stress*. https://www.yalemedicine.org/conditions/stress-disorder

Young, L. M., Pipingas, A., White, D. J., Gauci, S., & Scholey, A. (2019). A systematic review and meta-analysis of B vitamin supplementation on depressive symptoms, anxiety, and stress: Effects on healthy and 'at-risk' individuals. *Nutrients, 11*(9), 2232. https://www.mdpi.com/2072-6643/11/9/2232

Zuraikat, F. M., Wood, R. A., Barragán, R., & St-Onge, M. P. (2021). Sleep and diet: Mounting evidence of a cyclical relationship. *Annual Review of Nutrition, 41*, 309–332. https://doi.org/10.1146/annurev-nutr-120420-021719

10 Psychosocial Eating

Psychosocial eating involves various factors, both personal and environmental, that impact food choice and eating behavior. Influence on how we engage with food is present from our family beliefs and traditions around food, decades of advertising and rhetoric around what to eat as well as the impact of social influencers that keep us thinking constantly about food and eating. There are innumerable theories about how, when, what, and why we should eat certain foods. Our eating behavior is influenced by factors such our emotional state, cultural rules we learned about eating, information (and misinformation) we have learned about food, and food prices.

EMOTIONAL EATING

Emotional eating is all too familiar for most of us. During times of stress, we eat for reasons other than hunger, most notably to soothe difficult feelings. Camped in front of the television, happily left alone in our pajamas with our quart of ice cream, we find a little tranquility and a break from our worries. *Emotional eating* is defined as eating in response to emotions, positive or negative, to change those emotions (Albers, 2013a). It can affect our motivation to eat, our food choices, where and with whom we eat, and the speed at which we eat (Frayn & Knäuper, 2017; Taitz & Safer, 2012). Emotional eating is often an attempt to self-soothe or to experience momentary distraction from difficult emotions, and has been associated with cravings for foods high in fats and sugars, binge eating, weight gain, and obesity (Ruiz et al., 2023).

Emotional eating takes many forms, such as snacking when we are not hungry due to boredom or agitation. It also includes continuing to eat after we are full, so much so, that we end up feeling uncomfortably full at the end of the meal, even though we may still not feel fully satiated. Emotional eating often includes eating quickly, taking the next bite before we have finished chewing, tasting, or swallowing the previous bite, and is associated with boosting positive feelings and/or numbing or soothing negative feelings (Albers, 2013a; Taitz & Safer, 2012). The drive for momentary relief from uncomfortable feelings is so strong that we continue to eat even though we recognize we may experience regret or discomfort later due to indigestion or guilt about weight gain.

To gain a clearer understanding of the emotions and behaviors associated with emotional eating, Stanford University School of Medicine professors Arnow, Kenardy, and Agras developed the *Emotional Eating Scale (EES)* (Arnow et al., 1995). The EES helps quantify specific negative emotional states (anger/frustration, depression, anxiety) and overeating behaviors (primarily focused on binge eating). The EES was updated in 2003 as the Emotional Eating Scale-II (EES-II) (Ruiz et al., 2023).

Researchers have used the EES to study treatment for binge eating, to illuminate which treatment areas make the most difference. Binge eating episodes are often the result of people feeling out of control and helpless to stop emotional eating once they have started. Treatment for binge eating that includes mindfulness and acceptance skill building (e.g., acceptance and commitment therapy) helps reduce emotional eating and binge episodes. Tools such as mindful eating and deep breathing teach emotional eaters strategies for coping with and soothing negative emotions without overeating (Frayn & Knäuper, 2017).

TIMES OF CHANGE

Life transitions are often stressful, including both "positive" transitions like moving to a new home or having a child, and "negative" transitions like death of a loved one or a natural disaster. The increased stress of these transitions often results in changes to our eating behavior. Starting college

DOI: 10.1201/9781032647647-14

is one of those life transitions that brings with it a higher risk for emotional eating. Many first-year college students worry about gaining weight, jokingly referred to as the *Freshman Fifteen*. The combination of high stress and more freedom in food choices can result in significant changes in eating habits which can lead to weight gain. A study of first-year college women noted that most of the participants who gained weight (which in reality averaged closer to 4 pounds rather than 15 pounds) had ineffective coping strategies for managing these life changes, and would benefit from learning about emotional eating, stress management, and relaxation training during college orientation (Vella-Zarb & Elgar, 2009; Wilson et al., 2015).

Loneliness and Emotional Eating

It can be important to differentiate between biological or hedonic hunger and heart or emotional hunger to improve our food decision making. Loneliness is often a trigger for emotional hunger. When we eat because we feel lonely, we are trying to fill a need and satisfy a desire with food. Food can often provide comfort in the short term, distract from the pain, or even make you feel numb, but food will not solve the problem. Eventually, you will need to deal with the source of the emotion.

Author Martha Peaslee Levine (2012) reminds us that loneliness serves a purpose. In the same way that physical pain cues the body to take action to protect itself from injury, social pain helps protect us from the danger of getting used to being isolated. We are social beings with an inborn need for social bonds to feel safe. Feelings of loneliness remind us that we need to take action to create more social connections in our lives.

Increased awareness of how loneliness triggers emotional eating can help you ask yourself a few key questions. "Is this hedonic hunger, where the body wants to fill a nutritional need, or is it coming more from a place of emotional discomfort?" If it is a time when you would typically eat, then you are probably at least a little physically hungry, and it can be important to eat even if there is also an emotional aspect to why you are reaching for food so that you do not amplify your emotions by also being physically hungry. If you are not hungry, try to be curious about what you are thinking or feeling without judgement, even if you decide to eat (Matz et al., 2024). Remember, making peace with food is not about control, so you should feel permission to eat without criticism. As much as possible, maintain compassion, curiosity, and kindness while you gently explore the ways that you take care of your needs, including reaching for food.

If you are reaching for food to manage uncomfortable feelings, ask yourself what else you might be hungry for in addition to food. Are you lonely and hungry for connection with another? What might you be thinking or feeling if you do not eat right now? What else might you need? Do you need a hug, some intellectual stimulation, or something else? If you end up using food to cope, use it as information to notice that something is going on in your life that needs attention.

Mindfulness

Mindfulness is an important stress management skill and is very helpful in decreasing emotional eating. Based on Buddhist practices, mindfulness has gained tremendous popularity in psychotherapy to teach clients how to cope better with complex life events (see Chapter 16 for more details about mindfulness). The goal is to stay focused on the present moment, not the past or the future, just noticing different sensations and thoughts while maintaining an attitude of nonjudgment (i.e., nothing is good or bad, it just is). It involves being in the moment, focusing only on your current experience, both internal (e.g., stomach rumbling, tight neck) and external (e.g., a bird chirping, the air conditioning fan blowing). It sounds so simple, yet it is so hard to do consistently! Especially when a piece of cake is readily available, and we are busily running through our mental gymnastics of things that need to get done or ruminating about past events. Our busy brains have a hard time slowing down and just staying focused on what we feel right now – sights, sounds, sensations – without reference to the past or future and without judgment, just acceptance that we are feeling what we are feeling in this moment. For example, take a moment to look around the room and notice the different colors. Do you see anything blue, green, or red? Just notice, without judgment about how the room should be different or what you should be doing. Stay focused on being aware of colors. Notice how everything slows down as you gently survey the room simply paying attention to the colors.

In her book, *Mindful Eating 101: A Guide to Healthy Eating in College and Beyond*, psychologist Susan Albers, PsyD, discusses some of the behaviors associated with mindless eating (Albers, 2013b). Mindless eating can include: overeating to the point of feeling too full; skipping meals or eating on the run due to feeling too busy; obsessing about food or body image; and eating because you are under pressure (e.g., eating a bag of potato chips while rushing to finish writing a paper).

After periods of mindless eating, many students become concerned about weight gain and turn to dieting. Dieting often begins a cycle of food deprivation, craving "forbidden foods," and then overeating when they finally give in to the cravings and eat the forbidden foods. Dieting teaches students to stop listening to their body's cues around food, restrict their nutrition, and base their self-worth on the shape of their body. In contrast, mindful eaters consciously think about what they eat with awareness, flexibility, and a nonjudgemental attitude. They stay attentive to the physical, social, and emotional thoughts and sensations associated with their eating, and include a broad variety of foods, including forbidden foods. Eating mindfully helps ensure a person consumes adequate nutrition and improves self-esteem and overall physical and mental health (Albers, 2013a).

It is important to remember that emotional eating can serve an important function. For many people, emotional eating is a way of improving feelings of safety. They eat as a response to feeling stressed and uncomfortable. Therefore, telling someone to just stop emotional eating without offering other means of managing distress is unlikely to be successful. It is only after we learn other coping strategies like seeking support, exercise, and mindfulness that we have the coping skills necessary to let go of the less effective coping strategy of emotional eating (Murphy, 2024).

Of Note . . . A MINDFULNESS MOMENT

Take a moment to try this simple mindfulness exercise. Find a relaxed comfortable position sitting upright in a chair. Take three slow gentle breaths, slowly in and slowly out, fully emptying your lungs with each exhale. If it is comfortable, softly look down or close your eyes. Let yourself relax and become curious about your body. Notice any sensations, such as where your body is touching the chair and how your feet are resting on the floor. Notice and relax any areas of tightness or tension in your body. Just breathe and let go. No judgment, no effort, just allowing. Tune into your breath. Feel the natural flow of breath in and out. You do not need to change your breath, not long, not short, just natural. Notice where you feel your breath in your body. Is it in the rise and fall of your chest or belly? Or do you feel it more in your throat or nostrils? See if you can feel the sensations of breath, one breath at a time. When one breath ends, the next breath begins. As you do this, you might notice that your mind may start to wander. You may start thinking about other things. If this happens, it is not a problem. It is very natural. Just notice that your mind has wandered and softly say to yourself "thinking" or "wandering" in your head. And then gently redirect your attention back to your breathing. After a few minutes, once again notice your body, your whole body, seated here. Let yourself relax even more deeply and then offer yourself some appreciation for doing this practice today as you slowly open your eyes.

A lack of mindfulness is a common component of emotional eating. We love to multitask! When we eat food, it often happens at the same time we are watching television, reading social media, driving, or working. Did you ever notice how many cup holders are in new cars compared to old cars with no cup holders? How did people drive without a thermos full of their favorite hot beverage?

When we give only part of our attention to what we eat, we tend to eat more than planned and still do not feel satiated afterward. Eating while distracted can cause us to feel less pleasure from the experience and can leave us searching for more pleasure later. A study by Murphy et al. (2024) found that those who ate a meal while distracted watching a video or playing a video game reported lower enjoyment and satisfaction with their meal, which was associated with more snacking behavior later in the day and an increased drive to find further gratification, such as checking social media. The lack of satisfaction from the meal contributed to unconsciously seeking out other forms of pleasure to compensate for their unmet expectation of pleasure from the meal. In this way, overconsumption can be seen as the simple human desire to experience a certain amount of pleasure that remains just out of reach because of our constant distractions keeping us from really deeply enjoying our individual simple daily experiences such as eating a meal.

Eating while distracted also bypasses some important cues to our body that it is time to digest food. Chapter 5 introduces us to the fact that looking at and smelling our food activates our digestive juices, including increasing salivation, stomach acid, and digestive enzymes, which improve digestion. Mindfulness helps us slow down and pay attention to how the food feels in our mouth, throat, and stomach, which can help remind us to chew our food thoroughly before we swallow. Slowing down allows us to taste and savor the flavors in foods, and to appreciate the more complex and interesting flavors found in higher-quality foods and layered flavors. It also gives us time to notice when we are starting to feel comfortably full, which helps us stop eating before we continue into overeating where we will feel overfull.

When we increase the amount of time we spend chewing our food, the increased release of digestive juices helps us do a much better job digesting our food. This improved digestion decreases stomach upset and indigestion and increases nutrient absorption. As discussed in Chapter 4, micronutrient deficiencies can make us feel unwell. For example, low magnesium levels in the body contribute to feelings of nervousness and tension. When we support our body to better utilize all of the nutrients we consume in food through improved nutrient absorption, we provide what the body needs to run smoothly. This contributes to feeling more satisfied, more comfortable, and supports a better mood.

MINDFUL EATING

Mindful eating "involves cultivating a combination of 'inner wisdom' (awareness of how our body and mind are responding), and 'outer wisdom' (engaging nutrition information and recommendations to meet your own needs and preferences)" (Kristeller, 2024). It includes tuning into your natural physical hunger signals, really tasting your food, learning to know when you have had enough, and choosing foods for both satisfaction and health. Many treatment programs for disordered eating and weight management include mindful eating as an important component of the treatment (Tapper, 2022).

In her book *Eat.Q.: Unlock the Weight-loss Power of Emotional Intelligence*, Susan Albers discusses the importance of mindful eating and its relationship to emotional intelligence, which is the ability to perceive, use, understand, and manage emotions. Albers encourages readers to explore their current mindfulness and eating habits from the perspective of emotional intelligence by asking themselves key questions (Albers, 2013a, pp. 27–28) such as:

- Can I have an uncomfortable feeling and just notice it without doing anything about it?
- Can I identify specific feelings that typically prompt me to eat, such as boredom or stress?
- Can I distinguish between emotional and physical hunger?

Emotional eating is a common challenge for many people as a fast way to feel better when feeling distressed. Food surrounds us, so the temptation is never-ending. We end up paying the price for how and what we eat when we are feeling upset with later feelings of sadness, guilt, overwhelm, and hopelessness. This cycle becomes compounded by the nature of the foods we tend to choose during emotional eating, such as cookies and soda since these foods have properties that make us want to eat more and more of them (see Chapter 13) which can lead to having a stomachache, eventual sluggishness or feeling overfull in the moment with the potential for long-term weight gain.

CULTURAL EATING

How and why we eat happens within a social context. In addition to our physiological response to food, family and cultural values and environments significantly impact food choices. Our early experiences train the palate, meaning specific foods become connected to meanings and feelings from past events that can emotionally charge food and influence what foods we associate with a pleasurable eating experience. Mom's lasagna, with its positive memories of enjoyable family meals, is associated with comfort and nurturing that I then extend to my next eating experience when I order lasagna in a restaurant. Not only flavors and textures are part of this decision process, but also whether we associate those foods with health or illness, celebration or mourning, pleasure or discomfort.

FAMILY AND FOOD

Food can be a source of internal conflict. In families, purchasing and preparing food has traditionally been a woman-related activity. At the same time, there is tremendous societal pressure on women to be slender and attractive, resulting in pressure to think and interact with food a great deal while denying oneself the pleasure of enjoying all of the food. Women often use food as a measure of self-control, which increases the pressure and guilt associated with food choices. Teenage girls often are heavily influenced by peer pressure to avoid certain foods or to avoid eating altogether in an effort to be thin and feel harshly judged by their peers and themselves when they do eat. This intense focus on eating behavior as a measure of self-control extending to a perception of self-worth not only interferes with enjoying and finding satisfaction with eating but can become harmful in people with eating disorders (Ogden, 2010).

Food can communicate affection, family status, and desired behavior. Preferential treatment of a family member is given by choosing who gets the tastiest piece of meat or the last piece of cake. Sweet foods are often used to pacify children and are frequently viewed as signs of affection and reward. "Looks like you had a rough day. Here is a cookie to help you feel better." Typical is the agony suffered by parents who struggle with wanting to provide their children with healthy foods but also desiring family harmony in the face of child preferences for sweet and processed foods. Sugary foods surround children at every turn (school parties, sporting events, snack foods, stores) and are heavily marketed on television and in social media so that children are primed to always be on the lookout for sweet ultra-processed foods. Sometimes processed foods are the only real options for families (see food deserts in Chapter 14). The ability to afford enough high-quality food is often a core concern in families. Families with food insecurity often struggle with feelings of guilt and hopelessness around food options and family wellbeing.

For many families, the dinner table is the only place where the family gathers and shares experiences of the day. While this experience can span from pleasurable to torturous depending on the family dynamics, research suggests that overall having a higher frequency of family meals helps decrease the rate of eating problems (Neumark-Sztainer et al., 2008). For some families, mealtime has become a battleground of wills. Parents determined to have their child eat healthy foods often pressure, coerce, threaten, and bribe their child using the oft-repeated phrase "eat your vegetables." This pressure around food can become a problem, especially if the child is a picky eater, and can contribute to the child growing up with difficult feelings around food. In a fascinating study of 112 parent/child pairs, the researchers found that parents who attempted greater control of their child's diet reported that their child had higher intakes of snack foods and higher levels of body dissatisfaction. In comparison, the parents who focused on modeling healthy eating behavior rather than attempting to control what their child ate resulted in improvements in the healthfulness of their child's diet (Brown & Ogden, 2004).

Eating in College

College provides its own unique environment for food. Many students struggle with healthy eating at college for a variety of reasons. Factors that contribute to unhealthy eating include: alcohol use, cost, lack of time, and lack of healthy options on campus (Lacaille et al., 2011). Often all-you-can-eat buffets in dining halls tend to include many unhealthy food options, as well as the belief that you should eat more to "get your money's worth." Dorm rooms generally allow limited cooking and food storage compared to off-campus housing, which limits opportunities to cook for themselves and to make whole food choices at the grocery store. However, when students are feeling pressured by a high workload with limited free time, even if they had cooking facilities, they are more likely to opt for fast food and processed convenience foods to save time and energy.

In surveys of students about food choice and food purchasing behaviors, students defined healthy eating as consuming plenty of whole fruits, vegetables, and milk, and regularly eating a wide variety of foods that are high in vitamins and minerals. Positive influences on healthy eating include friends and family who eat healthy, and university support to decrease prices and increase availability of fruits and vegetables on campus. Cost and convenience of foods are some of the greatest determinants of food choice on college campuses (Tam et al., 2017). Universities can improve student nutrition by providing information about healthy food choice opportunities on campus and

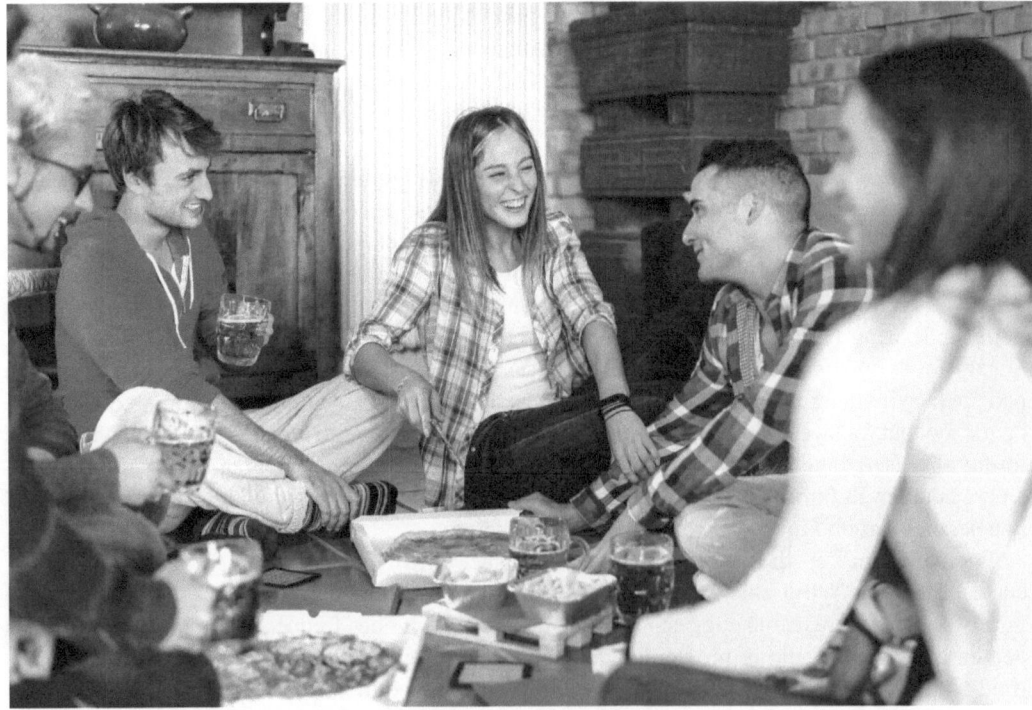

FIGURE 10.1   College eating. Credit: View Apart (Shutterstock).

making healthy foods convenient, such as providing vending machines with more healthy products (Deliens et al., 2014).

SOCIAL EATING

Communal eating where we eat a meal in the company of others, whether in feasts or everyday meals with family and friends, is a universal human experience. In a survey of 2000 adults, the data showed that people who regularly ate socially were more likely to have higher self-esteem, to feel they had a supportive social network, and believe that having a meal together is an important way of making or reinforcing friendships, with an emphasis on the importance of evening meals (Dunbar, 2017).

Not surprisingly, we eat differently in a group than we do when we are alone, where our dietary choices tend to converge with our close social connections. Eating norms are set by shared cultural expectations and environmental cues which can be a source of cultural cohesion and identity, making us feel more connected to each other. All cultures seem to value some forms of social eating (Herman et al., 2019).

Whether we follow the norms can depend on our immediate concerns about social acceptance, which might be higher during meals with added importance, such as a meal with work colleagues or clients. It might also be influenced by conflicting personal norms, such as following a vegetarian diet for health benefits or personal conviction when you are alone, which can be challenging in a social environment where there is pressure to meat (Higgs, 2015; Higgs & Thomas, 2016). When we dine with healthy eaters, we are more likely to make healthier food choices, which can be important if we are making dietary changes and experimenting with new eating behaviors (Mötteli et al., 2017).

CASE STUDY: A CLIENT FAR FROM HOME

Dr. Champion works with clients from many cultural backgrounds. One client came to her for help with a recent polycystic ovary syndrome (PCOS) diagnosis. Dr. Champion listened to her client's concerns about weight gain, blood sugar instability, and high cholesterol – a common trifecta of PCOS. When clients present with these three symptoms, Dr. Champion will often use a reduced carbohydrate diet to help rebalance the blood sugar and reduce unwanted weight. While no two clients ever receive exactly the same treatment, starting with a reduced carbohydrate diet is often effective for managing PCOS symptoms. The difference with this case was that this young woman was an Indian immigrant living in the U.S.

Indian cultural eating typically involves high carbohydrate, moderate fat, and low protein intake, especially if the individual is vegetarian or vegan. This client was fine eating meat and did not restrict her animal protein intake other than avoiding beef. As Dr. Champion and the client proceeded to work together, Dr. Champion noticed that the client's emotional status seemed to be declining. When asked, the client reported that this new way of eating made her feel less connected to her home country and her mom, which was difficult to maintain. She longed for the foods she enjoyed growing up because it was a way for her to celebrate her culture and hold on to her mom, especially while in a foreign country.

Instead of throwing away all the hard work that the client had done so far, Dr. Champion and the client created a plan to incorporate a cultural meal for her lunchtime and keep the rest of her meals with reduced carbohydrates. At the next follow-up session, the client reported feeling more energized about her plan and willing to make other changes. Restoring her emotional wellbeing through consuming cultural foods made all the difference. The client reported that she now felt committed to making other changes and felt more connected with her culture and community.

It is important to take into consideration a person's cultural background. Our DNA and upbringing help shape our dietary requirements. When we are upset, we may find ourselves craving something that was a favorite from our youth which we often used to comfort ourselves. Those cultural foods remind us, at a deeper level, of who we are and where we came from. Being able to incorporate those foods into our nutrition plan can help not only our physical wellbeing but also our emotional wellbeing. Comfort foods can be an important part of any food plan, as long as they are eaten in a quantity and manner that matches our body's needs. Chapter 15 discusses strategies for making healthy food choices, as well as some of the common pitfalls to be aware of.

FOOD RESEARCH

People eat food for many reasons. Some eating is for flavor, pleasure, and positive feelings. Other eating is for health and basic physiological needs. Food industry corporate interests have invested huge money to influence our thinking about both of these reasons to eat food.

BLISS POINT

Have you ever thought about what makes some foods taste really good, while other food just fills you up? Not all of that food pleasure can be attributed to Mother Nature. Some of it is carefully crafted and very much by design. When we consider the key drivers of our eating choices, we must include the influence of the processed food industry to guide our food decisions.

In his groundbreaking book *Salt, sugar, fat: How the food giants hooked us*, Michael Moss reports how the food industry deliberately designed their processed foods to create cravings to increase consumption. As a Pulitzer Prize-winning journalist, Moss uncovered confidential industry records that described food manufacturers using intricate charts and statistical analyses to create what industry insiders called the *bliss point*. The bliss point is the "precise amount of sugar or fat or salt that will send consumers over the moon." Moss met with different food scientists who walked him through the process of engineering a new soda, designing a new snack with just the right amount of fat-laden meat and cheese, and manipulating different levels of fat and salt to create new potato chip options. Each of these required remarkable efforts by company officials to "reduce the ideal snack to a mathematical equation of taste and convenience" (Moss, 2013, pp. xxv–xxvi).

According to Moss, food scientists have been altering the physical shape and structure of salt, sugar, and fat to boost their power to elicit a pleasurable response. For example, they have been pulverizing salt into a fine powder so that it hits the taste buds faster and harder and improves the "flavor burst." With sugar, they crystallized the sweetest component of simple sugar, fructose, to make foods more alluring, and create enhancers that "amplify the sweetness of sugar to two hundred times its natural strength." If they are marketing a food product as a healthier option, such as making it low fat, they quietly add more sugar and salt to compensate for the loss of fat to keep people hooked.

CORPORATE INTERESTS

Our understanding of what constitutes a healthy diet has also been heavily influenced by the food manufacturing industry. Diet recommendations are based on food research and information published by nutrition experts. This broad and changing field is full of often conflicting information about how to make good food choices, leaving many people feeling confused and overwhelmed. At least some of that confusion is not an accident. The food industry has been very active in funding nutrition research and shaping nutrition education and policy.

The U.S. food industry spends a lot of money on food research. In the last decade, food research expenditures reached an annual expense of around $5 billion, especially research focused on processed food products, which now make up more than half of the food products exported from the U.S. to other countries (Unnevehr, 2017). This funding raises concerns that the end-product of that research is biased by a financial conflict of interest for the authors, who are under pressure to demonstrate results that support food industry interests. Research comparing food-related articles funded by food manufacturers versus other funding sources found they were much more likely to result in findings that were favorable to the food industry (Mozaffarian, 2017; Sacks et al., 2020). Clearly, this difference skews the results of any food-related body of research.

Sometimes the argument is as subtle as whether or not there is sufficient evidence to call out a problem with a specific food type. A specific example of this bias was found in a study that analyzed research on the impact of sugar-sweetened beverages (SSBs) on body weight. The study found that industry-funded studies were more likely to find there was only weak evidence that SSBs contribute to weight gain, whereas non-industry-funded research found the evidence to be much stronger (Massougbodji et al., 2014). These findings raise questions about how best to manage food industry involvement in research that assesses the health profiles of mass-produced foods (Devenyns, 2020).

In a 2020 article in *The BMJ.*, Gyorgy Scrinis discussed the ways that food corporations have exploited nutrition science to defend and promote the perceived health benefits of their ultra-processed products (Scrinis, 2020). For example, in 2015, the *New York Times* (*NYT*) published a story reporting that Coca-Cola, the world's largest producer of SSBs, had begun promoting the idea that obesity was primarily due to a lack of exercise and only minimally influenced by nutrition by funding research to appear in medical journals, at conferences, and through social media (O'Connor, 2015). This industry influence was described in an analysis of research studies on the impact of SSB on obesity. The researchers found that studies where the authors had financial conflicts of interest (i.e., received funds from soda manufacturers for their research) were five times more likely to present a conclusion that there was no positive association between SSB consumption and obesity (Bes-Rastrollo et al., 2013). This was in contrast to research not funded by the food industry, which reported a clear connection between drinking SSBs and obesity.

According to the *NYT* article, health experts felt this message was misleading and an effort to deflect criticism about the role SSBs have played in the rapid rise of obesity and type 2 diabetes. Since that article, studies performed in multiple countries have demonstrated that a higher intake of ultra-processed foods, including SSBs, is clearly a driving factor for obesity after controlling for confounding variables such as exercise (Askari et al., 2020; Canella et al., 2014; Machado et al., 2020; Nardocci et al., 2019; Neri et al., 2022; Rauber et al., 2020).

Scrinis also argued that food manufacturing corporations use nutritionism to distort how we understand the properties of food to market ultra-processed foods. Nutritionism, as discussed in Chapter 4, reduces foods to the basic macronutrient, micronutrient, or ingredient, often with disregard for the complex interplay between the nutrients within that food item. Oranges become a source of vitamin C and celery becomes a source of fiber. Scrinis feels this approach has obscured the broader determinants of dietary health by intensely focusing on a single aspect of a food product (e.g., one micronutrient such as vitamin D or one macronutrient such as fat). This focus helps draw attention away from the impact of other ingredients like food additives (such as synthetic flavors, emulsifiers, hydrogenated oils, and soy protein isolates) and food processing techniques (pulverizing, high heat, chemical extractors) used to manufacture ultra-processed foods that have a less recognized negative impact on health (Scrinis, 2020).

Directly funding research is not the full picture. Food companies have also made large donations to academic institutions without transparency about how the funds were to be used. For example, one study found that from 2000 to 2016, of the $366 million in food industry donations, universities received about 68 percent of the total dollars given. About half of the donations did not include a reason for the donation, which raises concerns that the funds were used to influence research and publications produced by university faculty so the results were favorable to food industry interests (Bragg et al., 2020). "The longstanding influence of food industry funding on nutrition research, researchers, and professional societies threatens the credibility of nutrition science" (Nestle, 2016, p. 1). It is important to take steps to ensure that industry-funded research promotes public health, not the marketing claims of food products.

CHILDREN AND OBESITY

Misleading the public not only causes confusion, it also drains our resources by directing us to waste our efforts on ineffective treatments, such as obesity interventions that are not working, especially for children with obesity. A Cochrane systematic review of randomized controlled trials found that current health interventions for children that focus on eating less and exercising more have little to no effect on preventing weight gain and obesity in children and adolescents (Spiga, Davies, et al., 2024; Spiga, Tomlinson, et al., 2024). We need to think about obesity with a broader lens beyond just changing the eating and exercise behavior of the child.

The WHO Commission on Ending Childhood Obesity acknowledges that we need to focus not only on the individual who is struggling with obesity but also on those around them and the environment in which they live. Caregivers and communities create cultural norms related to eating, movement, sleep, body image, and health knowledge, all of which heavily impact the risk of childhood obesity. The WHO report states, "The evidence base is clear that the marketing of unhealthy, ultra-processed food is causally related to childhood obesity. Any attempt to tackle childhood obesity has, therefore, to include a reduction in the exposure of children and adolescents to such foods and their marketing" (WHO, 2016, p. 127).

FOOD MARKETING

Food marketing makes it really hard to understand the benefits and challenges of different foods. Here again, the food industry intentionally tantalizes us with exciting, tasty, hyper-palatable foods that light up our taste buds and our brain's pleasure center. Then they give us permission to eat this yummy food by putting out messages that this food is either healthy (because they added a few vitamins) or at least neutral because there is not enough evidence that it is bad for you. Both ideas minimize and confuse the reality that we have solid research showing that daily consumption of sweetened ultra-processed foods is associated with numerous chronic health issues including mental health challenges such as anxiety and depression. To add confusion, we see big billboards with athletes who we associate with health and vitality holding up and praising these ultra-processed foods (Clapp & Scrinis, 2017).

SOCIAL MEDIA FOOD MARKETING

But marketing is not just what we see on big billboards. It happens in many subtle ways, including TV, movies, and social media. A small study explored what adolescents see on social media related to food and found that over two-thirds of the images and messages focused on eating large quantities of highly processed foods like soft drinks, cake, fries, pizza, and sweets (Qutteina et al., 2019). When the researchers dug deeper, they found that many of the influencers who were posting positive images of branded foods did not disclose that these were paid endorsements designed to market these products to their followers. On television, advertising by food and beverage manufacturers target Black and Hispanic consumers by placing ads for the least healthy food options in their food production lines on TV programs predominantly watched by these ethnic groups. For example, the ads on these channels are much more likely to be for high-sugar cereal and chips than for healthier brand portfolios like unsweetened yogurt and whole fruit products (UConn Rudd Center for Food Policy & Health, 2022).

MARKETING TO CHILDREN

Of particular concern is the marketing of sugary beverages to children. These sweetened drinks often contain loads of sugar or artificial sweeteners. In a 2019 analysis performed by the Rudd Center for Food Policy and Health at the University of Connecticut, they found that 62 percent of the beverages marketed to children were sweetened, including fruit drinks and flavored water. Of those, 65 percent had added sugars, 74 percent had artificial sweeteners, 85 percent showed images of fruit on the packaging but only a third of those actually contained any real juice, and none of these products met dietary recommendations for drinks that should be served to children under 14 years old (Harris et al., 2019). Consumption of high quantities of sugar is problematic for children, even though it has become embedded as a normal part of the American diet.

Children and adolescents are constantly exposed to food and beverage marketing. On social media alone, they receive many exposures. One study estimated that children are exposed to food marketing through social media an average of 30 times per week, which is small compared to adolescents, who are exposed to food marketing around 189 times per week (Potvin Kent et al., 2019). But it is not just social media. Television advertising of calorie-dense low-nutrient foods like potato chips has a substantial impact. Exposure to food advertising during television viewing may contribute to obesity by triggering automatic (mindless) snacking behavior. In a study of elementary school-aged children, when exposed to food advertising while watching a cartoon, the children consumed 45 percent more snack food with food advertising compared to watching the same cartoon that marketed other products (Harris et al., 2009).

Marion Nestle, a long-time advocate for making changes to the U.S. food industry, argues for a food system approach to health and nutrition that considers food transportation, storage, retailing, preparing, eating, and, eventually, wasting (Nestle, 2019). This includes government and social action that curbs or supports food industry marketing practices. Nestle recognizes that food companies whose primary goal is to earn a profit end up influencing the food system in ways that are

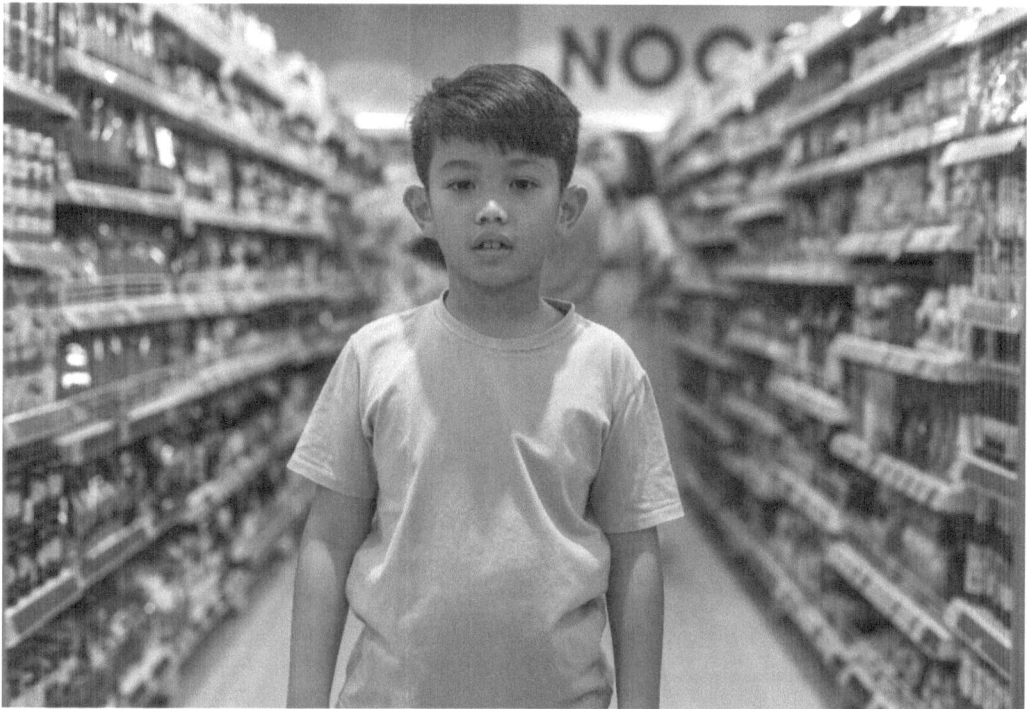

FIGURE 10.2 Marketing to children. Credit: BK Awangga (Shutterstock).

barriers to healthy eating. According to Nestle, as a society, we must take action to regulate some of these practices, like marketing ultra-processed foods to children, to improve the mental and physical health of our communities.

FOOD FOR THOUGHT: FOOD WASTE

A common source of family tension associated with food is the imperative to "clean your plate" and eat all the food served to you or that you served yourself. The sentiment behind this command is about food waste and the social, political, and economic concerns surrounding that issue. Food conservation is an issue of global importance, and children benefit when they learn to be mindful of food portion size and to not waste food. However, for many children, this directive sends the message that they should ignore their body's cues of feeling satiated and eat when they are not hungry in order to not waste food. During times of hardship, the pressure on this issue increases. Not surprisingly, a household with a lower-income has less food waste than a higher-income household. However, even for moderate-income households, an awareness and sensitivity to the high cost of quality food can lead many people to be overly cautious or demanding around food, with tremendous guilt for any uneaten or spoiled food (Thyberg & Tonjes, 2016).

Food waste looms as a pervasive issue in our current global food system. Researchers define food waste as "food which was originally produced for human consumption but then was discarded or was not consumed by humans," which includes "food that spoiled prior to disposal and food that was still edible when thrown away." Estimates report that over 30 percent of global food production remains entirely unconsumed, meaning that of all the food we grow, raise (in the case of animals), cook, or manufacture, a third of that food goes in the trash or is left out in the field (Schmidt, 2016). In the U.S. alone, 15 percent of all landfill waste is food, with food being disposed of at the rate of over half a pound of food waste per person per day (Thyberg & Tonjes, 2016).

There are different contributors to food waste, such as attitudes toward food, food industry norms and protocols, socioeconomic status, and culture. For example, it is common for restaurants to serve large helpings of food, even though consumers often do not eat the overly portioned food on their plates, nor do they take the food home. Food safety protocols are very restrictive around what the restaurants can do with the uneaten food. In California, for instance, food safety standards prohibit foods returned to the kitchen, even when completely untouched by customers, to be served again (California Health and Safety, 2019). So, an unfinished breadbasket must be thrown away.

Culture also plays a significant role in people's beliefs and perceptions about food waste. For example, in some cultures *nose-to-tail-eating* includes use of the entire animal while cooking. Have you ever been surprised to find open eyeballs on your plate when ordering a seafood dish? Some cultures utilize animal parts deemed "unfit" for consumption by others, feeling it is important to try to use the whole animal and discourage throwing away edible parts of the animal, even if they are less popular. For example, Menudo, a traditional Mexican dish, is made from the stomach lining of a cow. This part of the cow is not generally on the menu for a Standard American Diet, which usually only serves the muscles of the cow (i.e., steak, hamburger, ribs) and ignores the organs (liver, kidneys, tongue) that are eaten in many other cultures. Many cultures have culinary traditions that use all parts of an animal evolved from periods of food shortages that instilled a deep respect for using all food that is available and being wary about food waste (Heng & House, 2022).

The prevalence of food waste has become an international issue and anti-waste initiatives and policy changes have become more common. For example, the *Anti-food Waste Law of the People's Republic of China* enacted in 2021 targets food waste in the catering and restaurant industries. The policy prohibits excessive food waste in restaurants in an effort to "guarantee grain security, conserve resources, and protect the environment" (Feng et al., 2022, pp. 457–458). Policies like China's Anti-food Waste Law are indicative of the changing attitudes about the significant harm of food waste. Citizens around the world are demanding that governments get actively involved to prevent food waste by creating targeted policies aimed at the food and restaurant industries (Corrado & Sala, 2018), as well as educating the general public regarding methods for reducing individual food waste (Schmidt, 2016).

REFERENCES

Albers, S. (2013a). *Eat.Q.: Unlock the weight-loss power of emotional intelligence*. Harper Collins.

Albers, S. (2013b). *Mindful eating 101: A guide to healthy eating in college and beyond*. Routledge.

Arnow, B., Kenardy, J., & Agras, W. S. (1995). The emotional eating scale: The development of a measure to assess coping with negative affect by eating. *The International Journal of Eating Disorders, 18*(1), 79–90. https://doi.org/10.1002/1098-108X(199507)18:1<79::AID-EAT2260180109>3.0.CO;2-V

Askari, M., Heshmati, J., Shahinfar, H., Tripathi, N., & Daneshzad, E. (2020). Ultra-processed food and the risk of overweight and obesity: A systematic review and meta-analysis of observational studies. *International Journal of Obesity, 44*(10), 2080–2091. https://doi.org/10.1038/s41366-020-00650-z

Bes-Rastrollo, M., Schulze, M. B., Ruiz-Canela, M., & Martinez-Gonzalez, M. A. (2013). Financial conflicts of interest and reporting bias regarding the association between sugar-sweetened beverages and weight gain: A systematic review of systematic reviews. *PLoS Medicine, 10*(12), e1001578.

Bragg, M., Elbel, B., & Nestle, M. (2020). Food industry donations to academic programs: A cross-sectional examination of the extent of publicly available data. *International Journal of Environmental Research and Public Health, 17*(5), 1624.

Brown, R., & Ogden, J. (2004). Children's eating attitudes and behaviour: a study of the modelling and control theories of parental influence. *Health Education Research, 19*(3), 261–271. https://doi.org/10.1093/her/cyg040

California Health and Safety. (2019). *California retail food code*. Division 104 Environmental Health. https://www.cdph.ca.gov/Programs/CEH/DFDCS/CDPH%20Document%20Library/FDB/FoodSafetyProgram/MEHKO/CALIFORNIA%20RETAIL%20FOOD%20CODE%202019.pdf

Canella, D. S., Levy, R. B., Martins, A. P. B., Claro, R. M., Moubarac, J. C., Baraldi, L. G., Cannon, G., & Monteiro, C. A. (2014). Ultra-processed food products and obesity in Brazilian households (2008–2009). *PLoS One, 9*(3), e92752.

Clapp, J., & Scrinis, G. (2017). Big food, nutritionism, and corporate power. *Globalizations, 14*(4), 578–595. https://doi.org/10.1080/14747731.2016.1239806

Corrado, S., & Sala, S. (2018). Food waste accounting along global and European food supply chains: State of the art and outlook. *Waste Management, 79*, 120–131. https://doi.org/10.1016/j.wasman.2018.07.032

Deliens, T., Clarys, P., De Bourdeaudhuij, I., & Deforche, B. (2014). Determinants of eating behaviour in university students: A qualitative study using focus group discussions. *BMC Public Health, 14*(1), 53. https://doi.org/10.1186/1471-2458-14-53

Devenyns, J. (2020). Study: Food industry funding can influence research. *Food Dive*, (December *18*, 2020). https://www.fooddive.com/news/study-food-industry-funding-can-influence-research/592343/

Dunbar, R. I. M. (2017). Breaking bread: The functions of social eating. *Adaptive Human Behavior and Physiology, 3*(3), 198–211. https://doi.org/10.1007/s40750-017-0061-4

Feng, Y., Marek, C., & Tosun, J. (2022). Fighting food waste by law: Making sense of the Chinese approach. *Journal of Consumer Policy, 45*(3), 457–479. https://doi.org/10.1007/s10603-022-09519-2

Frayn, M., & Knäuper, B. (2017). Emotional eating and weight in adults: A review. *Current Psychology, 37*(4), 924–933. https://doi.org/10.1007/s12144-017-9577-9

Harris, J. L., Bargh, J. A., & Brownell, K. D. (2009). Priming effects of television food advertising on eating behavior. *Health Psychology, 28*(4), 404.

Harris, J. L., Romo-Palafox, M., Choi, Y.-Y., & Kibwana, A. (2019). *Children's drink facts 2019: Sales, nutrition, and marketing of children's drinks*. University of Connecticut Rudd Center for Food Policy and Obesity. https://uconnruddcenter.org/wp-content/uploads/sites/2909/2020/09/FACTS2019-1.pdf

Heng, Y., & House, L. (2022). Consumers' perceptions and behavior toward food waste across countries. *International Food and Agribusiness Management Review, 25*(2), 197–210. https://doi.org/10.22434/IFAMR2020.0198

Herman, C. P., Polivy, J., Pliner, P., & Vartanian, L. R. (2019). Effects of social eating. In C. P. Herman, J. Polivy, P. Pliner, & L. R. Vartanian (Eds.), *Social influences on eating* (pp. 215–227). Springer International Publishing. https://doi.org/10.1007/978-3-030-28817-4_13

Higgs, S. (2015). Social norms and their influence on eating behaviours. *Appetite, 86*, 38–44. https://doi.org/10.1016/j.appet.2014.10.021

Higgs, S., & Thomas, J. (2016). Social influences on eating. *Current Opinion in Behavioral Sciences, 9,* 1–6. https://doi.org/10.1016/j.cobeha.2015.10.005

Kristeller, J. (2024). *Mindful eating.* https://www.mb-eat.com/

Lacaille, L. J., Dauner, K. N., Krambeer, R. J., & Pedersen, J. (2011). Psychosocial and environmental determinants of eating behaviors, physical activity, and weight change among college students: A qualitative analysis. *Journal of American College Health, 59*(6), 531–538. https://doi.org/10.1080/07448481.2010.523855

Levine, M. P. (2012). Loneliness and eating disorders. *The Journal of Psychology, 146*(1-2), 243–257. https://doi.org/10.1080/00223980.2011.606435

Machado, P. P., Steele, E. M., Levy, R. B., da Costa Louzada, M. L., Rangan, A., Woods, J., Gill, T., Scrinis, G., & Monteiro, C. A. (2020). Ultra-processed food consumption and obesity in the Australian adult population. *Nutrition & Diabetes, 10*(1), 39. https://doi.org/10.1038/s41387-020-00141-0

Massougbodji, J., Le Bodo, Y., Fratu, R., & De Wals, P. (2014). Reviews examining sugar-sweetened beverages and body weight: Correlates of their quality and conclusions. *The American Journal of Clinical Nutrition, 99*(5), 1096–1104. https://doi.org/10.3945/ajcn.113.063776

Matz, J., Pershing, A., & Harrison, C. (2024). *The emotional eating, chronic dieting, binge eating & body image workbook.* PESI Publishing, Inc.

Moss, M. (2013). *Salt, sugar, fat: How the food giants hooked us.* Random House.

Mötteli, S., Siegrist, M., & Keller, C. (2017). Women's social eating environment and its associations with dietary behavior and weight management. *Appetite, 110,* 86–93. https://doi.org/10.1016/j.appet.2016.12.014

Mozaffarian, D. (2017). Conflict of interest and the role of the food industry in nutrition research. *Jama, 317*(17), 1755–1756.

Murphy, E. (2024). *Emotional eating is about safety.* https://www.linkedin.com/pulse/emotional-eating-safety-emma-murphy-miacp-udfte

Murphy, S. L., van Meer, F., van Dillen, L., van Steenbergen, H., & Hofmann, W. (2024). Underwhelming pleasures: Toward a self-regulatory account of hedonic compensation and overconsumption. *Journal of Personality and Social Psychology.* https://doi.org/10.1037/pspa0000389

Nardocci, M., Leclerc, B. S., Louzada, M. L., Monteiro, C. A., Batal, M., & Moubarac, J. C. (2019). Consumption of ultra-processed foods and obesity in Canada. *Canadian Journal of Public Health, 110*(1), 4–14. https://doi.org/10.17269/s41997-018-0130-x

Neri, D., Steele, E. M., Khandpur, N., Cediel, G., Zapata, M. E., Rauber, F., Marrón-Ponce, J. A., Machado, P., da Costa Louzada, M. L., Andrade, G. C., Batis, C., Babio, N., Salas-Salvadó, J., Millett, C., Monteiro, C. A., & Levy, R. B., for the NOVA Multi-Country Study Group on Ultra-Processed Foods, Diet Quality and Human Health (2022). Ultraprocessed food consumption and dietary nutrient profiles associated with obesity: A multicountry study of children and adolescents. *Obesity Reviews, 23*(S1), e13387. https://doi.org/10.1111/obr.13387

Nestle, M. (2016). Corporate funding of food and nutrition research: Science or marketing? *JAMA Internal Medicine, 176*(1), 13–14.

Nestle, M. (2019). A food lover's love of nutrition science, policy, and politics. *European Journal of Clinical Nutrition, 73*(12), 1551–1555.

Neumark-Sztainer, D., Eisenberg, M. E., Fulkerson, J. A., Story, M., & Larson, N. I. (2008). Family meals and disordered eating in adolescents: Longitudinal findings from project EAT. *Archives of Pediatrics & Adolescent Medicine, 162*(1), 17–22. https://doi.org/10.1001/archpediatrics.2007.9

O'Connor, A. (2015). Coca-Cola funds scientists who shift blame for obesity away from bad diets. *New York Times.* https://archive.nytimes.com/well.blogs.nytimes.com/2015/08/09/coca-cola-funds-scientists-who-shift-blame-for-obesity-away-from-bad-diets/

Ogden, J. (2010). *The psychology of eating: From healthy to disordered behavior* (2nd ed.). Wiley-Blackwell.

Potvin Kent, M., Pauzé, E., Roy, E. A., de Billy, N., & Czoli, C. (2019). Children and adolescents' exposure to food and beverage marketing in social media apps. *Pediatric Obesity, 14*(6), e12508.

Qutteina, Y., Hallez, L., Mennes, N., De Backer, C., & Smits, T. (2019). What do adolescents see on social media? A diary study of food marketing images on social media. *Frontiers in Psychology, 10,* 2637.

Rauber, F., Steele, E. M., Louzada, M. L. D. C., Millett, C., Monteiro, C. A., & Levy, R. B. (2020). Ultra-processed food consumption and indicators of obesity in the United Kingdom population (2008-2016). *PLoS One, 15*(5), e0232676.

Ruiz, M. C., Devonport, T. J., Chen-Wilson, C. H., Nicholls, W., Cagas, J. Y., Fernandez-Montalvo, J., Choi, Y., Gan, Y., & Robazza, C. (2023). Brief emotional eating scale: A multinational study of factor structure, validity, and invariance. *Appetite, 185,* 106538. https://doi.org/10.1016/j.appet.2023.106538

Sacks, G., Riesenberg, D., Mialon, M., Dean, S., & Cameron, A. J. (2020). The characteristics and extent of food industry involvement in peer-reviewed research articles from 10 leading nutrition-related journals in 2018. *PLoS One, 15*(12), e0243144.

Schmidt, K. (2016). Explaining and promoting household food waste-prevention by an environmental psychological based intervention study. *Resources, Conservation and Recycling, 111*, 53–66.

Scrinis, G. (2020). Ultra-processed foods and the corporate capture of nutrition—an essay by Gyorgy Scrinis. *BMJ, 371*, m4601. https://doi.org/10.1136/bmj.m4601

Spiga, F., Davies, A. L., Tomlinson, E., Moore, T. H. M., Dawson, S., Breheny, K., Savović, J., Gao, Y., Phillips, S. M., Hillier-Brown, F., Hodder, R. K., Wolfenden, L., Higgins, J. P., & Summerbell, C. D. (2024). Interventions to prevent obesity in children aged 5 to 11 years old. *Cochrane Database of Systematic Reviews, 5*(5), CD015328. https://doi.org/10.1002/14651858.CD015328.pub2

Spiga, F., Tomlinson, E., Davies, A. L., Moore, T. H. M., Dawson, S., Breheny, K., Savović, J., Hodder, R. K., Wolfenden, L., Higgins, J. P. T., & Summerbell, C. D. (2024). Interventions to prevent obesity in children aged 12 to 18 years old. *Cochrane Database of Systematic Reviews, 5*(5), CD015330. https://doi.org/10.1002/14651858.CD015330.pub2

Taitz, J. L., & Safer, D. L. (2012). *End emotional eating using dialectical behavior therapy skills to cope with difficult emotions and develop a healthy relationship to food.* New Harbinger Publications.

Tam, R., Yassa, B., Parker, H., O'Connor, H., & Allman-Farinelli, M. (2017). University students' on-campus food purchasing behaviors, preferences, and opinions on food availability. *Nutrition, 37*, 7–13. https://doi.org/10.1016/j.nut.2016.07.007

Tapper, K. (2022). Mindful eating: What we know so far. *Nutrition Bulletin, 47*(2), 168–185. https://doi.org/10.1111/nbu.12559

Thyberg, K. L., & Tonjes, D. J. (2016). Drivers of food waste and their implications for sustainable policy development. *Resources, Conservation and Recycling, 106*, 110–123.

UConn Rudd Center for Food Policy & Health. (2022). *Targeted food and beverage advertising to Black and Hispanic consumers: 2022 update.* https://uconnruddcenter.org/research/food-marketing/targetedmarketing/

Unnevehr, L. (2017). *Economic contribution of the food and beverage industry: A report by the Committee for Economic Development of The Conference Board.* https://www.ced.org/pdf/Economic_Contribution_of_the_Food_and_Beverage_Industry.pdf

Vella-Zarb, R. A., & Elgar, F. J. (2009). The 'freshman 5': A meta-analysis of weight gain in the freshman year of college. *Journal of American College Health, 58*(2), 161–166. https://doi.org/10.1080/07448480903221392

WHO. (2016). *Consideration of the evidence on childhood obesity for the Commission On Ending Childhood Obesity: Report of the ad hoc working group on science and evidence for ending childhood obesity.* World Health Organization.

Wilson, S. M., Darling, K. E., Fahrenkamp, A. J., D'Auria, A. L., & Sato, A. F. (2015). Predictors of emotional eating during adolescents' transition to college: Does body mass index moderate the association between stress and emotional eating? *Journal of American College Health, 63*(3), 163–170. https://doi.org/10.1080/07448481.2014.1003374

Section V

Eating Behaviors

11 Weight Loss

The topic of weight loss is complicated and confusing. Misinformation abounds as people struggle to understand what constitutes a healthy weight for their body and the best path to achieve that weight. Obesity has become a frequent topic of conversation in the healthcare world due to its associated health risks. Unfortunately, the focus on obesity has increased anti-fat sentiments and stigma associated with living in a larger body. People with higher amounts of body fat are blamed and shamed for the composition of their body, with little recognition of the vast role the current food industry plays in creating unhealthy communities that are at the root of the rapid rise of obesity.

OBESITY

The term obesity is often heard in the news, on social media, and in the healthcare system as a measure of health. There is now general agreement that the term is defined as a person who falls within a weight and height category on the *body mass index (BMI)*. The BMI is based on an equation developed in the 1830s by Lambert Adolphe, a Belgian astronomer, mathematician, statistician, and sociologist. Adolphe created the equation for measuring body composition in populations. It was never designed to calculate an individual person's health; however, its use changed in the 1970s. The application of BMI calculation for individuals became popular beginning in 1972 when the modern term "body mass index" was established by Ancel Keys. The current BMI scale describes adults aged 20 years and older using five main weight status categories: Underweight (<19), Healthy weight (19–24), Overweight (25–29), Obese (30–39), and Extremely Obese (≥40) (see Figure 11.1). These categories are the same for men and women of all body types and ages.

The World Health Organization (WHO) developed additional cut-off points to further break down the weight status categories (see Table 11.1). The Underweight category was expanded to include mild, moderate, and severe thinness, and the Obese category was expanded to include Pre-obese and Obese class I, II, and III (also known as Grade or Class 1, 2, or 3 Obesity). Class 3 Obesity is sometimes referred to as severe obesity or morbid obesity.

The usage of the BMI as a tool to simplify and provide objective terms to discuss body composition relies on estimating a person's proportion of body fat compared to their lean mass (muscle, bone, organs) based on their height and weight. Research and medical practitioners use the BMI as an objective measure of body composition to understand the impact of BMI on potential health problems associated with weight gain and weight loss.

The BMI does not specifically measure body fat (also called *adiposity*) like more direct measures of body fat such as using calipers to measure a fold of skin, underwater weighing (since increased adiposity is more buoyant), and bioelectrical impedance (the rate at which an electrical current travels through the body, which is slowed more by adipose tissue compared to lean mass). These direct measures of adiposity are generally less accessible and more expensive, which makes them less practical to use, however, they are often more accurate measures of body composition. The BMI is considered a fast and easy approximation of body composition, although less helpful for lean athletes who generally have a high muscle-to-fat ratio; therefore, their BMI score is misleadingly high relative to their body-fat percentage.

A great deal of focus with the BMI has been on the obesity weight category. Many people assert that obesity has become an epidemic in the U.S. Approximately two in five Americans fall in the current category described as obese, often at the same time demonstrating nutritional deficiencies (e.g., vitamin D), so we have an issue with people being overfed yet undernourished (CDC, 2024a; Fryar et al., 2018). As people continue to feed a hunger that cannot be satisfied with nutrient-deficient food, waist sizes expand. In this chapter, we explore the connection between weight, weight loss,

DOI: 10.1201/9781032647647-16

Height \ Weight	lbs	90	100	110	120	130	140	150	160	170	180	190	200	210	220	230	240	250	260	270	280	290
	kgs	41	45	50	54	59	64	68	72	77	82	86	91	95	100	104	109	113	118	122	127	132
ft/in	cm																					
4 ft 8 in	142.2	20	22	25	27	29	31	34	36	38	40	43	45	47	49	52	54	56	58	61	63	65
4 ft 9 in	144.7	19	22	24	26	28	30	32	35	37	39	41	43	45	48	50	52	54	56	58	61	63
4 ft 10 in	147.3	19	21	23	25	27	29	31	33	36	38	40	42	44	46	48	50	52	54	56	59	61
4 ft 11 in	149.8	18	20	22	24	26	28	30	32	34	36	38	40	42	44	46	48	51	53	55	57	59
5 ft 0 in	152.4	18	20	21	23	25	27	29	31	33	35	37	39	41	43	45	47	49	51	53	55	57
5 ft 1 in	154.9	17	19	21	23	25	26	28	30	32	34	36	38	40	42	43	45	47	49	51	53	55
5 ft 2 in	157.4	16	18	20	22	24	26	27	29	31	33	35	37	38	40	42	44	46	48	49	51	53
5 ft 3 in	160.0	16	18	19	21	23	25	27	28	30	32	34	35	37	39	41	43	44	46	48	50	51
5 ft 4 in	162.5	15	17	19	21	22	24	26	27	29	31	33	34	36	38	39	41	43	45	46	48	50
5 ft 5 in	165.1	15	17	18	20	22	23	25	27	28	30	32	33	35	37	38	40	42	43	45	47	48
5 ft 6 in	167.6	15	16	18	19	21	23	24	26	27	29	31	32	34	36	37	39	40	42	44	45	47
5 ft 7 in	170.1	14	16	17	19	20	22	24	25	27	28	30	31	33	34	36	38	39	41	42	44	45
5 ft 8 in	172.7	14	15	17	18	20	21	23	24	26	27	29	30	32	33	35	37	38	40	41	43	44
5 ft 9 in	175.2	13	15	16	18	19	21	22	24	25	27	28	30	31	33	34	35	37	38	40	41	43
5 ft 10 in	177.8	13	14	16	17	19	20	22	23	24	26	27	29	30	32	33	34	36	37	39	40	42
5 ft 11 in	180.3	13	14	15	17	18	20	21	22	24	25	27	28	29	31	32	33	35	36	38	39	40
6 ft 0 in	182.8	12	14	15	16	18	19	20	22	23	24	26	27	28	30	31	33	34	35	37	38	39
6 ft 1 in	185.4	12	13	15	16	17	18	20	21	22	24	25	26	28	29	30	32	33	34	36	37	38
6 ft 2 in	187.9	12	13	14	16	17	18	19	21	22	23	24	26	27	28	30	31	32	33	35	36	37
6 ft 3 in	190.5	11	13	14	15	16	18	19	20	21	23	24	25	26	28	29	30	31	33	34	35	36
6 ft 4 in	193.0	11	12	13	15	16	17	18	19	21	22	23	24	26	27	28	29	30	32	33	34	35
6 ft 5 in	195.5	11	12	13	14	15	17	18	19	20	21	23	24	25	26	27	28	30	31	32	33	34
6 ft 6 in	198.1	10	12	13	14	15	16	17	18	20	21	22	23	24	25	27	28	29	30	31	32	34
6 ft 7 in	200.6	10	11	12	14	15	16	17	18	19	20	21	23	24	25	26	27	28	29	30	32	33
6 ft 8 in	203.2	10	11	12	13	14	15	16	18	19	20	21	22	23	24	25	26	27	29	30	31	32
6 ft 9 in	205.7	10	11	12	13	14	15	16	17	18	19	20	21	24	24	25	26	27	28	29	30	31
6 ft 10 in	208.2	9	10	12	13	14	15	16	17	18	19	20	21	22	23	24	25	26	27	28	29	30
6 ft 11 in	210.8	9	10	11	12	13	14	15	16	17	18	19	20	21	22	23	25	26	27	28	29	30

Underweight   Healthy   Overweight   Obese   Extremely Obese

FIGURE 11.1   Body Mass Index (BMI) Chart. Credit: Abhijeet Bhosale (ShutterStock).

and mental health, and elucidate potential causes of obesity that mental health challenges may exacerbate. First, however, let us consider some of the metrics and theories about obesity.

BMI AND HEALTH

The BMI is one of the most common tools used to study health problems associated with a high percentage of body fat, especially as a risk factors for chronic disease and early death. Most practitioners learned to correlate high BMI scores with a wide range of chronic illnesses, including high blood pressure, high cholesterol, type 2 diabetes, cardiovascular disease, stroke, arthritis, sleep apnea, chronic inflammation, cancer, and depression. Childhood obesity is associated with an increased risk of anxiety and depression, low self-esteem, social problems such as bullying and stigma, and obesity as an adult.

Yet the BMI is controversial and there is disagreement in the field about its accuracy for predicting health issues. For example, early research identified that anybody whose weight was outside of the healthy weight range (BMI 19–24) was at higher risk of death from all types of diseases and injuries (known as *all-cause mortality*). Then, a 2013 systematic review found that increased all-cause mortality was really only a risk for people who were underweight or with class 2 or class 3 obesity, and that class 1 obesity was not associated with higher risk and people in the overweight category were at signficantly *lower* risk of mortality (Flegal et al., 2013).

TABLE 11.1
Body Mass Index (BMI) Classification Cut-Off Points

Classification	BMI (kg/m²) Principal Cut-Off Points
Underweight	*<18.50*
Severe thinness	<16.00
Moderate thinness	16.00–16.99
Mild thinness	17.00–18.49
Normal range	*18.50–24.99*
Overweight	*≥25.00*
Pre-obese	25.00–29.99
Obese	*≥30.00*
Obese class I	30.00–34.99
Obese class II	35.00–39.99
Obese class III	≥40.00

Source: Adapted from Table 3.1: WHO classification of adult underweight, overweight, and obesity according to BMI including additional cut-off points recommended by the WHO Expert Consultation (p. 22) (WHO Global InfoBase Team, 2005).

This assertion was challenged in a 2016 meta-analysis of 239 prospective studies with participants from Asia, Australia, New Zealand, Europe, and North America (The Global BMI Mortality Collaboration, 2016). The results demonstrated that participants in the underweight, overweight, and class 1 obesity groups were associated with increased all-cause mortality, with a rising level of risk at higher levels of obesity (class 2 and 3 obesity). This study challenges previous suggestions in the field that overweight and class 1 obesity are not associated with higher mortality and provides evidence that people with these more moderate BMI scores are still at increased risk of mortality. In 2018, a very large study in the UK confirmed that there is a "J-shaped" association between BMI and mortality, where people with a BMI who are overweight have only a slightly increased risk of all-cause mortality, while people who are underweight or obese have a higher risk, with increasing risk for people in the severely underweight, and the class 2 and class 3 obesity categories (Bhaskaran et al., 2018).

The BMI became popular because people in the 20th century became thicker, and the development of health problems and death related to obesity became more common. The prevalence of adults with a BMI in the obese range has dramatically increased. Obesity rates in the U.S. have doubled over the last 25 years, rising from an average rate of 15.8 percent in 1995 to 31.9 percent in 2020, while rates for overweight adults remain stable (CDC, 2022b).

Currently, nearly one in five children and adolescents in the U.S. ages 2–19 years are obese. For this group, we have data from 1971, which recounts an even more disturbing trend, with pediatric obesity rates more than tripling over the last 50 years from 5.2 percent in 1971 to 19.7 percent in 2020. The hardest hit has been teens ages 12–19 (22.2 percent), non-Hispanic Black children (24.8 percent), and Hispanic children (26.2 percent). Medical conditions associated with childhood obesity include high blood pressure, high cholesterol, type 2 diabetes, breathing problems (such as asthma and sleep apnea), and joint problems (CDC, 2022a; Fryar et al., 2020).

VISCERAL AND SUBCUTANEOUS FAT

There is ample evidence that how a person stores fat in the body significantly impacts the association between body fat and health problems. *Subcutaneous fat* grows just under the skin and plays a significant role in body temperature regulation. It also serves as cushioning for the body and protects the organs. Typically, subcutaneous fat is not associated with chronic disease. *Visceral fat* typically creates an apple-shaped body with the majority of the fat stored in the abdomen. This fat surrounds the organs and is more intimately associated with increased chronic illness and all-cause mortality.

It is also important to discuss fat as a source of inflammation (Karczewski et al., 2018). Researchers suspect that visceral fat makes more of certain proteins that inflame the body's tissues and organs, narrowing blood vessels, increasing blood cholesterol levels, increasing blood pressure, and contributing to inflammation-related chronic diseases (Frysh, 2024). Evidence is accumulating that increased visceral fat promotes systemic low-grade inflammation and has been strongly linked to heart disease, Alzheimer's disease, type 2 diabetes, stroke, and depression. (see Chapter 7 for more on inflammation and mental health.)

However, the BMI does not distinguish between subcutaneous fat and visceral fat, so there is concern it does not accurately portray a person's body composition and health risks. We need to look at a wider range of health markers than just the BMI, such as blood chemistry, stool, organic acids, hormones, gut health, and lifestyle habits, to more accurately determine a person's health risks.

CASE STUDY: BODY ACCEPTANCE AND THE BMI CLASSIFICATIONS

Lana struggled with obesity for years. She decided to lose weight and chose to follow a strict regimen of consuming only 700 calories a day, along with spending hours at the gym every day doing what was classically celebrated to lose weight – eat less and exercise more. But even after losing 200 pounds, the BMI still classified her as obese. Lana felt demoralized and continued to have negative feelings about her body, despite how her body was changing, which she felt went unacknowledged.

Over time, she learned that if she did not drink or eat anything before a doctor's appointment, she could stave off the disapproving glances from the nurse taking her vitals. They focused only on the weight she was carrying, not the weight she had lost. She limited her food intake as much as she could until she could no longer take the growling cries from her stomach. She often ate in secret where no eyes could witness her desperate feasting. Anxiety and disappointment were her constant emotions.

In her youth, she visited the doctor frequently with concerns about her upset digestive system. For each visit, she was weighed and shown the representation of her weight on the BMI chart. With each appointment, her BMI increased, and the caloric allotment from the doctor decreased. Eat less and move more was the slogan she heard repeatedly growing up. However, it just never seemed to work for her, and by the time she turned 22, she weighed over 350 pounds and was very unhappy.

She received societal messaging that added up to, "Just lose weight and all of your problems will go away." This mantra rang in her ears. When she began losing weight, she wondered when her problems would go away. Even though she had lost significant weight, the BMI chart consistently still put her in the overweight category. At the same time that she lost fat, she had also gained significant muscle mass from all of her time at the gym, which kept her body weight and BMI at a higher number. At times she would stare at the scale, unable to come to terms with the fact that the number on the scale remained unchanged even though her body composition was significantly changing. She had gained muscle and lost fat, exactly the way she had been told to go about weight loss, yet the BMI and the health professionals who used it as their most relied on measure, still scolded her for being overweight.

For a long time, when looking in the mirror Lana still saw the same morbidly obese person she was two years before starting her journey. It did not seem to matter how much weight she had lost. The shame and disapproving looks she had experienced for so many years were slow to let go. It took several more years for her to accept her body the way it is and to not allow the BMI chart to dictate her self-worth.

Waist-to-Hip Ratio

The *Waist-to-Hip Ratio (WHR)* is seen by many as a more accurate way of assessing health risk. This method determines how much fat is stored in the waist, hips, and glutes. Not all excess weight is the same. Those who carry excess weight around the belly carry the greatest risk of cardiovascular disease due to the inflammatory nature of visceral fat. Those who carry excess weight around the hips and thighs are at a lower risk of disease. To calculate the WHR, measure the *waist circumference (WC)* just above the belly button and the *hip circumference (HC)* at the widest part of the hips. Divide the WC by the HC. For example, a person with a 31-inch waist and 40-inch hips has a 0.78 WHR. Table 11.2 depicts the potential cardiovascular risk as determined by WHR.

This is an important measurement because more fat around the midsection (apple-shaped body) means a person has larger visceral fat deposits, which puts a person at higher risk for chronic disease than someone who carries more of their fat in the hips and thighs (pear-shaped body). Where we carry fat on our bodies not only impacts physical health risks, it also increases mental health risks. According to a study done in 2009 by Susan Everson-Rose et al., those with a higher WHR are more likely to develop depression (Everson-Rose et al., 2009). The authors speculate that those who are overweight or obese, with the preponderance of the excess weight being visceral fat, are more likely to experience depression, which also compounds the cardiovascular risk. Those with more subcutaneous fat and less visceral fat were less likely to experience depression.

The correlation between BMI and percentage of body fat is reasonably strong, but their fat distribution and body composition may differ even if two people have the same BMI. In general, at the same BMI: women tend to have more body fat than men; the amount of body fat may be higher or lower depending on the racial/ethnic group; older people tend to have more body fat than younger adults, and athletes generally have less body fat than do non-athletes. For many people, an alternative measure of body composition such as the WHR provides more accurate information regarding health risks associated with body composition.

While there is generally good alignment between the BMI and the WHR, for a subset of the population, the BMI is not as effective as the WHR in predicting the risk of chronic disease based on body composition. A large Australian study with over 40,000 participants studied the risk of mortality associated with BMI and WC scores. A WC greater than 35 inches (88 cm) for women and 40 inches (102 cm) for men indicates obesity and a higher risk for heart disease and type 2 diabetes. In this sample, over one-quarter of the population had obesity, as defined by the BMI or WC. They found a 6% discordance between the BMI and the WC, where participants were identified as obese with one score but not the other. When the participant was identified as obese by the WC but not by the BMI, they were at increased risk of all-cause mortality and cardiovascular disease mortality, which demonstrated that assessing a person's adiposity using the BMI alone will fail to identify risk factors for a portion of the population (Tanamas et al., 2016). Therefore, it would be beneficial for the healthcare industry to include WC or WHR to help patients better understand their chronic disease and death risk.

TABLE 11.2
Waist-to-Hip Ratio (WHR) and
Risk of Cardiovascular Disease

Health Risk	Women	Men
Low	0.80 or lower	0.95 or lower
Moderate	0.81–0.85	0.96–1.0
High	0.86 or higher	1.0 or higher

SOCIAL STIGMA

Social stigma around body fat continues to be a challenging problem. Many people who are obese struggle with disliking their bodies and suffer social stigma associated with their appearance, such as assumptions that they are lazy, unsuccessful, and don't care how they look because they live in a large body. Even if they do not meet the full diagnostic criteria for body dysmorphic disorder, where their concerns about the appearance of their body interfere with their ability to function adequately, they can still feel significantly unhappy with their body and inhibited in their life due to the shape of their body and their concerns about how others view them.

Despite the ongoing increase in obesity prevalence in the U.S., the level of obesity stigmatization continues to be a problem across a number of areas including social media, advertising, news, and public health (Westbury et al., 2023). This discrimination occurs at both system levels (e.g., career opportunities) as well as in their interpersonal lives with friends and families, with some of the most frequent sources of discriminatory comments and treatment coming from family members and physicians. This frequent onslaught increases the likelihood of isolating and avoiding seeking medical treatment. In a study of over 800 U.S. young adults who completed the *Attitudes Toward Obese Persons Scale*, results indicated that 92.5 percent of respondents held at least one stigmatizing belief about obesity (Ambwani et al., 2014). The participants shared common negative beliefs, such as "obese people are inferior," and harbored negative attitudes toward obese persons which were pervasive across different characteristics, including body size and gender.

There is a tendency to blame someone who is obese for being lazy, unhealthy, and undisciplined. However, new research is starting to illuminate the complexity of obesity and the many factors associated with eating behavior and weight gain. A growing body of data has demonstrated a physiologic component to eating behavior associated with obesity. It identifies that some people are more susceptible to developing unhealthy eating patterns when they regularly eat highly processed foods due to how their body responds to those hyper-palatable substances, leading to behavior that is sometimes termed *food addiction* due to the similarity in symptoms to other addictive processes (see more on this in Chapter 13).

GENETICS

People often blame their genes when their BMI score declares that they are obese, which has some scientific backing. Twin studies have demonstrated an inherited component to a person's BMI, making some people genetically vulnerable to obesity (Kim et al., 2022). So, our genes are one factor that makes us more vulnerable to weight gain when exposed to certain environments, but it is not the whole story. Weight gain and obesity are complex issues.

In 1962, James Neel introduced the "thrifty gene" concept to help explain the growing prevalence of obesity and diabetes in the U.S. population (Neel, 1962). The hypothesis was that, during times of feast-or-famine, it was beneficial to have genes that made the body more likely to hang onto stored fat to survive famines which was an advantage that helped you procreate and pass on your genes. However, in our current culture, where cheap, highly processed foods are abundant and famines are rare, this same genetic makeup is a disadvantage in that it increases the likelihood of becoming obese compared to someone with different genes who eats the same food and does not gain weight. From this perspective, an environment filled with enticing foods may be more brutal to resist for someone who has genes that make them susceptible to craving those types of food and more vulnerable to becoming obese. While the thrifty gene theory has remained popular, there is some pushback about how to interpret and utilize this concept. In the current science of genetics, the specific genes for obesity have not been identified across populations (Reddon et al., 2018).

Another perspective comes from the field of epigenetics, where it is argued that, in addition to whether a person carries a specific gene, we also must acknowledge the impact of the environment on whether that gene is activated so that it produces a specific effect in the body. Therefore, a range of genes may make us genetically vulnerable to obesity, and if those genes interact with an environment that preys upon that vulnerability and causes the genes to be activated, a person is more likely to struggle with weight gain and increased adiposity. For example, a 2022 literature review presented evidence that epigenetic changes affect immune cell function in obesity and type 2 diabetes, contributing to the inflammation that underlies much of the negative impact of both of these issues (Zatterale et al., 2022).

The rate of obesity in the U.S. has been consistently rising since the 1950s across all income levels, racial/ethnic backgrounds, and educational attainments (Banas et al., 2024). The fact that there has been such a dramatic increase in obesity in such a short period of time indicates it is unlikely a change in our genetic makeup and more a factor of our environment. There are various factors that have made the environment more "obesogenic" for many people including increased portion sizes, readily available ultra-processed foods, sedentary lifestyles, chronic stress, and environmental toxins (Garvey, 2022; Heindel et al., 2023). Which implies that changing the environment to be less obesogenic an essential component to decreasing the number of people who are obese.

CONVENTIONAL APPROACHES TO WEIGHT LOSS

Weight loss is big business! The U.S. weight-loss market grew to a historic peak of $90 billion in 2023 (up from $73 billion in 2021), largely due to the rapidly rising popularity of prescription GLP-1 weight-loss drugs, which have outcompeted all non-medical segments of the market (Research and Markets, 2024; Wood, 2022). Sadly, the amount of money thrown at the obesity epidemic has not reduced the prevalence. In fact, the prevalence of obesity in adults has increased from 30.9 percent in 2018 to 41.9 percent in 2023 (CDC, 2024b; NIH, 2018).

WEIGHT-LOSS DRUGS

The history of weight-loss drugs is a testament to humanity's enduring struggle with obesity and the desire for quick fixes. In the 1930s, researchers realized that dinitrophenol (DNP), initially used in explosives manufacturing, could increase metabolic rate and promote weight loss. DNP works by uncoupling oxidative phosphorylation in mitochondria, causing the body to burn fat quickly. However, its use was marred by severe side effects, including hyperthermia, cataracts, and even death, leading to its ban by the FDA in 1938 (Grundlingh et al., 2011).

Amphetamines became popular in the post-World War II era for their appetite-suppressing effects. Phentermine, a sympathomimetic amine, emerged in the 1950s and was widely prescribed as an appetite suppressant. It stimulates the release of norepinephrine, a neurotransmitter that reduces hunger. Phentermine gained significant popularity and remains in use today, often in combination with topiramate as part of the drug Qsymia. Despite its effectiveness, concerns about addiction and cardiovascular side effects have tempered its use (Rasmussen, 2015).

The 1990s brought a new wave of weight-loss drugs, most notably the fen-phen combination (fenfluramine and phentermine). Initially hailed as a breakthrough, fen-phen was linked to severe heart valve problems, leading to its withdrawal from the market in 1997. This event underscored the importance of rigorous safety evaluations for weight-loss medications (Wadden et al., 1998). An importance that is often overlooked in an eagerness to profit off of acts of desperation by those who deal with excess weight.

By the late 1990s, the development of weight-loss drugs shifted toward targeting specific metabolic pathways. Orlistat, approved in 1999, inhibits pancreatic lipase, reducing fat absorption in the intestines. While effective, its gastrointestinal side effects, including intractable constipation and explosive diarrhea coupled with incontinence, have limited its popularity (Guarino, 2005). Another notable drug is lorcaserin, approved in 2012, which targets serotonin receptors to promote satiety. However, it was withdrawn in 2020 due to concerns about an increased cancer risk, irreversible erectile dysfunction, and pulmonary hypertension (DiNicolantonio et al., 2014; Greenway et al., 2016).

A supposed significant breakthrough came with the advent of GLP-1 (glucagon-like peptide-1) inhibitors, which were initially developed for diabetes management. Drugs like liraglutide and semaglutide mimic the action of GLP-1 in the body, a hormone that enhances insulin secretion, slows gastric emptying, and reduces appetite. These medications have shown impressive weight-loss results, with semaglutide leading to substantial weight reductions in clinical trials. The dual benefit of glycemic control and weight loss has made GLP-1 inhibitors a promising option for obese individuals, particularly those with type 2 diabetes.

However, as with their predecessors, these drugs come with risks. There is concern that when patients stop taking the medication, they are likely to regain the weight they lost (Wilding et al., 2022). Also, the manufacturers of semaglutide are under litigation at the time of this publication for failure to provide informed consent to recipients with details about potential side effects such as increased thyroid cancer risk, gastrointestinal tract diseases, gallbladder disease, increase in heart rate, acute kidney injury, diabetic retinopathy, and allergic reaction. Proper informed consent delivered by the administering healthcare provider is an essential part of making an informed decision about the pros and cons of these medications (Smits & Van Raalte, 2021).

The quest for effective and safe weight-loss drugs continues, with current research exploring novel mechanisms and combinations. For instance, a bupropion-naltrexone medication combines an antidepressant with an opioid antagonist to reduce appetite and cravings, reflecting a multi-faceted approach to weight management. This antidepressant is often used successfully with smoking cessation, which may have some shared mechanisms that drive continued use, like cravings.

Overall, the history of weight-loss drugs is marked by innovation and caution. While early efforts were often fraught with dangerous side effects, modern drugs will hopefully offer safer and more effective solutions. The evolution from crude metabolic stimulants like DNP to sophisticated hormonal modulators like GLP-1 inhibitors illustrates the progress made in understanding and addressing obesity. However, the quest for a safe and effective weight-loss drug remains ongoing, driven by the complex interplay of biological, psychological, and social factors that contribute to obesity.

BARIATRIC SURGERY

Bariatric surgery includes gastric bypass and other types of weight-loss surgeries that make permanent changes to your digestive system to help you lose weight. It is designed to aid significant weight loss for individuals with extreme obesity and presents both mental health benefits and risks. On the positive side, many patients experience improved psychological wellbeing post-surgery, which is generally a time of substantial weight loss that often leads to enhanced self-esteem, reduced symptoms of depression, and improved quality of life (Dawes et al., 2016). The social stigma associated with obesity diminishes, allowing individuals to engage more confidently in social activities and professional settings. Additionally, the alleviation of obesity-related health issues, such as diabetes and hypertension can reduce stress and anxiety, contributing to a more positive mental state.

However, bariatric surgery is not without its risks, both physical and mental. The sudden dramatic weight loss and reduced ability to absorb and utilize nutrients as a result of the surgery can cause significant nutrient deficiencies that can lead to hair loss, tooth loss, and mental health challenges. The rapid physical changes and lifestyle adjustments required post-surgery can be overwhelming, potentially leading to emotional distress (Kubik et al., 2013). Some patients may experience a "bariatric surgery honeymoon period," followed by disappointment or frustration if weight loss plateaus. There is also the risk of developing or exacerbating eating disorders, as individuals must adhere to strict dietary guidelines, which can trigger unhealthy eating behaviors (Brode & Mitchell, 2019;

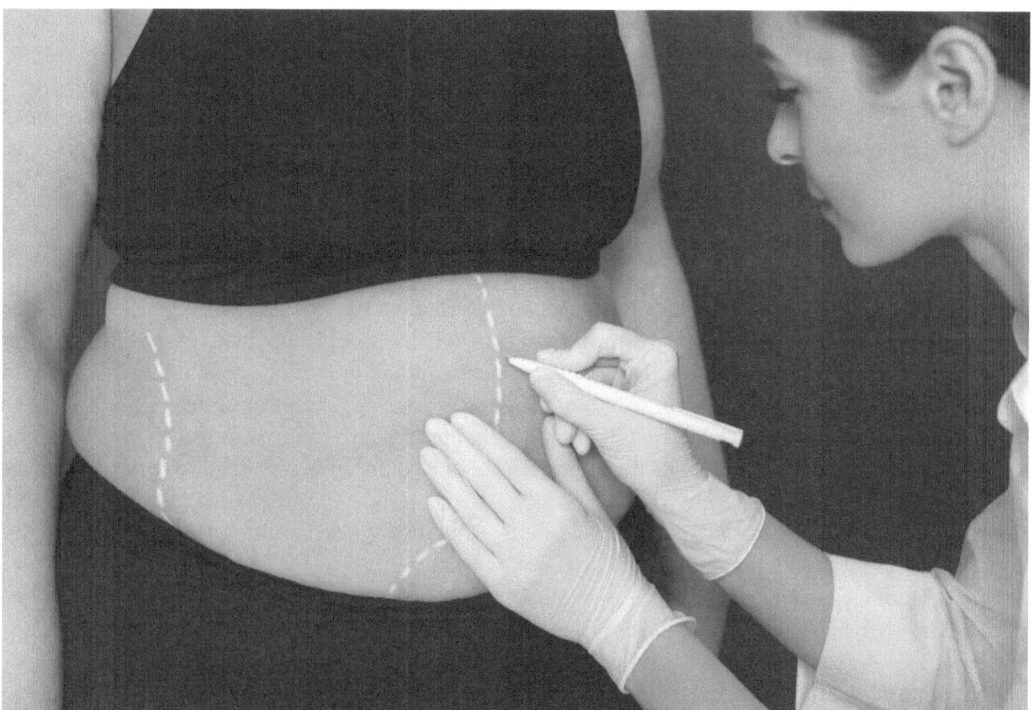

FIGURE 11.2 A doctor preparing a patient for bariatric surgery. Credit: New Africa (Shutterstock).

Conceição et al., 2015). Body image dissatisfaction may persist or even intensify for some, despite significant weight loss. Furthermore, the psychological impact of potential complications or surgical failures can be profound, leading to feelings of regret or guilt.

It is crucial for individuals considering bariatric surgery to undergo a comprehensive psychological evaluation and to receive ongoing mental health support before and after the procedure. Limited research has studied bariatric surgery recipients beyond 6–12 months after the surgery. However, one study that interviewed patients ten years after bariatric surgery found their mental health had worsened significantly compared to pre-operative levels (Canetti et al., 2016). It is important with bariatric surgery to take a holistic approach to care that ensures patients are mentally prepared for the changes and can address any psychological challenges that arise, maximizing the mental health benefits while mitigating the risks.

OBSTACLES TO WEIGHT LOSS

The healthcare field has tried to distill the diet and nutrition industry down to a one-size-fits-all approach, which has never worked. Over the last few years, bio-individuality, set-point theory, and epigenetics have risen to the forefront as a more effective approach to weight loss. As a society, we are gradually moving away from the simplistic "eat less and exercise more" approach to health and moving toward environmental and lifestyle modifications as key components to achieving optimal overall health.

Bio-individuality looks at the whole person and accounts for cultural background, lifestyle factors, genetics, and epigenetics. Each component plays a significant role in determining all-cause morbidity and mortality risk more than BMI. For example, a person struggling with depression that was triggered by a difficult life event has been struggling with poor sleep and increased consumption of caffeine and sweets. They begin using medications to help manage their depressive symptoms. Because of this person's genetic makeup, they are affected by the side effects of those medications including weight gain and nutrient deficiencies, as well as some other small discomforts. The nutrient deficiencies, side effects, and weight gain can also worsen depression symptoms – trapping a person in a cycle of torment. In this case, a holistic weight-loss approach would need to consider the initial drivers of the depression and modify the medication and/or lifestyle factors (e.g., improved nutrition) to better manage the medication side effects and resulting weight gain.

SET-POINT THEORY

Set-point theory is based on the idea that the body maintains a set weight based on our DNA and is hard-wired into the hypothalamus within the brain. The hypothalamus plays many critical roles in the body, including hormone regulation, heart rate and blood pressure regulation, and body temperature regulation, which all work to maintain homeostasis (a state of equilibrium) in the body. The body may experience several pound fluctuations but typically returns to the set-point weight, which is higher for some individuals than it is for others who are the same height. Trying to change our weight to be something either higher or lower than the set-point means we are fighting with the body's determined functional weight and helps account for the fact that most people who lose significant weight eventually gain it back without ongoing rigor.

The set-point changes over the course of our lifetime and can also be altered by life events (e.g., childbirth, medical crisis, menopause). There is some evidence that yo-yo dieting increases the set-point to a higher weight, which is why with traditional low-calorie dieting, people often lose weight and then gain it back plus a few more pounds. Obesity medications help with weight loss but do not appear to change the set-point, so the weight is regained when the medication is discontinued. There is some evidence that bariatric surgery changes the set-point for some people, which may be due to alterations in ghrelin and leptin levels that decrease hunger and increase satiety, although there is a high rate of weight regain over time even with these initial hormone changes (Garvey, 2022).

While all of this sounds like a reliable tool, the set-point theory does come with potential issues. First of all, it cannot explain certain phenomena such as why many college students gain the "Freshman 15," why those who are sedentary tend to gain weight since set-point speaks to the body being able to maintain the weight on its own, those who gain weight after getting in a relationship or getting married, and those who are in lower socioeconomic groups who tend to fall in the obese category.

SLOW BURN, METABOLISM, AND FAD DIETING

For those trying to lose weight, there is no shortage of information online and in bookstores. Some of the information is beneficial, but most leads to confusion. One day we are told that eggs are bad for us and then good for us and, finally, back to being bad again. There is no nutrition and label reading training in school – life skills for which we typically have to do our own research.

The human body is not designed to have dramatic increases and decreases in weight. In fact, the human body is designed to maintain homeostasis – a relatively stable balance of physiological processes. Metabolism is one of these systems within the body that requires homeostasis. The more yo-yo dieting an individual participates in, the greater the movement away from metabolic homeostasis. Fortunately, all is not lost! If you have tried various diets to lose weight or have had drastic changes in weight over a short time, the body can heal. One of the most important things to remember is that healing takes time. We do not typically get to an unhealthy weight overnight; getting back out of it will also take time.

Fad dieting is one sure way to throw the metabolism off. While many popular eating styles are labeled as fad dieting, true fad dieting is more along the lines of the baby food, cabbage, volumetrics, and grapefruit diets. Let us examine each one.

Baby Food Diet	This diet suggests replacing one or two meals daily with baby food. Each jar of baby food contains about 20–100 calories. This diet reduces the number of calories consumed daily and can also lead to multiple nutrient deficiencies since adults need to have higher nutrient concentrations than babies.
Cabbage Soup Diet	This is an extremely low-calorie diet that involves eating only cabbage soup for one week. Unfortunately, this weight loss is going to be mostly water and the weight will come back. Not to mention, when we restrict foods and calories, our bodies will strongly compel us to rebound and eat more food than if we had simply balanced our meals and ate whole, real food to begin with.
Volumetrics Diet	This diet focuses on eating foods that are mostly made of water as the primary food source. While no food is off-limit, it does reduce the consumption of healthy fats, which are essential for mental health and hormonal balance. It is also very calorie focused, can be boring due to eating the same foods, and does not allow for eating out easily.
Grapefruit Diet	This is one of the oldest fad diets out there, having its origins in the 1930s. According to the theory, there is a fat burning enzyme in the grapefruit and by consuming half of a grapefruit with each meal weight loss should occur. What we really see happening is a goal of about 800 calories consumed daily so it is more likely the dramatic calorie reduction than an enzyme.

Society has always placed so much pressure on losing weight and keeping a slim figure that people become desperate. Despite our ongoing obsession with being thin, the U.S. population's adiposity and waist size has increased yearly.

ROLLERCOASTER RIDES AND YO-YO DIETING

Human blood sugar (glucose) levels are designed to stay within a narrow range of stability. When it exceeds or drops below this range, a host of symptoms, from physical to mental and emotional, may occur. Each time we eat simple carbohydrates without fat or protein, they are rapidly digested and enter the bloodstream in a surge. The body responds to this glucose spike with an insulin spike to store extra glucose in the fat cells, which immediately drops glucose levels and increases hunger as the brain demands renewed glucose for fuel. This can create a "glucose rollercoaster" throughout the day as we fluctuate between glucose spikes and rapid drops. These rapid fluctuations caused by eating too many simple carbohydrates for your personal metabolism can make you feel unstable, tired, or anxious, and increase insulin resistance (Ede, 2024).

Walking after a meal can help reduce the glucose rollercoaster ride by reducing the glucose spike after the consumption of simple carbohydrates. When we exercise, even just a 15-minute walk, the muscles use some of the glucose in the bloodstream for energy to power them. Using some of the immediately available glucose right after a meal by moving leaves less glucose in the bloodstream to be cleaned up by a surge of insulin and then stored as fat. It can also reduce the crash that follows a glucose spike, which helps smooth out emotions and energy.

Remember that these symptoms do not often immediately appear, but emerge from years of yo-yo dieting, starvation, and overindulgence. Cohen et al. (2006) demonstrated a 7 percent increase in hyperglycemia (high blood sugar levels) and 14.5 percent increase in type 2 diabetes in those with schizophrenia and schizoaffective disorders. In addition, the psychotropic medications used to treat psychiatric disorders often cause weight and blood sugar fluctuations (Akinola et al., 2023; Haupt & Newcomer, 2001; Liao & Phan, 2014; Lindenmayer et al., 2001). Unfortunately, many individuals are then prescribed a blood sugar-lowering medication to help protect their brains and bodies from the ill effects of elevated blood sugar levels without addressing the other possible negative impacts of the medication, such as constant hunger, weight gain, and the development of other chronic diseases.

WEIGHT AS A REFLECTION OF TRAUMA

There is a connection between experiencing trauma and gaining weight, although the mechanisms are still being explored. One theory is that extra layers of fat provide some cushioning and protection from the outside world, creating both a physical and often emotional barrier that maintains some distance from other people to stay safe (Brewster, 2022). Other theories associated with research about ACEs (adverse childhood experiences) include mechanisms such as disruption of social bonds, early changes in health behaviors (e.g., smoking), a chronic stress response, as well as the social stigma and bullying linked to childhood obesity (Wiss & Brewerton, 2020). Some data suggests that food addiction (see Chapter 13) may be involved in the pathway from trauma to obesity since there is a positive association between childhood trauma and food addiction (Imperatori et al., 2016; Mason et al., 2013).

Food is often viewed as a source of comfort, an entity that is there in your time of need and lacks the ability to judge. When we are having a tough day at work or school, a fight with a loved one, the loss of a relationship, or a resurgence of the darkest feelings within us, food often becomes the one thing we turn to. Food is also that one drug we cannot live without. In this way, it becomes an acceptable addiction hidden in plain sight because we must eat to live. Yet, for those who turn to food for emotional comfort, recognizing that point where food is more than just fuel can be tricky.

OBESITY AND VITAMIN DEFICIENCIES

With the increasing number of individuals facing obesity, it is also important to connect the dots between obesity and vitamin deficiencies. According to a research study conducted in 2019, the study authors noted that those who were obese were also more likely to experience a vitamin D deficiency (Vranic et al., 2019). Vranic et al., continued on to say that the likelihood of vitamin D deficiency may be attributed to its dilution into fat stores, blood, and liver. They also reported that, according to their research, they believed that vitamin D deficiency was partly to blame for the increased body weight. In addition, a 2023 study demonstrated a connection between visceral adiposity (belly fat) and vitamin A deficiency (Goes et al., 2023).

FOOD FOR THOUGHT: HAES AND BODY POSITIVITY

There has been a growing movement around body acceptance, especially for people in larger bodies. The *body positivity movement* has been gaining momentum since it emerged in social media in 2012, where it aimed to confront the unrealistic expectations and portrayals of women in popular media and advertising (Gelsinger, 2021). An important part of this movement has been the *Health at Every Size (HAES)* approach that started in the 1990s. HAES principles include compassionate and comprehensive healthcare regardless of body size, improved community care such as equitable access to food, and actively raising awareness of and reducing anti-fat bias and fatphobia in our communities. The HAES approach promotes shifting from a weight-centered to a weight-neutral approach to healthcare where people of all body sizes are encouraged to practice healthier behaviors without focusing on losing weight (ASDAH, n.d.). The idea is to focus on building pleasurable and sustainable physical activity and eating behaviors that respond to body cues of hunger, satiety, nutritional needs, and pleasure (Dimitrov Ulian et al., 2022).

The weight-loss industry has focused on a one-size-fits-all approach that dictates specific behaviors that are believed to help all people lose weight and improve their health. Moreover, since it is indeed an industry, it has also been an approach that is profitable for the companies who provide and promote these weight-loss health practices, be they pills, exercise plans, or meal programs. Unfortunately, they have not been very successful at actually helping people lose weight and stay healthy long-term. Instead, they are often a source of increased stigma and shame that promote weight gain and poor health behaviors.

Body acceptance has been a fight to stop the culturally sanctioned widespread practice of criticizing people for the shape of their body in the name of good health. For example, someone who carries fat around their hips and thighs and has relatively little visceral fat in their abdomen may be told they need to lose weight but in reality, they are not necessarily at a higher risk of chronic disease even if their BMI falls in the overweight category. We cannot assume poor health based on a person's weight and body shape. If we want to help people be healthier, it is important to shift our focus away from physical appearance and look instead to other markers of health that facilitate a better understanding of how to support and guide individuals to feel their best. Better markers include both physical measures such as blood glucose and blood pressure, as well as psychological measures such as optimism, life satisfaction, and pleasurable activities. Weight loss is often not the first step toward improving health. It is more often the outcome of improved self-esteem and confidence from taking progressively bigger lifestyle enhancing steps to create a life where we can be our best selves.

Body positivity does not mean we close our eyes to the health risks associated with obesity. Many people want to make changes to their body that allows them to have more energy and flexibility. Shaming a person for their current body shape is counterproductive to creating any lasting change. So, we need to start with acceptance and then support people how they prefer so they can create dietary and other lifestyle changes that feel good and honor their individual needs.

REFERENCES

Akinola, P. S., Tardif, I., & Leclerc, J. (2023). Antipsychotic-induced metabolic syndrome: A review. *Metabolic Syndrome and Related Disorders*, *21*(6), 294–305. https://doi.org/10.1089/met.2023.0003

Ambwani, S., Thomas, K. M., Hopwood, C. J., Moss, S. A., & Grilo, C. M. (2014). Obesity stigmatization as the status quo: Structural considerations and prevalence among young adults in the U.S. *Eating Behaviors*, *15*(3), 366–370. https://doi.org/10.1016/j.eatbeh.2014.04.005

ASDAH. (n.d.). *About Health at Every Size® (HAES®)*. Association for Size Diversity and Health. https://asdah.org/haes/

Banas, J., McDowell Cook, A., Raygoza-Cortez, K., Davila, D., Irwin, M. L., Ferrucci, L. M., & Humphries, D. L. (2024). United States long-term trends in adult BMI (1959-2018): Unraveling the roots of the obesity epidemic. *International Journal of Environmental Research and Public Health*, *21*(1). https://doi.org/10.3390/ijerph21010073

Bhaskaran, K., dos-Santos-Silva, I., Leon, D. A., Douglas, I. J., & Smeeth, L. (2018). Association of BMI with overall and cause-specific mortality: A population-based cohort study of 3.6 million adults in the UK. *The Lancet Diabetes & Endocrinology*, *6*(12), 944–953. https://doi.org/10.1016/S2213-8587(18)30288-2

Brewster, K. (2022). *What's eating you? A step-by-step guide to finally take control of your emotional eating*. WestBow Press.

Brode, C. S., & Mitchell, J. E. (2019). Problematic eating behaviors and eating disorders associated with bariatric surgery. *Psychiatric Clinics*, *42*(2), 287–297.

Canetti, L., Bachar, E., & Bonne, O. (2016). Deterioration of mental health in bariatric surgery after 10 years despite successful weight loss. *European Journal of Clinical Nutrition*, *70*(1), 17–22.

CDC. (2022a). *Body mass index (BMI)*. Centers for Disease Control and Prevention. https://www.cdc.gov/bmi/about/?CDC_AAref_Val=https://www.cdc.gov/healthyweight/assessing/bmi/index.html

CDC. (2022b). *BRFSS prevalence & trends data: Overweight and obesity (BMI)*. Center for Disease Control and Prevention. https://nccd.cdc.gov/BRFSSPrevalence/rdPage.aspx?rdReport=DPH_BRFSS.ExploreByTopic&irbLocationType=StatesAndMMSA&islClass=CLASS14&islTopic=TOPIC09&islYear=2020&rdRnd=72140

CDC. (2024a). *Adult obesity facts*. Centers for Disease Control and Prevention. https://www.cdc.gov/obesity/adult-obesity-facts/

CDC. (2024b). *High obesity program*. Centers for Disease Control and Prevention. https://www.cdc.gov/hop/php/about/

Cohen, D., Stolk, R. P., Grobbee, D. E., & Gispen-de Wied, C. C. (2006). Hyperglycemia and diabetes in patients with schizophrenia or schizoaffective disorders. *Diabetes Care*, *29*(4), 786–791. https://doi.org/10.2337/diacare.29.04.06.dc05-1261

Conceição, E. M., Utzinger, L. M., & Pisetsky, E. M. (2015). Eating disorders and problematic eating behaviours before and after bariatric surgery: Characterization, assessment and association with treatment outcomes. *European Eating Disorders Review*, *23*(6), 417–425.

Dawes, A. J., Maggard-Gibbons, M., Maher, A. R., Booth, M. J., Miake-Lye, I., Beroes, J. M., & Shekelle, P. G. (2016). Mental health conditions among patients seeking and undergoing bariatric surgery: A meta-analysis. *The Journal of the American Medical Association*, *315*(2), 150–163.

Dimitrov Ulian, M., Pinto, A., Morais Sato, P., Benatti, F., Lopes de Campos-Ferraz, P., Coelho, D., Roble, O., Sabatini, F., Perez, I., Aburad, L., Vessoni, A., Fernandez Unsain, R., Rogero, M., Sampaio, G., Gualano, B., & Scagliusi, F. (2022). Health At Every Size®-based interventions may improve cardiometabolic risk and quality of life even in the absence of weight loss: An ancillary, exploratory analysis of the health and wellness in obesity study. *Frontiers in Nutrition, 9.* https://doi.org/10.3389/fnut.2022.598920

DiNicolantonio, J. J., Chatterjee, S., O'Keefe, J. H., & Meier, P. (2014). Lorcaserin for the treatment of obesity? A closer look at its side effects. In (Vol. 1, p. e000173): Archives of Disease in childhood.

Ede, G. (2024). *Change your diet, change your mind: a powerful plan to improve mood, overcome anxiety, and protect memory for a lifetime of optimal mental health* (1st ed.). Balance.

Everson-Rose, S. A., Lewis, T. T., Karavolos, K., Dugan, S. A., Wesley, D., & Powell, L. H. (2009). Depressive symptoms and increased visceral fat in middle-aged women. *Psychosomatic Medicine, 71*(4), 410–416. https://doi.org/10.1097/PSY.0b013e3181a20c9c

Flegal, K., Kit, B., Orpana, H., & Graubard, B. (2013). Association of All-Cause Mortality With Overweight and Obesity Using Standard Body Mass Index Categories. *JAMA: The Journal of the American Medical Association, 309*(1), 71–82. https://doi.org/10.1001/jama.2012.113905

Fryar, C. D., Carroll, M. D., & Afful, J. (2020). *Prevalence of overweight, obesity, and severe obesity among children and adolescents aged 2–19 years: United States, 1963–1965 through 2017–2018. NCHS Health E-Stats.* National Center for Health Statistics. https://www.cdc.gov/nchs/data/hestat/obesity-child-17-18/obesity-child.htm

Fryar, C. D., Carroll, M. D., & Ogden, C. L. (2018). *Prevalence of overweight, obesity, and severe obesity among adults aged 20 and over: United States, 1960–1962 through 2015–2016. NCHS Health E-Stats.* National Center for Health Statistics. https://stacks.cdc.gov/view/cdc/58670

Frysh, P., & Morgan, K. K. (2024). *Visceral fat: What is it?* Nourish by WebMD. Retrieved January 29, 2025 from https://www.webmd.com/diet/what-is-visceral-fat

Garvey, W. T. (2022). Is obesity or adiposity-based chronic disease curable: The set point theory, the environment, and second-generation medications. *Endocrine Practice, 28*(2), 214–222. https://doi.org/10.1016/j.eprac.2021.11.082

Gelsinger, A. S. (2021). A critical analysis of the body positive movement on Instagram: How does it really impact body image? *Spectra Undergraduate Research Journal, 1*(1), 4.

Goes, E., Cordeiro, A., Bento, C., & Ramalho, A. (2023). Vitamin A deficiency and its association with visceral adiposity in women. *Biomedicines, 11*(3). https://doi.org/10.3390/biomedicines11030991

Greenway, F., Shanahan, W., Fain, R., Ma, T., & Rubino, D. (2016). Safety and tolerability review of lorcaserin in clinical trials. *Clinical Obesity, 6*(5), 285–295.

Grundlingh, J., Dargan, P. I., El-Zanfaly, M., & Wood, D. M. (2011). 2, 4-Dinitrophenol (DNP): A weight loss agent with significant acute toxicity and risk of death. *Journal of Medical Toxicology, 7*, 205–212.

Guarino, A. H. (2005). Treatment of intractable constipation with orlistat: A report of three cases. *Pain Medicine, 6*(4), 327–328.

Haupt, D. W., & Newcomer, J. W. (2001). Hyperglycemia and antipsychotic medications. *Journal of Clinical Psychiatry, 62*(Suppl 27), 15–26; discussion 40–11. https://www.ncbi.nlm.nih.gov/pubmed/11806485

Heindel, J. J., Alvarez, J. A., Atlas, E., Cave, M. C., Chatzi, V. L., Collier, D., Corkey, B., Fischer, D., Goran, M. I., Howard, S., Kahan, S., Kayhoe, M., Koliwad, S., Kotz, C. M., La Merrill, M., Lobstein, T., Lumeng, C., Ludwig, D. S., Lustig, R. H., & Blumberg, B. (2023). Obesogens and obesity: State-of-the-science and future directions summary from a healthy environment and endocrine disruptors strategies workshop. *American Journal of Clinical Nutrition, 118*(1), 329–337. https://doi.org/10.1016/j.ajcnut.2023.05.024

Imperatori, C., Innamorati, M., Lamis, D., Farina, B., Pompili, M., Contardi, A., & Fabbricatore, M. (2016). Childhood trauma in obese and overweight women with food addiction and clinical-level of binge eating. *Child Abuse & Neglect, 58*, 180–190. https://doi.org/10.1016/j.chiabu.2016.06.023

Karczewski, J., Sledzinska, E., Baturo, A., Jonczyk, I., Maleszko, A., Samborski, P., Begier-Krasinska, B., & Dobrowolska, A. (2018). Obesity and inflammation. *European Cytokine Network, 29*(3), 83–94. https://doi.org/10.1684/ecn.2018.0415

Kim, S. Y., Yoo, D. M., Kwon, M. J., Kim, J. H., Kim, J. H., Bang, W. J., & Choi, H. G. (2022). Differences in nutritional intake, total body fat, and BMI score between twins. *Nutrients, 14*(17). https://doi.org/10.3390/nu14173655

Kubik, J. F., Gill, R. S., Laffin, M., & Karmali, S. (2013). The impact of bariatric surgery on psychological health. *Journal of Obesity, 2013*(1), 837989.

Liao, T. V., & Phan, S. V. (2014). Acute hyperglycemia associated with short-term use of atypical antipsychotic medications. *Drugs, 74*(2), 183–194. https://doi.org/10.1007/s40265-013-0171-7

Lindenmayer, J. P., Nathan, A. M., & Smith, R. C. (2001). Hyperglycemia associated with the use of atypical antipsychotics. *Journal of Clinical Psychiatry*, *62*(Suppl 23), 30–38. https://www.ncbi.nlm.nih.gov/pubmed/11603883

Mason, S., Flint, A., Field, A., Austin, S. B., & Rich-Edwards, J. (2013). Abuse victimization in childhood or adolescence and risk of food addiction in adult women. *Obesity*, *21*(12), undefined-undefined. https://doi.org/10.1002/oby.20500

Neel, J. V. (1962). Diabetes mellitus - A "thrifty" genotype rendered detrimental by "progress"? *American Journal of Human Genetics*, *14*(4), 353–362.

NIH. (2018). *Prevalence of overweight and obesity*. https://www.niddk.nih.gov/health-information/health-statistics/overweight-obesity#:~:text=the%20above%20table-,Nearly%201%20in%203%20adults%20(30.7%25)%20are%20overweight.,9.2%25)%20have%20severe%20obesity.

Rasmussen, N. (2015). Amphetamine-type stimulants: The early history of their medical and non-medical uses. *International Review of Neurobiology*, *120*, 9–25.

Reddon, H., Patel, Y., Turcotte, M., Pigeyre, M., & Meyre, D. (2018). Revisiting the evolutionary origins of obesity: Lazy versus peppy-thrifty genotype hypothesis. *Obesity Reviews*, *19*(11), 1525–1543. https://doi.org/10.1111/obr.12742

Research and Markets. (2024). *The U.S. weight loss market: 2024 status report & forecast*. https://www.researchandmarkets.com/report/united-states-weight-loss-industry-market?utm_code=fc8z39&utm_exec=elco286prd

Smits, M. M., & Van Raalte, D. H. (2021). Safety of semaglutide. *Frontiers in Endocrinology*, *12*, 645563.

Tanamas, S. K., Ng, W. L., Backholer, K., Hodge, A., Zimmet, P. Z., & Peeters, A. (2016). Quantifying the proportion of deaths due to body mass index- and waist circumference-defined obesity. *Obesity*, *24*(3), 735–742. https://doi.org/10.1002/oby.21386

The Global BMI Mortality Collaboration. (2016). Body-mass index and all-cause mortality: individual-participant-data meta-analysis of 239 prospective studies in four continents. *The Lancet*, *388*(10046), 776–786. https://doi.org/10.1016/S0140-6736(16)30175-1

Vranic, L., Mikolasevic, I., & Milic, S. (2019). Vitamin D deficiency: Consequence or cause of obesity? *Medicina*, *55*(9), 541. https://doi.org/10.3390/medicina55090541

Wadden, T. A., Berkowitz, R. I., Silvestry, F., Vogt, R. A., Sutton, M. G. S. J., Stunkard, A. J., Foster, G. D., & Aber, J. L. (1998). The Fen-Phen finale: A study of weight loss and valvular heart disease. *Obesity Research*, *6*(4), 278–284.

Westbury, S., Oyebode, O., van Rens, T., & Barber, T. M. (2023). Obesity stigma: Causes, consequences, and potential solutions. *Current Obesity Reports*, *12*(1), 10–23. https://doi.org/10.1007/s13679-023-00495-3

WHO Global InfoBase Team. (2005). *The SuRF report 2. Surveillance of chronic disease risk factors: Country-level data and comparable estimates*. World Health Organization. https://apps.who.int/iris/bitstream/handle/10665/43190/9241593024_eng.pdf?sequence=1&ua=1

Wilding, J. P. H., Batterham, R. L., Davies, M., Van Gaal, L. F., Kandler, K., Konakli, K., Lingvay, I., McGowan, B. M., Oral, T. K., Rosenstock, J., Wadden, T. A., Wharton, S., Yokote, K., Kushner, R. F., & Group, S. S. (2022). Weight regain and cardiometabolic effects after withdrawal of semaglutide: The STEP 1 trial extension. *Diabetes, Obesity and Metabolism*, *24*(8), 1553–1564. https://doi.org/10.1111/dom.14725

Wiss, D. A., & Brewerton, T. D. (2020). Adverse childhood experiences and adult obesity: A systematic review of plausible mechanisms and meta-analysis of cross-sectional studies. *Physiology & Behavior*, *223*, 112964. https://doi.org/10.1016/j.physbeh.2020.112964

Wood, L. (2022). Overview of the $58 billion U.S. weight loss market 2022. *Globe Newswire Research and Markets*. https://www.globenewswire.com/en/news-release/2022/03/23/2408315/28124/en/Overview-of-the-58-Billion-U-S-Weight-Loss-Market-2022.html

Zatterale, F., Raciti, G. A., Prevenzano, I., Leone, A., Campitelli, M., De Rosa, V., Beguinot, F., & Parrillo, L. (2022). Epigenetic reprogramming of the inflammatory response in obesity and type 2 diabetes. *Biomolecules*, *12*(7). https://doi.org/10.3390/biom12070982

12 Eating Disorders

The DSM characterizes an *Eating Disorder (ED)* as having a persistent disturbance of eating-related behaviors that results in distorted food consumption and significantly impairs physical health and/or social functioning (American Psychiatric Association, 2022). Obesity is not included as a mental disorder since there are a range of genetic, physiological, behavioral, and environmental factors that contribute to obesity.

EDs include symptoms that reflect the Four Ds of psychopathology discussed in Chapter 1, deviance, dysfunction, distress, and danger. For example, a person with a restrictive ED such as anorexia (discussed below) may eat far fewer calories compared to the general population (deviance) often associated with intense fear around gaining weight (distress), so much that they are frequently unable to attend to or participate in daily activities and events (dysfunction), and perhaps even fail to consume enough food to fuel basic functioning for the body's survival (danger).

EDs are mental health conditions that can significantly harm an individual's psychological, physical, and emotional wellbeing. They are dangerous in their ability to cause physical harm, even though they often are met with approval or praise from others for losing weight or meeting certain physical standards, such as those body types preferred in modeling, ballet, or gymnastics. They can lead to organ damage due to malnutrition or on the other end of the spectrum, cardiovascular disease due to weight gain and obesity. Some clinicians include EDs as a form of non-suicidal self-harm like cutting and hair pulling, which recognizes that people experiencing an ED may be in quiet distress and at a higher risk for other forms of self-injury.

As discussed in Chapter 2, there are advantages and disadvantages to the process of using the DSM to diagnose a psychiatric illness, including EDs. For example, individuals with an ED may find comfort in their diagnosis to help understand the powerful thoughts and behaviors associated with their ED. It can help them understand what is driving their behavior and why they are drawn to, even compelled to continue them even though these actions can cause self-harm. However, the rigidity of defining and diagnosing EDs may lead to trouble for some individuals, since many people meet at least some criteria for multiple EDs or meet criteria for more than one ED at different times in their lives. This can limit their access to treatment if their symptoms do not fully match the diagnostic criteria for a specific disorder.

THE BIG THREE EATING DISORDERS

While there are a variety of ED differences for children and adults, this chapter only focuses on the three most commonly diagnosed EDs: anorexia nervosa, bulimia nervosa, and binge-eating disorder.

ANOREXIA NERVOSA

Anorexia nervosa (AN), referred to as anorexia, is an ED in the DSM characterized by a distorted body image and excessive dieting that often leads to severe weight loss with a pathological fear of becoming fat. The diagnostic criteria for AN include caloric restriction, low body weight, intense fear of gaining weight or becoming fat, preoccupation with physical appearance, and distorted self-evaluation of body weight (American Psychiatric Association, 2022). It is also common for these individuals to experience isolation, a preoccupation with food and dieting, and use of exercise as a compensatory behavior for eating even normal amounts of food (Eating Recovery Center, 2024a).

Restrictive EDs such as AN often focus on maintaining control in an environment that feels chaotic or unpredictable. In her book *Eating Disorders: Decode the Controlled Chaos*, author Erica

DOI: 10.1201/9781032647647-17

Ives, an ED specialist, reveals EDs as an attempt to adapt and cope when the sufferer feels they have few, if any, other options to manage their world. While EDs can provide short-term comfort, ultimately, they end up causing harm. "The sufferer seeks control through food, but the truth of the matter is that the food is actually controlling them, and they are therefore 'losing control.'" As the disorder progresses, a person becomes more disconnected from "their voice, their story, their thoughts, and their feelings" (Ives, 2013, pp. 2–3).

Starvation places tremendous pressure on the body, which makes AN a particularly dangerous mental health disorder. There are numerous health risks and medical consequences associated with AN including: low blood pressure, slow resting heart rate (bradycardia), fatigue, dizziness, the absence of menstruation (amenorrhea), hair loss, dehydration, disruption to the gastrointestinal system (e.g., bloating and constipation), damage to bones (osteoporosis), seizures, blood problems (anemia), infertility, and heart disease. AN also significantly increases a person's risk of suicide. A person with AN is almost 3 times more likely to attempt suicide, and 18 times more likely to die by suicide than a comparable group in the general population (Smith et al., 2018).

While the start of AN symptoms can vary widely by individual, research suggests that the median age of onset of significant and challenging behaviors is 18 years old (NIMH, 2023; Volpe et al., 2016). Even before it is a full-blown mental health disorder, many children display early warning signs. When surveyed, a large portion of elementary school-aged children claimed a desire to be thinner and/or reported engaging in disordered eating behavior such as not eating for fear of gaining weight (Martin, 2010). This includes children from a wide range of communities.

Early warning signs for AN include a preoccupation with food, such as continually trying new diets and distinguishing foods as "good" and "bad," known as dichotomous thinking toward food. Other signs are unusual eating behaviors and food rituals, such as spreading food around the plate to create the perception that they have eaten more food. Spitting out chewed food without swallowing, cutting food into tiny pieces (microtearing), and taking very little bites of food (micobiting) are also

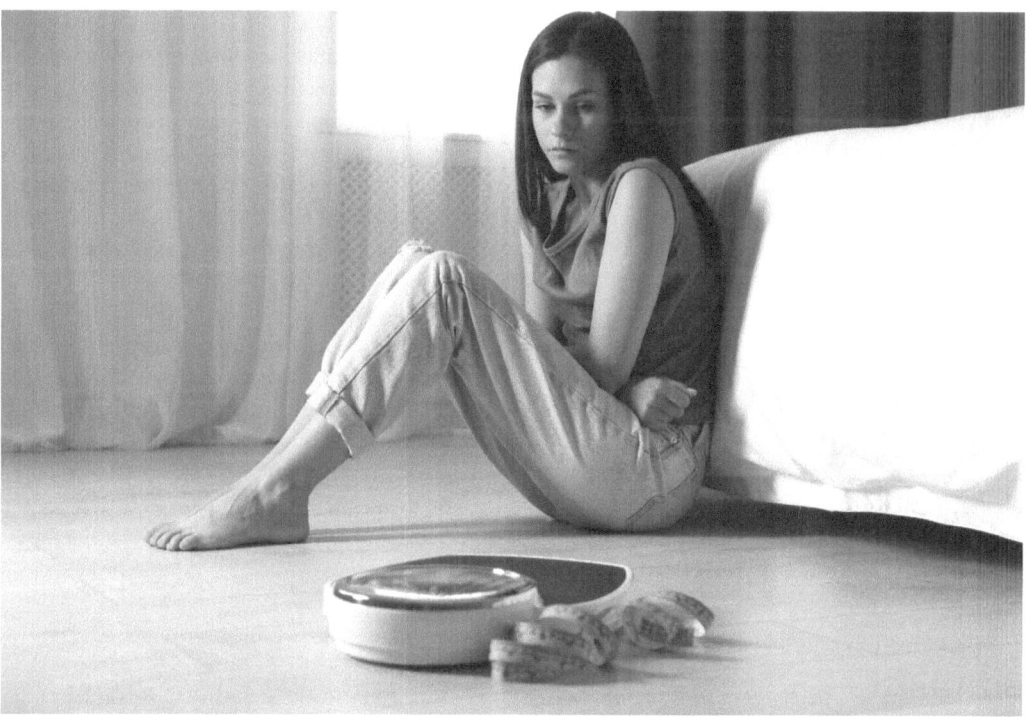

FIGURE 12.1 Preoccupation with weight. Credit: New Africa (Shutterstock).

common behaviors to avoid actually consuming food. A preoccupation with weight, body shape, and appearance is also a warning sign, with behaviors such as constantly looking in the mirror or pinching or measuring parts of the body (body checking), weighing oneself, and negatively comparing oneself to others (Ives, 2013).

The DSM describes two types of anorexia: *anorexia nervosa restricting type (AN-R)* and *anorexia nervosa binge-eating/purging type (AN-B/P)*. Both AN-R and AN-B/P include the attributes described above, can span a range in their degree of severity and functional disability, and are characterized by weight loss primarily through dieting, fasting, and/or excessive exercise. What differentiates them is the purging or compensatory behaviors associated with AN-B/P, including self-induced vomiting, and/or the misuse of laxatives, diuretics, or enemas. These compensatory behaviors can be performed with or without being preceded by a binge-eating episode, and often follow eating a regularly portioned meal. The driver behind the behavior is not the quantity of food eaten as much as the emotional need to regain a sense of control around what they believe impacts body weight or shape (American Psychiatric Association, 2022). While AN-B/P has bingeing and/or purging symptoms similar to bulimia nervosa, there are a few key differences which are discussed below.

Bulimia Nervosa

Bulimia nervosa (BN), referred to here as bulimia, is characterized by at least weekly binge-eating episodes followed by compensatory behaviors. A binge-eating episode is eating a large amount of food in a short period of time (e.g., within a two-hour period) and feeling a lack of control around eating. Episodes of bingeing often begin during plating food where large quantities of food are served piled high or spread across larger plates, or even during planning for a binge before the food is present or available. Similar to AN-B/P, compensatory behaviors associated with BN are recurrent and unhealthy attempts to prevent weight gain including self-induced vomiting, compulsive exercise, and misuse of laxatives, diuretics or other medications (American Psychiatric Association, 2022). BN also includes an excessive focus on body shape and weight as the primary measure applied to evaluating self-worth.

The major difference between AN-B/P and BN is low body weight. People diagnosed with both types of AN fall within the BMI-classified underweight category, whereas those with BN are generally in the healthy to overweight BMI category (Federici, 2021). What they have in common is the act of bingeing as a coping mechanism in response to stress as an attempt to feel more relaxed or by numbing themselves by doing something momentarily pleasurable. Unfortunately, that pleasurable feeling is short-lived and the person goes from feeling pleasure and relief to feeling out of control, ashamed, and desperate to feel in control again, which is what drives the compensatory purging behavior (Kelvas, 2023).

Similar to AN, the median age of onset for BN is 21 years old. Also similar is that BN is associated with health risks and medical consequences. Nutritional deficiencies and disrupted function of the digestive system from compensatory behaviors such as induced vomiting over time lead to symptoms such as bradycardia, low blood pressure, tooth decay and discoloration, throat inflammation, face swelling, or more immediately to electrolyte imbalances, dehydration, water retention (edema), constipation, and fatigue, and then at an advanced stage to stomach ulcers and ruptured stomach lining (NIMH, n.d.). Although AN is found to be the deadliest ED to date as a result of the body's inability to sustain itself during starvation, BN also deserves caution due to the tremendous trauma to the body at every level and with increasing severity.

Binge-Eating Disorder

The DSM added the *binge-eating disorder (BED)* classification in 2013 in the DSM-5. BED has since become recognized as the most common ED in the United States (Galmiche et al., 2019). Diagnostic criteria for BED include at least weekly binge-eating episodes associated with rapid

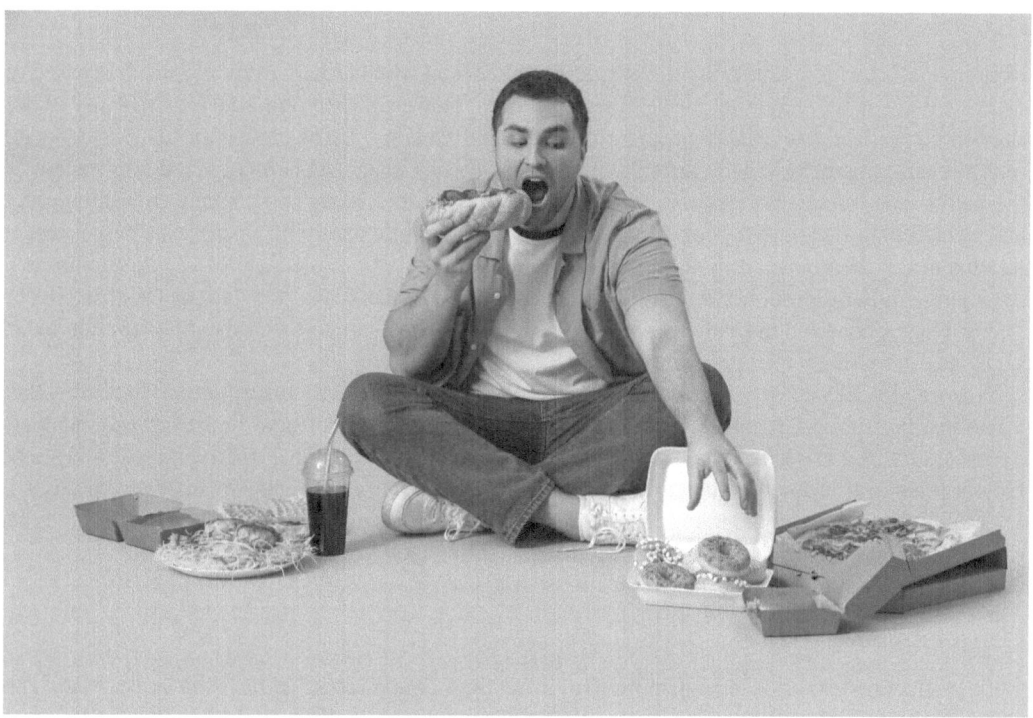

FIGURE 12.2 Binge eating. Credit: Pixel-Shot (Shutterstock).

eating, feeling out of control before and during eating, intense feelings of distress, eating beyond fullness, eating without hunger, eating in secret due to shame, and feelings of self-loathing and guilt following food consumption (American Psychiatric Association, 2013).

Again, there are similarities between BED, AN, and BN in that symptoms are most likely to start when a person is a young adult (average BED onset is 21 years old) and can lead to significant and severe medical problems. Common medical risks associated with BED include stomach and intestinal perforation, insomnia, gout, weight gain, heart disease, high cholesterol, and type II diabetes (Ekern, 2023). In addition, since there is tremendous stigma around binge eating and weight gain, a person with BED is at a heightened risk of facing discrimination, especially if they are in a larger body. Weight stigma makes diagnosis and access to treatment challenging as the ED and its associated symptoms are often neglected by the healthcare system and misdiagnosed as an obesity issue without understanding the significant psychological underpinnings that can be related to weight gain. Unlike individuals with EDs who are viewed as underweight or normal weight, when those with BED and its associated weight gain meet with a medical professional, the provider is more likely to recommend dieting and maybe seeing a nutritionist rather than recognizing that the person is struggling with a mental health disorder and making a referral to an evidence-based ED treatment program (Chastain, 2023).

PREVALENCE OF EATING DISORDERS

At least 9 percent (nearly 29 million) of Americans will have an ED at some time in their life (ANAD, 2024). On an annual basis, that means, for example, that in 2019, around 2 percent of the U.S. population – almost 5.5 million people – experienced an ED. In order of frequency of diagnosis, BED is the most common, followed by AN, and then BN (Davison & Adams, 2024; Gerhardt, 2024).

DEMOGRAPHICS

Research tells us there are racial and ethnic differences in who is likely to develop an ED based on examinations of ED diagnoses in healthcare records. However, there are concerns that the data is skewed by the fact that Caucasians are more frequently recognized as having an ED than a person in a minority population. This difference impacts whether their ED is recognized and treated by the healthcare system. For example, Caucasian people with AN are more likely to be diagnosed and treated than Indigenous people and people of color. While receiving a diagnosis and access to treatment may be impacted by a person's race and ethnicity, the trajectory of ED development is not significantly different between White, Hispanic, Asian, and Black populations (Within Health, 2023). Thus, Caucasian individuals are more likely to seek and receive treatment but are not necessarily any more likely to experience an ED.

Historically, EDs have been associated with SWAG (skinny, white, affluent girls). In reality, they affect people from all demographics, are prevalent among people of both high and low socioeconomic status, and arise from a combination of biological, psychological, interpersonal, and social factors (Gerhardt, 2024). Statistically, females are more likely than males to suffer from any ED (NIMH, n.d.), and transgender and other LGBTQIA+ identities are also at heightened risk for experiencing disordered eating, EDs, and body dissatisfaction (ANAD, 2024; Davison & Adams, 2024).

COLLEGE STUDENTS

College students experience higher rates of EDs than similar-aged adults who are not students (ANAD, 2024; Eating Recovery Center, 2024c; Gerhardt, 2024; Within Health, 2023). Although EDs can develop or return throughout the lifespan, people between the ages of 18 and 21 are especially susceptible. The transition to college comes as a culture shock for some people and is a stressful milestone in one's life, complete with newfound independence, change in structure, social pressures, campus food culture, and access to drugs, alcohol, sexual experimentation, and social events. Thus, it does not come as a surprise that 28 percent of college students screened positive for an ED, especially among younger, female, and Hispanic students, and the numbers are going up. The Healthy Minds Study examined trends in ED risk among U.S. college undergraduate and graduate students and found the prevalence of EDs increased from 15 percent to 28 percent from 2013 to 2021 (Daly & Costigan, 2022) and that ED rates were higher for students who self-identified as having a lower family socioeconomic status, Latinx, bisexual, and lesbian (Burke et al., 2022).

Disordered eating is culturally normalized and remains rampant on college campuses. For example, students may regard food as a reward for completing assignments attached to being such a dedicated student as shown by "not having enough time to eat," rather than seeing food as a necessary daily requirement to maintain their energy and health. Food restriction can stem from perfectionistic attitudes and mask itself as prioritizing work over other needs in order to appear perfect, and therefore worthy. Compounded with that may be the desire to gain a sense of control when they are feeling chaotic and surrounded by competing priorities and social and academic pressures. There is often peer pressure for both eating too little and eating too much, especially when it is combined with dating culture, drinking alcohol, and partaking of cannabis. The high pressure of college life causes many students to struggle with mood issues like depression and anxiety that can be exacerbated by irregular eating habits and can spiral into an ED (Li et al., 2022).

OTHER MENTAL HEALTH CONDITIONS

EDs are highly comorbid with other mental health disorders. For example, nearly 60 percent of those with AN have a comorbid psychiatric disorder, most often an anxiety disorder. Obsessive-compulsive disorder (OCD) is also common among people with AN, which is not surprising since they share an underlying motivation to control uncomfortable emotions by performing dysfunctional behaviors. BN and BED are also commonly diagnosed alongside other mental health disorders. Over 80 percent of people with BN and BED have been diagnosed with a comorbid disorder, most often an anxiety disorder (NIMH, n.d.).

EDs impact many aspects of an individual's life. When a person engages in some of the intense symptoms of an ED, such as secretive-induced vomiting, it creates tremendous strain on inter-personal relationships. In addition, many people with EDs struggle to manage their emotions and experience big highs and lows that feel chaotic and out of control (known as emotion dysregulation). This dysregulation contributes to extreme behaviors and ineffective coping strategies, such as binge eating, in an attempt to relieve their anxiety and gain a sense of control. Their inability to manage their emotions and feelings of overwhelm impedes their ability and desire to engage socially and to seek out or accept support from others (Ekern, 2023).

MORTALITY AND EATING DISORDERS

The National Association of Anorexia and Associated Disorders (ANAD) makes the bold statement that "eating disorders are among the deadliest mental illnesses," only second behind opioid addiction (ANAD, 2024). The organization also states on its website that "10,200 deaths each year are the direct result of an eating disorder – that's one death every 52 minutes." These deaths are due to both the physical damage caused by both restrictive and binge eating disorders, as well as the result of suicide, as people with any ED are at an increased risk for suicidality (Kelvas, 2023).

AN has the highest mortality rate of any mental illness and alone annually kills nearly 3000 people as the result of malnutrition, medical complications, and suicide (Gerhardt, 2024). One in five of those deaths is a direct result of suicide, which is a rate 18 times higher than the general population (Harold, 2023; Hudson et al., 2007). Malnutrition causes tremendous physical damage, including organ failure (e.g., cardiac arrest known commonly as a heart attack) and changes in brain structure that impair cognitions (the ability to think clearly) and dysregulate neurotransmitter function (which impacts emotion regulation) (Curzio et al., 2020). These changes can decrease the brain's reward center process, which makes it harder to feel good and may help explain the correlation between restrictive EDs and suicidality.

Suicidality and medical complications are not limited to AN. Suicidal behavior remains frequent across the BN and BED populations as well (Conti et al., 2017). People struggling with BN are seven times more likely to die by suicide than the general population (Smith et al., 2018). Heart failure as a result of electrolyte imbalance and dehydration due to severe purging behaviors is also a risk for individuals with BN (Kelvas, 2023). Risk of a gastric (stomach) rupture due to eating extremely large quantities of food in a short period (a binge) has been associated with the frequent binge-eating episodes that are a part of BN and BED (Youm et al., 2015).

Please remember that if you or someone you know is having frequent thoughts about suicide, help is available, and it is possible to feel better with the appropriate care. Feeling suicidal is a treatable condition for most people. It is important to ask for help. The National Suicide Prevention Lifeline is available in the U.S. at 1-800-273-8255 or you can dial the 988 Suicide & Crisis Lifeline for free and confidential crisis support 24/7/365.

THE FORGOTTEN NERVOSA: ORTHOREXIA

Orthorexia nervosa, or orthorexia, a term coined in 1996 by Steven Bratman, centers around an obsessive focus on eating healthy food (Mahoney, 2021). Stemming from the Greek word *orthos* which describes moral or ethical correctness, orthorexia has come to mean "righteous eating." Healthy eating becomes a way to achieve a positive sense of self through "pure" or "clean" living. Eating and exercise often become regimens with strict rules that must be adhered to to avoid facing intense feelings of fear and shame. Self-worth can become attached to a self-righteous dedication to eating correctly that becomes rigid and isolating.

Although ED professionals identify orthorexia as a form of disordered eating that can be as debilitating as any other classified ED, the American Psychiatric Association has yet to include orthorexia as a recognized ED diagnosis in the DSM. The inability to diagnose clients with this condition means treatment is often not reimbursed by insurance, which creates barriers to people accessing treatment for orthorexia. Currently, groups of ED professionals have proposed potential criteria for the diagnosis of orthorexia, including a fixation on limiting food variety to what an individual considers "clean" or "healthy" that results in serious physical and/or psychological complications, impaired functioning, and clinically significant distress (Bhattacharya et al., 2022).

ATYPICAL ANOREXIA

A cultural myth is that people in larger bodies do not suffer from restrictive EDs simply based on the size of their bodies. When we think of AN and BN, we imagine underweight bodies. However, the National Eating Disorder Association (NEDA) debunks this belief, and notes that "most people with an eating disorder are not underweight…[and] you can't tell whether someone has an eating disorder just by looking at them" (NEDA, n.d.-a). This myth is often perpetuated in the AN research, which generally focuses on smaller bodies to stay in alignment with the requirement that a person must be underweight to meet the diagnostic criteria for AN as currently described in the DSM (Hazzard et al., 2020). Thus, a DSM ED diagnosis is at times a poor fit when assessing someone's relationship with food and body. For example, people in larger bodies are often overlooked as ED patients and mistakenly seen as someone who needs to try harder and care more so that they can lose weight.

Atypical anorexia nervosa falls under the DSM ED subcategory *other specified feeding or eating disorders (OSFED)*. The primary difference between AN and atypical anorexia concerns body weight. People diagnosed with AN must meet the diagnostic criteria of being underweight (a BMI of 17 or less), whereas people diagnosed with atypical anorexia can have a BMI score ranging from 18.5 to 30 showing they are normal weight, overweight, or obese. Except for weight categorization, atypical anorexia shares identical symptomatology and harm as AN, including fatality and other serious medical complications due to the disorder and its associated behaviors. In fact, 25–40 percent of patients in inpatient ED treatment centers have atypical anorexia (Harrop et al., 2021). Yet, because people diagnosed with atypical anorexia are not categorized as underweight, they are not as likely to receive treatment as those diagnosed with AN (Eating Recovery Center, 2024b).

RESEARCH LIMITATIONS

Cultural stigma about EDs often distorts our ability to understand the population that struggles with the scope of these symptoms. For example, much of our current research notes a significant disparity between genders and indicates that women are much more likely than men to suffer from an ED. However, often women are the predominant participants of these studies, with men making up a significantly smaller proportion of the research participant population, thereby skewing the data toward women (Ulfvebrand et al., 2015).

This conclusion is also drawn from cultural gender roles and expectations, such as the concept of toxic masculinity. This view of masculinity contributes to an unwillingness to acknowledge the presence of an ED because it is seen as a sign of weakness and unmanliness, and because EDs are seen as a women's disease (ED Hope, 2024). In contrast, women often receive praise for their control around food that results in thinness and who are considered more socially acceptable recipients of an ED diagnosis. This disconnect supports the myth narrative that men do not suffer from EDs.

Additionally, this research scope is often limited to a binary gender lens by primarily including people who identify as either men or women, and excluding the transgender and non-binary gender populations (Heiden-Rootes et al., 2023). However, as discussed in earlier sections of this chapter, other gender identities, including transgender individuals, have a heightened risk for ED development, yet the transgender population remains underrepresented in current research (ANAD, 2024; Davison & Adams, 2024).

Recently, people in the ED field have called for further investigation of the etiology and development of EDs to better understand these fatal illnesses (Halbeisen et al., 2022). The majority of the research has focused on AN, BN, and BED, which has led to a lack of awareness and understanding of other EDs. For example, the DSM-5 also identifies avoidant restrictive food intake disorder (ARFID), OSFED, pica, and rumination syndrome as EDs, yet research on these EDs remains limited.

CONTRIBUTORY FACTORS FOR EATING DISORDER DEVELOPMENT

ED development is associated with a range of risk factors, including biological, psychological, social, and cultural. There are no known "causes" of EDs. There are, however, multiple known factors that appear to correlate with the onset of an ED (Hilbert et al., 2014).

BIOLOGICAL

Genetic predisposition is one of the key biological risk factors for the development of any ED. A person is at higher risk if they have a biological parent or sibling who has been diagnosed with an ED, demonstrates ongoing efforts to control their weight (such as through constant dieting), or intentionally consumes insufficient calories to sustain a healthy body (NEDA, n.d.-b). Other risk factors include childhood obesity and early puberty.

PSYCHOLOGICAL

Known psychological risk factors associated with EDs include perfectionism, body dissatisfaction, a comorbid mental health diagnosis, and rigidity in rule-following. Low self-esteem is a common thread among all EDs and includes characteristics such as negative mood, poor body image, feeling inadequate, withdrawal from social situations, and unrealistically high expectations. Certain personality traits can make an individual more vulnerable to an ED, such as having an intense response to emotional stimuli and a slow return to emotional baseline once emotionally aroused. This natural sensitivity can be exacerbated by abuse, trauma, and teasing, which can lead to impairment of the ability to identify and appropriately communicate about emotions (Ives, 2013).

The experience of trauma is significantly correlated with the development of EDs. Upwards of 40 percent of people diagnosed with an ED have experienced a traumatic event. A history of trauma may lead to more intense ED symptoms, such as greater frequency of binging and purging cycles compared to people with no trauma history (Vidaña et al., 2020).

EDs are recognized as ineffective and maladaptive coping strategies associated with avoidance of difficult emotions (Mahoney, 2021). There are clear correlations between individuals with a trauma history and development of a mental health disorder (e.g., depression, PTSD, or anxiety), which then increases the risk of also developing an ED. In particular, sexual trauma is commonly associated as a risk factor preceding the onset of an ED. Experiences of sexual violence can foster a disconnection between self and body, suppression of negative emotions, and the drive to control one's physical space to feel safe, which can manifest as ED symptomology.

DISORDERED EATING

Disordered eating describes a wide range of food encounters and eating behaviors that negatively affect a person's physical and emotional wellbeing. These include cutting out entire food groups without a medical reason, acting on feeling out of control at times with food such as in binge eating, feeling guilt and disgust around eating, following strict food rules, and a preoccupation with food. Many people live with one or more of these behaviors, and while they can be uncomfortable at times, they are understood and defined as disordered unless and until they are life-threatening or impair a person's ability to function. However, disordered eating does put a person at a higher risk of developing the more intense and life-altering symptoms associated with an ED.

Healthy or non-disordered eating is when one mindfully consumes food when they are hungry, stops eating when they feel full, and incorporates variety into their diet. In contrast, disordered eating takes the form of an unhealthy relationship with food. For many, this looks like yoyo dieting where there are periods of restrictive eating (e.g., low calorie or low carb) followed by periods of being "off my diet" where a broader range of foods are eaten, including "forbidden foods" and cheat days. Disordered eating is present when a person frequently feels distressed about eating correctly and imposes rules such as earning food through exercise or following a highly restrictive fad diet. Disordered eating can also include creating food rituals, such as only being able to eat at certain times of the day or having periods of excessive eating where a person eats significantly past their point of comfort in response to stress (Dennis, n.d.).

Body Dysmorphia

Body dysmorphia is often associated with disordered eating, where a person becomes preoccupied with flaws in their physical appearance which feeds more extreme and problematic eating behavior in an attempt to relieve their distress about how they look. The person battles with food driven by misinformed and unrealistic personal or societal standards to attain healthy eating habits and an acceptable physical appearance. They frequently spend time in different forms of body checking, such as weighing themselves daily, staring at themselves in the mirror, and measuring parts of their body. The societal pressure to have an ideal body appearance can skew a person's perception of themselves and, if left unchecked, can evolve into an ED.

Preoccupation with weight loss, appearance, and maintaining a controlled dietary plan leads many individuals to form disordered relationships with food and exercise where their identity and sense of wellbeing get overly tied to these issues. These unhealthy relationships and behaviors can remain longstanding despite them being uncomfortable and unrealistic. Unchecked, they can develop into a DSM-classified ED diagnosis where they become destructive and cause disability.

Not all EDs center around an obsession to achieve a certain physical appearance. The ED ARFID, for example, has symptoms that are not rooted in a preoccupation to obtain a desired physical shape or weight. Symptoms of ARFID focus instead on avoidance of certain foods based on the sensory characteristics (e.g., discomfort with how it feels in their mouth) and concerns about aversive consequences of eating such as indigestion or bloating.

SOCIAL ISSUES ASSOCIATED WITH DISORDERED EATING

Genetic factors and exposure to traumatic life events are not the only known risk factors associated with the development of an ED. EDs and disordered eating are recognized as pervasive social issues that distort and confuse what it means to have a normal or healthy relationship with food. We are surrounded by inaccurate and harmful information about food, health, and body weight that creates pressure and expectations for how we eat and how we look. As discussed in Chapter 11, there is massive pressure through modern media to diet and look thin, much of which is driven by a capitalist motivation to sell diet-related foods, supplements, and equipment. Even systemic racism has been identified as an underlying belief system that contributes to the prevalence of fatphobia and idolizing thinness.

The History of the American Body Image

Beliefs and attitudes toward body size are socially constructed. They change over time and are influenced by many factors. Between the 16th and 20th centuries, a larger body was perceived as the common body size and was often recognized as beautiful in art work (Hollander, 1977). Since the early 1900s there has been a shift in how we view bodies and what body style we identify as beautiful and healthy, with a belief system that also attaches an identity to body size as a measure of success and moral correctness (Howard, 2018).

The Flapper Era in early 20th-century U.S. culture began the shift toward slender bodies as the ideal body shape. This era also featured more body exposure as women began to test their newfound position in society following gaining the right to vote, which came for many with a desire for more self-expression. The dawn of filmmaking and the admired lives of early actresses, now viewed for the first time by the masses, perpetuated a preference toward slender bodies.

Each decade of the 20th century featured a new slender look, perpetuated by the promise of prosperity, a carefree life, and the ability to attract the attention of a "suitable" mate forged a perfect self-image storm enhanced by advertising, marketing and the allure of easy-living and glamour. Add to that the advent of television, fashion magazines, and billboard advertising, image-making became big business promoting ideals that were neither attainable nor representative

PROFITING FROM THE THIN IDEAL

The *thin ideal* is the idea that people should strive to obtain physical thinness because it satisfies the Western ideal bodily aesthetic. The thin ideal can be harmful in that it encourages individuals to strive toward thinness even if that is not the natural shape of their body. Some people's bodies naturally hold more body fat in a way that is very healthy for their bodies (butt and thighs versus belly fat). The thin ideal ignores individual differences in body type emphasizing the same standard of thinness as optimal for all bodies. When pursuing the thin ideal, sometimes a person's psychological and physical wellbeing are sacrificed in the pursuit of unhealthy beauty standards.

Dieting is big business! The weight loss industry has continuously taken a power position in marketing and sales since the 1950s. A lot of money is spent on activating and promoting the drive toward perfection. This marketplace pressure has been a huge contributor to perpetuating the thin ideal which keeps anyone who aspires to it in a cycle of repeated strivings. Bodies have become commodities to be molded at will and changed through the purchase of goods and services. Advertisements repeatedly communicate to consumers that they are flawed and the only way to repair those flaws is to purchase products, be they diet books, exercise programs, nutrition bars, or weight loss retreats. These goods are marketed as health regimens that will "fix" you and make you a better person (Van Horne, 2019).

Diet culture promotes products to consumers promising to assist you to achieve the ideal body. This harmful messaging encourages rigid beliefs around food and health and can lead to unhealthy behaviors in a desperate attempt to make the diet work. The messaging can easily be interpreted that consumers who are unsuccessful at achieving the desired dieting goal are at fault, rather than the inherently flawed and unsustainable diet as the more obvious culprit that needs to be changed. For example, the slogan "fat makes you fat" stemmed from the anti-fat tirade of the 1980s that took the food industry by storm when low-fat diets were promoted as the ultimate health elixir. The food industry used this slogan to create fear around eating the macronutrient fat and quickly began promoting low-fat products that were less expensive to manufacture. As mentioned in Chapter 4, fat is a vital component of our diet and promotes healthy organ and brain function and hormone regulation. Yet diet culture demonized fat, and to an extent, continues to do so today. People are still encouraged to count calories and choose low-fat food options.

Calorie restriction is known to contribute to ED development but is still promoted and practiced across contexts. Often driven by commercial interests that profit from people's desperate desire to lose weight, people are told to eat less (i.e., fewer calories) and exercise more, even if there is no evidence of that plan working long-term to keep off the weight (Memon et al., 2020). Diet culture marketing often aims to persuade consumers to buy their products by using tactics that shame and scare people and that reinforce dieting and the thin ideal, even though they are known contributors to EDs (Jovanovski & Jaeger, 2022).

EATING DISORDER TREATMENT

EDs require highly specialized treatment programs. Without treatment, people with EDs are significantly more likely to experience life-threatening consequences of their disorder. Engaging in recovery from an ED diminishes the gap between the ED and the risk of death (Center for Discovery, 2019).

LEVELS OF CARE

ED treatment comes in a range of intensities based on the severity of the ED. A person with a serious ED who is at physical risk of harm or death starts at the most intensive treatment and then follows a step-down approach as their symptoms improve. The appropriate level of care is determined by medical and psychological examinations which are coordinated by an ED treatment program. The goal is to situate a person in the level of care that is most supportive for them and takes into consideration the severity of the ED. For example, a person with more intense ED symptoms, such as bradycardia or heightened ED behaviors (e.g., severe restriction) is at higher risk of suffering from a medical complication or a suicide attempt and therefore needs more intensive treatment where the staff can carefully monitor their food intake and their body's physical response to treatment.

ED treatment often begins with a client seeing a therapist or medical professional in an outpatient setting, such as going to a clinic or doctor's office. If the severity of the ED warrants more intensive treatment, the client is referred to a specialized higher-level ED program. After a client completes a higher-level treatment program that includes some level of residential or inpatient care, they are often encouraged to participate in outpatient therapy with an ED therapist where they attend sessions in an office or clinic.

There are four levels of ED care, listed below from most to least intensive. The duration of time spent in each level of care is determined by the ED treatment team who assesses the risk and needs of the patient while developing a treatment plan that recommends a term of care and potential discharge date based on the client's individual needs. Assessment of needs includes the severity of their ED behaviors, medical stability, and response to treatment both before admittance and throughout their treatment plan.

Inpatient care (also referred to as inpatient hospitalization) is the highest level of ED treatment and predominantly treats clients with anorexia. Clients live at a treatment facility and receive around-the-clock care to learn emotional regulation and coping skills, supported mealtimes, and individual and group activities (e.g., relapse prevention work, art therapy, and nutrition information). Clients in these programs have severe limitations in their ability to appropriately care for their basic needs without constant care that disrupts the ED behaviors and other forms of self-harm. Many clients in these programs are considered medically unstable due to being severely underweight or having blood work that indicates they are at risk of a medical event such as a heart attack and receive daily medical care and monitoring.

Residential care is similar to inpatient care in that it is also provided at a live-in facility where clients receive daily care; however, the focus is on long-term recovery rather than managing a medical crisis. Clients in these programs are more medically and clinically stable than inpatient clients but are not stable enough for independent living. Stays at these facilities are usually longer than inpatient care, and the environment is less medical and more comfortable and home-like.

Partial hospitalization programs (PHP) do not offer a live-in facility. Clients are medically stable enough to spend the days at the program and then return home at the end of each day. They still need frequent care to assist in disrupting their ED behaviors. Clients in these programs spend their days at the treatment program held in a medical or psychiatric clinic six to eight hours per day, five to seven days per week, and then return home at night and on non-program days.

Intensive outpatient programs (IOP) vary in the number of days and daily hours depending on the individual needs of the client. For example, a client might spend three hours per day, three days per week at the clinic engaged in treatment. These clients are medically and clinically stable but still need some additional support to recover from the ED.

GOALS OF TREATMENT

For all levels of higher care, clients are assigned to a treatment team, which consists of a therapist, dietitian, counselors, and the program's clinical supervisor. Inpatient, residential, and PHP care also include a medical doctor, psychiatrist, and nurses. Treatment goals focus on attaining medical and clinical stability, such as normal blood panels and blood pressure, normal heart rate, re-establishing hunger and fullness cues, and weight restoration for those categorized as underweight.

Clinical stability includes decreased engagement with ED behaviors such as bingeing, restricting, purging, or other compensatory behaviors like over-exercising, and improved belief systems around food and body centered choices and acceptance. Since lying and compulsive behaviors are integral parts of an ED, treatment goals include honesty about engagement with ED thoughts and behaviors, and a decrease in body checking, while holding accountable inappropriate eating behaviors such as hiding, microtearing, or microbiting food. Cognitive-behavioral therapy (CBT), dialectical behavior therapy (DBT), and acceptance and commitment therapy (ACT) are common modalities utilized in ED treatment to help clients better understand their distorted thinking, improve their emotion regulation, and assist in redirecting disordered behaviors.

RECOVERY AND RELAPSE

Recovery from an ED looks different from client to client based on their needs, experiences, and goals. Recovery is ongoing. The term "in recovery" is used to describe the active process of overcoming the ED and may be ongoing, even after completion of the treatment process. Recovery may include a transition from being "in recovery" to becoming "fully recovered," meaning that the individual considers themselves completely unconfined by their ED (Monte Nido, 2019).

Although treatment for EDs has been proven effective, EDs are known for high relapse rates and the return of ED behavior even following completion of treatment. Unfortunately, relapse is common, with 35 percent of people with anorexia resuming ED behaviors within 18 months of treatment completion, and 41 percent of people with bulimia experiencing relapse within two years of recovery (Berg, 2023). Leaving treatment before the clinical recommendation or integrating oneself back into society with a lack of support following treatment heightens the risk for relapse. Other major life changes (e.g., ending a relationship) also commonly act as a trigger for the return of ED behaviors, even in individuals who completed treatment.

CASE STUDY: A COLLEGE EXPERIENCE WITH ANOREXIA

A 21-year-old undergraduate student from California's East Bay shared her story about grappling with an ED.

I was diagnosed with my ED at age 20. I had just completed my sophomore year of college and returned home for the summer. In college, my friends did not understand my desperate need to control my eating by staying distracted and intensely focusing on my schoolwork. I can recall friends and peers, even after they knew of my condition, joking, "Chem for breakfast." Not eating was a normal part of my college life and culture. Sometimes it became a game and a competition. Who can study more as justification for eating less?

I remember sitting in the medical office with my primary care physician as she broke the news. Hearing the diagnosis – *anorexia nervosa* – was devastating. I was in shock. How could I have an ED, something I'd only ever heard about in tabloids?

My clinical team recommended I enter an IOP program, but I refused. My ED tried to convince me it did not exist. I was blinded by denial of the severity of my physical condition and mental wellbeing. At the time, treatment felt like a blockade to my life.

Early symptoms of my ED manifested as a fear of high calorie (energy dense) foods, rigidly following a highly restrictive meal plan, meal planning obsessiveness, stringent calorie counting, and limited food choice, exercising to "earn" my food and constant body checking (weighing myself, obsessively looking at my body in the mirror). On days when I struggled with body image, I felt greater distress and consequently more severely restricted my food intake and isolated myself from others. I also experienced anxiety, depression, and symptoms of OCD.

My focus turned to what I considered healthy eating, which ED specialists later diagnosed as orthorexia nervosa. My orthorexia manifested at the same time as my anorexia, and I quickly became obsessive, misinformed, and unhealthy. The information plastered across my social media from "fitness influencers" exacerbated my symptoms. I tracked my daily macronutrients (fat, protein, carbohydrates), checked food labels to identify and strictly avoid "unhealthy" foods, and cut out entire food groups out of fear of disrupting my gut microbiome. I avoided nutrient-rich foods that my body needed because inconsistent and inaccurate diet culture messages communicated the need to do so.

As the summer progressed, my ED symptoms got worse, and my poor physical health drew great concern from the people around me. The AN (restricting type) from which I suffered led to major calorie and ingredient restrictions, which spiraled me into drastic and rapid weight loss. As my ED continued to dominate my life, I experienced a plethora of other physically and emotionally damaging symptoms. The physical symptoms included: hair loss, lightheadedness, fatigue, skin bruising, disruption to hunger and fullness cues (no longer sensed), dry skin, slowed heart rate (bradycardia), temperature dysregulation (constantly either overly hot or cold), loss of menstruation, low blood pressure, dehydration, electrolyte imbalances and other troubling lab results that indicated poor health. The mental and emotional symptoms included being intensely fixated on "flaws" in my physical appearance (body dysmorphia), obsession with food and thoughts of food, interpersonal relationship hardships, emotional numbness, increased perfectionism, and self-loathing.

I was initially very resistant to treatment, however, when I finally understood it as a necessity, I fully engaged and completed the ED step-down treatment process from Residential to PHP for seven months, then IOP care. Between all levels of care, treatment taught me the importance of finding food freedom, learning how to eat intuitively, and the harm posed by diet culture and unattainable social ideals.

Today, I am fully recovered from my ED. Which is not to say that I have everything figured out. Living as a person fully recovered from an ED is challenging due to our culture and the normalization of damaging social ideas about food, health, and the thin ideal. After undergoing treatment, I started to recognize how normal, everyday interactions can be harmful to people's self-esteem. We, as a society, are immersed in diet culture which can often feel inescapable.

Treatment was challenging and required a commitment to strip my ED of its power. This journey toward regaining my life and regaining myself felt terrifying at times. After all, EDs are tremendous coping mechanisms. Now that I am fully recovered, I recognize that without treatment my ED would have taken my life. Freedom from my ED saved me.

FOOD FOR THOUGHT: ADVICE FROM AN EATING DISORDER SURVIVOR

The student whose story you just read now actively works to share her experience with others and offers advice about how to support someone you know who has or is displaying symptoms of an ED.

An ideal starting place to support someone with an ED is to become informed and active. Massive misinformation exists pertaining to EDs. Look for credible sources such as NEDA and the National Association of Anorexia Nervosa and Associated Disorders (ANAD) that provide truthful information for ED professionals and survivors. Important things to look for include: sensitive use of terminology, quality research-based statistics, and general information about symptoms and what recovery and treatment might look like. Get information about how you can get involved to support survivors. ED awareness week is an awesome place to start!

It is essential to be open minded. Social discourse often runs the risk of participating in diet culture. Beware of social interactions that support negative talk about bodies, food, and health. Be flexible in learning about what might be triggering for people and how you can avoid contributing to that source of discomfort. For example, do not make comments about other people's bodies, and instead, ask for permission from others when talking about their appearance, even for compliments.

A gentle approach is so important to help a person with an ED feel safe. EDs are devastating and traumatic diseases that strip away a person's independence, safety, and internal bliss. Thus, be gentle but proactive in sharing concern for others. Come from a place of nonjudgment. It could save someone's life!

Remember to ask how best you can support someone. No article, website, or other outside source knows the exact support someone may be seeking from their loved ones. ED recovery is highly variable, and there is no singular right or wrong way to support someone. So, ask what you can do to help and accept that there may not be a clear answer. Make an effort to respect recovery-conducive requests. It may be something as simple as avoiding mention of calories.

REFERENCES

American Psychiatric Association. (2013). *Diagnostic and statistical manual of mental disorders: DSM-5* (5th ed.). American Psychiatric Association. http://dsm.psychiatryonline.org/doi/book/10.1176/appi.books.9780890425596

American Psychiatric Association (2022). *Diagnostic and statistical manual of mental disorders: DSM-5-TR* (5th ed., text revision). American Psychiatric Association.

ANAD. (2024). *Eating disorder statistics.* National Association of Anorexia Nervosa and Associated Disorders. https://anad.org/eating-disorders-statistics/

Berg, B. (2023). *Eating disorder relapse is common: Here's why.* Eating Recovery Center. https://www.eatingrecoverycenter.com/resources/eating-disorder-relapse-common

Bhattacharya, A., Cooper, M., McAdams, C., Peebles, R., & Timko, C. A. (2022). Cultural shifts in the symptoms of anorexia nervosa: The case of orthorexia nervosa. *Appetite, 170,* 105869.

Burke, N. L., Hazzard, V. M., Schaefer, L. M., Simone, M., O'Flynn, J. L., & Rodgers, R. F. (2023). Socioeconomic status and eating disorder prevalence: at the intersections of gender identity, sexual orientation, and race/ethnicity. *Psychological Medicine, 53*(9), 4255–4265. https://doi.org/10.1017/S0033291722001015

Center for Discovery. (2019). *Expectations after treatment: Statistics on eating disorders.* https://centerfordiscovery.com/blog/statistics-on-eating-disorders/

Chastain, R. (2023). *Recognizing and resisting diet culture.* National Eating Disorders Association. https://www.nationaleatingdisorders.org/recognizing-and-resisting-diet-culture/

Conti, C., Lanzara, R., Scipioni, M., Iasenza, M., Guagnano, M. T., & Fulcheri, M. (2017). The relationship between binge eating disorder and suicidality: A systematic review. *Frontiers in Psychology.* https://doi.org/10.3389/fpsyg.2017.02125

Curzio, O., Calderoni, S., Maestro, S., Rossi, G., De Pasquale, C. F., Belmonti, V., Apicella, F., Muratori, F., & Retico, A. (2020). Lower gray matter volumes of frontal lobes and insula in adolescents with anorexia nervosa restricting type: Findings from a brain morphometry study. *European Psychiatry, 63*(1). https://doi.org/10.1192/j.eurpsy.2020.19

Daly, M., & Costigan, E. (2022). Trends in eating disorder risk among U.S. college students, 2013–2021. *Psychiatry Research, 317,* 114882. https://doi.org/10.1016/j.psychres.2022.114882

Davison, G., & Adams, M. (2024). *Bulimia facts and statistics.* Within Health. https://withinhealth.com/learn/articles/bulimia-facts-and-statistics

Dennis, A. B. (n.d.). *Disordered eating vs. eating disorders.* National Eating Disorders Association (NEDA). https://www.nationaleatingdisorders.org/what-is-the-difference-between-disordered-eating-and-eating-disorders/

Eating Disorder Hope. (2024). *Males, masculinity & shame in eating disorders.* https://www.eatingdisorderhope.com/information/eating-disorder/males-masculinity-shame-in-eating-disorders

Eating Recovery Center. (2024a). *Anorexia nervosa.* https://www.eatingrecoverycenter.com/conditions/anorexia

Eating Recovery Center. (2024b). *Atypical anorexia.* https://www.eatingrecoverycenter.com/conditions/atypical-anorexia

Eating Recovery Center. (2024c). *Types of eating disorders.* https://www.eatingrecoverycenter.com/conditions/eating-disorders

Ekern, J. (2023). *Dealing with the consequences of binge eating disorder.* Eating Disorder Hope. https://www.eatingdisorderhope.com/information/binge-eating-disorder/diagnosis-effects-consequences

Federici, A. (2021). *What is the difference between anorexia nervosa with a binge/purge subtype and bulimia nervosa?* The Centre for Psychology + Emotion Regulation. https://www.psychology-emotionregulation.ca/2021/01/18/what-is-the-difference-between-anorexia-nervosa-with-a-binge-purge-subtype-and-bulimia-nervosa/

Galmiche, M., Déchelotte, P., Lambert, G., & Tavolacci, M. P. (2019). Prevalence of eating disorders over the 2000–2018 period: A systematic literature review. *The American Journal of Clinical Nutrition, 109*(5), 1402–1413. https://doi.org/10.1093/ajcn/nqy342

Gerhardt, L. (2024). *Anorexia statistics and studies.* Center for Discovery. https://centerfordiscovery.com/blog/anorexia-statistics-and-studies/

Halbeisen, G., Brandt, G., & Paslakis, G. (2022). A plea for diversity in eating disorders research [Perspective]. *Frontiers in Psychiatry, 13.* https://doi.org/10.3389/fpsyt.2022.820043

Harold, L. (2023). *Why intervention is necessary to prevent eating disorder deaths.* Verywell Mind. https://www.verywellmind.com/yes-eating-disorders-can-be-deadly-1138269#:~:text=Dehydration&text=Dehydration%20is%20often%20responsible%20for,electrolyte%20levels%20in%20the%20body

Harrop, E. N., Mensinger, J. L., Moore, M., & Lindhorst, T. (2021). Restrictive eating disorders in higher weight persons: A systematic review of atypical anorexia nervosa prevalence and consecutive admission literature. *International Journal of Eating Disorders, 54*(8), 1328–1357.

Hazzard, V. M., Loth, K. A., Hooper, L., & Becker, C. B. (2020). Food insecurity and eating disorders: A review of emerging evidence. *Current Psychiatry Reports, 22,* 1–9.

Heiden-Rootes, K., Linsenmeyer, W., Levine, S., Oliveras, M., & Joseph, M. (2023). A scoping review of the research literature on eating and body image for transgender and nonbinary adults. *Journal of Eating Disorders, 11*(1), 111.

Hilbert, A., Pike, K. M., Goldschmidt, A. B., Wilfley, D. E., Fairburn, C. G., Dohm, F.-A., Walsh, B. T., & Weissman, R. S. (2014). Risk factors across the eating disorders. *Psychiatry Research, 220*(1-2), 500–506.

Hollander, A. (1977). When fat was in fashion. *The New York Times.* https://www.nytimes.com/1977/10/23/archives/when-fat-was-in-fashion-abundant-flesh-was-a-thing-of-beauty-to.html#:~:text=For%20about%20400%20years%2C%20roughly,natural%20to%20look%20physically%20substantial

Howard, J. (2018). The ever-changing "ideal" of female beauty. *CNN.* https://www.cnn.com/2018/03/07/health/body-image-history-of-beauty-explainer-intl/index.html

Hudson, J. I., Hiripi, E., Pope, H. G. Jr, & Kessler, R. C. (2007). The prevalence and correlates of eating disorders in the national comorbidity survey replication. *Biological Psychiatry, 61*(3), 348–358.

Ives, E. (2013). *Eating disorders: Decode the controlled chaos.* Balboa Press.

Jovanovski, N., & Jaeger, T. (2022). *Demystifying 'diet culture': Exploring the meaning of diet culture in online 'anti-diet' feminist, fat activist, and health professional communities.* Women's studies international Forum.

Kelvas, D. (2023). *Examining the bulimia death rate.* Within Health. https://withinhealth.com/learn/articles/examining-the-bulimia-death-rate

Li, W., Zhao, Z., Chen, D., Peng, Y., & Lu, Z. (2022). Prevalence and associated factors of depression and anxiety symptoms among college students: A systematic review and meta-analysis. *Journal of Child Psychology and Psychiatry, 63*(11), 1222–1230.

Mahoney, B. (2021). *Overview of orthorexia.* Center for Discovery Eating Disorder Treatment. https://centerfordiscovery.com/blog/overview-of-orthorexia/#:~:text=The%20term%20orthorexia%20was%20first,conflicts%20within%20the%20inner%20self.

Martin, J. B. (2010). The development of ideal body image perceptions in the United States. *Nutrition Today, 45*(3), 98–110.

Memon, A. N., Gowda, A. S., Rallabhandi, B., Bidika, E., Fayyaz, H., Salib, M., & Cancarevic, I. (2020). Have our attempts to curb obesity done more harm than good? *Cureus, 12*(9), e10275.

Monte Nido. (2019). *Fully recovered vs. in recovery: A discussion of the similarities and differences.* https://www.montenido.com/blog/fully-recovered-vs-in-recovery

NEDA. (n.d.-a). *Busting the myths about eating disorders.* National Eating Disorders Association. https://www.nationaleatingdisorders.org/toolkit/parent-toolkit/eating-disorder-myths

NEDA. (n.d.-b). *Risk factors*. National Eating Disorders Association. https://www.nationaleatingdisorders.org/risk-factors/

NIMH. (2023). *Mental illness*. National Institute of Mental Health. https://www.nimh.nih.gov/health/statistics/mental-illness

NIMH. (n.d.). *Eating disorders*. National Institute of Mental Health. https://www.nimh.nih.gov/health/statistics/eating-disorders

Smith, A. R., Zuromski, K. L., & Dodd, D. R. (2018). Eating disorders and suicidality: What we know, what we don't know, and suggestions for future research. *Current Opinion in Psychology*, *22*, 63–67.

Ulfvebrand, S., Birgegård, A., Norring, C., Högdahl, L., & von Hausswolff-Juhlin, Y. (2015). Psychiatric comorbidity in women and men with eating disorders results from a large clinical database. *Psychiatry Research*, *230*(2), 294–299.

Van Horne, C. (2019). *The capitalist machine aka diet culture*. Omni Counseling and Nutrition. https://www.omnicounselingandnutrition.com/blog/2019/3/12/diet-culture-weight-stigma-and-the-capitalist-machine

Vidaña, A. G., Forbush, K. T., Barnhart, E. L., Chana, S. M., Chapa, D. A., Richson, B., & Thomeczek, M. L. (2020). Impact of trauma in childhood and adulthood on eating-disorder symptoms. *Eating Behaviors*, *39*, 101426.

Volpe, U., Tortorella, A., Manchia, M., Monteleone, A. M., Albert, U., & Monteleone, P. (2016). Eating disorders: What age at onset? *Psychiatry Research*, *238*, 225–227.

Within Health. (2023). *Anorexia nervosa statistics: Gender, race and socioeconomics*. https://withinhealth.com/learn/articles/anorexia-nervosa-an-statistics-gender-race-and-socioeconomics

Youm, S. M., Kim, J. Y., & Lee, J. R. (2015). Acute gastric dilatation causing fatal outcome in A young female with eating disorder: A case report. *Korean Journal of Anesthesiology*, *68*(2), 188–192.

13 Food Addiction

Is food addiction real? This controversial question challenges deeply held beliefs about what it means to be addicted to something. Defined broadly, addiction is the continued and compulsive consumption of a substance despite its harm to self or others. Addiction includes *tolerance,* where a person needs to consume increasing amounts of a substance over time to achieve the same effect, and *dependence,* where a person continues to consume a substance even with conscious knowledge and recognition that the substance is in some way harmful to them. Addiction includes cravings, recurrent use that interferes with other obligations or puts a person in a hazardous situation, and repeated unsuccessful attempts to cut down or quit.

THE NATURE OF ADDICTION

Ironically, when we look at the nature of the addictive process, we see that while the goal of an addiction is to experience pleasure, the reality is that the resulting behaviors associated with the addiction often increase overall pain. Current neuroscience tells us that pleasure and pain are processed in overlapping brain regions that balance each other to maintain equilibrium (homeostasis), identified as the *pleasure–pain balance.* The body ferociously works to be in balance, so it responds to the intense release of dopamine associated with substance use by counterbalancing with pain. As the old saying goes, "What goes up must come down." Typically, this falls under the heading of "hangover"; however, it is more than just the immediate discomfort of the morning after. After intense bursts of dopamine, an aftermath of low dopamine levels can persist for prolonged periods (Ifland et al., 2012).

Long-Term Use

Long-term substance use can change our natural experience of pleasure and pain through neuroadaptation, which creates chronically low dopamine levels and changes in dopamine brain receptors. This neuroadaptation changes our natural pleasure set-point, meaning that something that used to give us pleasure will no longer make us feel good because the set-point to release dopamine has been raised. And as the body seeks balance, we may also become more vulnerable to experiencing pain. Eventually, nothing feels good anymore, and we are easily irritated, distressed, or not quite sure what we feel (Volkow et al., 2002). "The paradox is that hedonism, the pursuit of pleasure for its own sake, leads to anhedonia, which is the inability to enjoy pleasure of any kind" (Lembke, 2021, p. 57).

When the drug or behavior no longer provides a state of euphoria or feeling high, people often stop using it and feel symptoms of withdrawal, including anxiety, irritability, insomnia, and dysphoria (feeling very unhappy, uneasy, or dissatisfied). To escape the painful state of withdrawal, we crave the drug or behavior to feel "normal," which is often a neutral place of feeling neither good nor terrible, just a tolerable state where we can survive. The good news is that if we wait long enough without using the substance, our brain adjusts and returns to our baseline homeostasis (i.e., normal dopamine levels and dopamine sensitivity). This is a more balanced state with less intense levels of pain and pleasure and a greater ability to experience milder levels of pleasure from common stimuli such as going for a walk.

The long-term daily exposure to a substance that causes big dopamine spikes eventually makes us feel very unhappy most of the time. This is true with addictive foods as well. The key is to give your brain a break from the addictive foods to allow your dopamine response to reset to normal.

                    DOI: 10.1201/9781032647647-18

Once you are back in homeostasis, you can enjoy treat foods as a treat, meaning an occasional occurrence that brings delight, without paying the heavy price of living with a neuroadapted brain that keeps us miserable. When our dopamine system returns to normal, we can begin experiencing more pleasure in simple everyday activities like time spent with friends or being out in nature.

THE INTERSECTION OF PHYSIOLOGY AND PSYCHOLOGY

One of the challenges to changing addictive behavior is that triggers for cravings are not just physiological but also psychological. Situational cues make us think about our positive feelings connected to a substance and increase our cravings, known as *cue-dependent learning* or classical conditioning. Like Pavlov's dog being taught to salivate at the sound of a bell, humans can be taught to anticipate positive emotions tied to ingesting a substance. When we anticipate feeling good it increases how our body responds when we actually consume the substance and increases the dopamine release. Anticipation that is unfulfilled, because we thought about but did not consume the substance, causes our dopamine levels to fall well below our baseline level. So, if we were planning all day on eating that piece of chocolate cream pie after work and it turns out the diner that sells our favorite pie was sold out, our dopamine will plummet and increase our cravings and discomfort, which can result in feelings of anxiety and depression.

Imagine someone traveling to their favorite coffee house. They can already smell the coffee and pastries as they long for that first warm sip of coffee while they sink into a comfortable chair and release a deep sigh of contentment. When they arrive at the coffee house, there is a large sign on the door, "Closed for repairs." Immediately, they feel frustrated, disappointed, and disoriented. Their whole day feels knocked out of balance without their usual morning routine. Rather than taking this opportunity to explore a new coffee house, they grab a take-out cup of coffee from a nearby market. However, it is unsatisfying, and they find themselves craving their usual morning blend and feeling sad and irritable throughout the day. At night they fret about where to get coffee the following day and how to fill that desire so that they can have a decent day. They wake up tired and stressed, unfocused and miserable. The addictive urges not only for the taste and feel of the coffee, but the full experience associated with coffee, has been given the power to set the tone for their day.

DEFINING FOOD ADDICTION

So, where do we draw the line when it comes to food? In the Diagnostic and Statistical Manual of Mental Disorders (DSM-5) section on substance-related and addictive disorders, they list alcohol and caffeine with other known addictive substances, namely opioids, stimulants, and tobacco. When discussing food addiction, should we only talk about alcohol and caffeine, or is there enough evidence to also discuss the addictive properties of sugar and ultra-processed foods? And, do we consider other foods we eat so routinely that we miss them if they are absent from our day?

Let's consider what all these substances have in common. First, they all share the risk of excessive use, where people tend to use more of the substance despite the negative consequences associated with ongoing usage. For example, a person who struggles with insomnia continues to drink six cups of coffee throughout the day even though they are feeling anxious and making mistakes at work due to their lack of sleep.

Second, early definitions of addiction have focused on substances that directly promote intense activation of the brain reward system (Di Chiara & Imperato, 1988). When this reward system is activated, we crave the substance and are driven to consume more, even if that requires neglecting other important activities in our lives (American Psychiatric Association, 2013). Current definitions of addiction include preoccupation, temporary satiation, loss of control, and suffering negative consequences (Sussman & Sussman, 2011). In addition to substances that you ingest, the DSM-5 also includes "behavioral addictions" such as gambling and internet gaming, which reflects the evidence

TABLE 13.1

The Evolution of the Food Addiction Model

1956	Theron Randolph, M.D., coined the term food addiction (Randolph, 1956)
1960	Overeaters Anonymous founded when a member identified similarities between gambling and food addiction
1975	Book *Sugar Blues* argued sugar is addictive (Dufty, 1975)
1985	Book *Fat is a Family Affair: How Food Obsessions Affect Relationships* based on Hollis's work as an addiction counselor (Hollis, 1985)
1986	Glenbeigh Psychiatric Hospital opened a food addicts treatment unit as an addition to their Drug and Alcohol Rehab Centre
1989	Book *Food Addiction: The Body Knows* based on Sheppard's clinical experience working with food addicts (Sheppard, 1989)
1990	Book *Love Hunger: Recovery from Food Addiction* discussed treatment for food dependency (Minirth, 1990)
2001	Study demonstrating the similarity between obesity and drug addiction using neuroimaging that showed changes in dopamine receptors in the brain's reward pathway similar to substance dependence (Wang et al., 2004)
2005	Food Addiction Institute (FAI) founded as a nonprofit organization whose mission is to support the availability of abstinent-based resources and treatment for food addiction recovery
2008	Study showing that rats can become addicted to sugar (Avena et al., 2008)
2009	Book *The End of Overeating: Taking Control of the Insatiable North American Appetite* explained the brain chemistry behind food cravings and compulsive eating (Kessler, 2009)
2009	Development of the Yale Food Addiction Scale (YFAS) (Gearhardt et al., 2009)
2011	American Society of Addiction Medicine (ASAM) officially defined food addiction as a brain disorder

that these behaviors activate brain reward systems in ways like drugs of abuse and produce similar behavioral symptoms such as lying and risk-taking to continue the addictive behavior.

Therefore, the field of psychology has already accepted the idea that addiction includes more than drugs of abuse. An addictive substance or behavior is defined by how it affects the brain and the ways it activates the brain reward systems that drive addictive behavior like craving and feeling out of control. This brings us back to our original question about whether or not we can be addicted to sugar and ultra-processed foods. Since these foods have a similar effect on the brain to drugs of abuse and addictive behaviors, then there is evidence that food addiction to certain types of food is real (Bartoshuk, 2011; SHiFT, n.d.).

A BRIEF HISTORY OF FOOD ADDICTION RESEARCH

Food addiction as a theoretical model has been evolving since the 1950s (Meule, 2015). Table 13.1 provides a brief history of the research and arguments used to define this field.

HIGHLY PROCESSED FOODS

The *brain reward system* is a key driver of behavior, with dopamine as one of the most critical neurotransmitters. Rapid rises in dopamine levels are associated with the pleasurable response to addictive substances and behaviors. Addiction research measures the *addictive potential* of a substance or behavior by analyzing the amount and speed of dopamine released into the brain's reward pathway upon exposure. For example, in a study of what would have the strongest impact on the dopamine levels of rats, the researchers found that dopamine in the rats' brains was increased 55 percent by chocolate, 100 percent by sex, 150 percent by nicotine, 225 percent by cocaine, and 1000 percent by amphetamines, thereby ranking those items from lowest to highest in their addictive potential (Lembke, 2021).

When we compare the dopamine response of foods found in their whole form in nature (e.g., sugar cane) to those same foods after they have been manufactured and processed into the foods on our grocery shelves (e.g., table sugar), we see that the processed foods elicit a much stronger dopamine response. The artificial high from processed foods (e.g., a tablespoon of sugar in oatmeal) is far more powerful than the high found in nature (e.g., chewing on a piece of sugar cane), so the rewards are more intense and concentrated, which can make it a more potent stimulant than the brain was designed to handle (Tarman, 2019).

In an article in Scientific American titled *The Food Addiction*, the authors reported that foods high in fat and sugar trigger the brain to release endorphins and dopamine which influence decision making and motivate binge-eating behavior. These powerful chemicals can overpower conscious attempts to stop eating when full (Kenny, 2013).

Evidence of the addictive nature of processed foods was shown through the work at the Sleep, Eating, and Affect (SEA) Lab at the University of California San Francisco. SEA developed the *Reward Eating Drive (RED)* scale to explore if food addiction is associated with the influence of specific foods on opioid receptors (Epel et al., 2014; Lustig, 2021). Their research showed that some people experience a loss of control over specific foods and that bingeing episodes tend to focus on processed foods high in sugar and fat, such as cookies and crackers, which exhibit a strong influence on the brain reward system by activating opioid receptors.

An interesting parallel can be drawn between our country's history with tobacco and the current status of processed foods. Historically, tobacco was legal, cheap, easily accessible, and socially acceptable. The use of tobacco did not result in significant intoxication that impaired functioning like alcohol or heroin, but research eventually demonstrated that nicotine is both addictive and significantly harmful with long-term use. Similarly, processed foods are legal, cheap, easily accessible, and socially acceptable. We are just beginning to understand how truly addictive these foods are for some people and to appreciate the negative long-term consequences of eating these foods (Gearhardt & Corbin, 2012).

In her book *Food Junkies* (Tarman, 2019), Tarman's message is one of hope. The recent increased awareness of how specific foods can hijack our ability to regulate our appetite and the reward circuitry of the brain has prompted concern about the food industry's role in designing and promoting foods that target this weakness. With awareness that some foods can be addictive, people become empowered to experiment with abstaining from those foods and potentially feeling fewer cravings, greater satiety, and improved overall wellbeing.

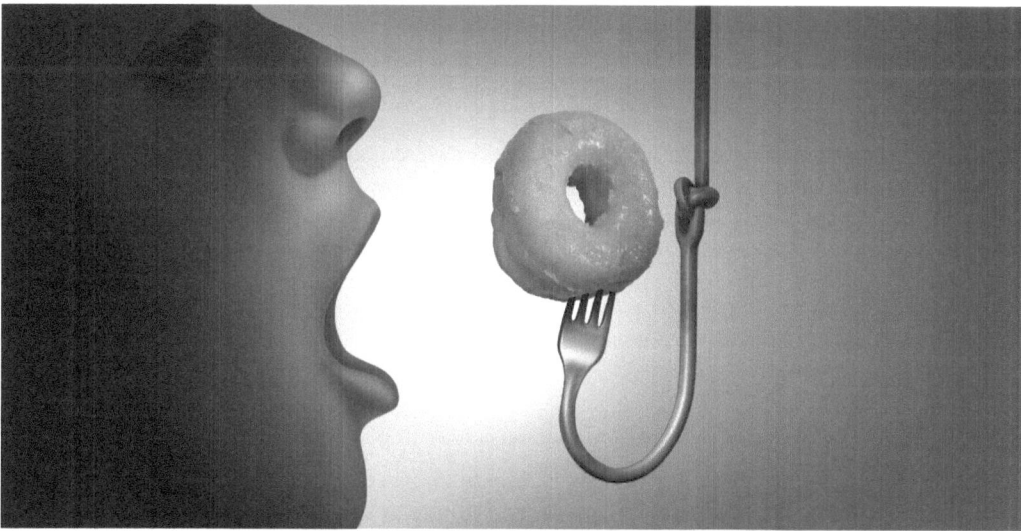

FIGURE 13.1   Food addiction. Credit: Lightspring (Shutterstock).

MEASURING FOOD ADDICTION

A 2018 systematic review evaluated 52 empirical studies and found there was sufficient evidence to demonstrate a clear association between some foods and addiction characteristics, such as risky use, impaired control, and symptoms of tolerance and withdrawal (Gordon et al., 2018). Processed foods with added sweeteners and fats showed the greatest addictive potential. Therefore, an argument can be made that, even though they have not yet been identified in the DSM-5 as drugs of abuse, processed foods are addictive for some people.

The *Yale Food Addiction Scale (YFAS)* (Gearhardt et al., 2009) marks an early step toward professional acceptance of the concept of food addiction. The YFAS was written to match the diagnostic criteria for substance abuse in the DSM-IV, and then revised as the YFAS 2.0 (Gearhardt et al., 2016) to reflect the updated criteria in the DSM-5. This scale has demonstrated clear markers of food addiction, and identified which foods are more likely to cause addictive behavior when consumed.

PREVALENCE OF FOOD ADDICTION

Approximately one in five people meet the YFAS criteria for struggling with a food addiction, especially to soda, starchy foods, and fast foods which have been associated with addictive tendencies (Pursey et al., 2014). This prevalence of food addiction is similar to the 16.5 percent prevalence of people in the U.S. diagnosed with a DSM-5 substance use disorder (SAMHSA, 2023).

For clients receiving treatment for an eating disorder, the prevalence is higher, with rates as high as 53 percent for anorexia nervosa (AN), 63 percent for binge-eating disorder (BED), and 84 percent for bulimia nervosa (BN) (Praxedes et al., 2022, 2024). Individuals who are either underweight or obese have higher rates of food addiction than those in the normal weight or overweight BMI categories (Schulte & Gearhardt, 2018). This paints the picture that, based on the results of studies using the YFAS, someone with food addiction is more likely to have an eating disorder and is at higher risk of being underweight or obese.

Tolerance and withdrawal are 2 of the 11 diagnostic criteria in the YFAS (Examine.com, 2024) and appear to be more prevalent in obese individuals. Rats fed high-fat sweet food showed a decrease in dopamine receptors (a marker of tolerance) the more they gained weight (Johnson & Kenny, 2010). Human studies resulted in a similar dopamine response. A comparison of dopamine function in obese human study participants versus normal-weight subjects found that obese participants had fewer dopamine receptors, which meant they needed to eat more food, especially foods with higher sugar and fat, to get the same feelings of satisfaction that a leaner person feels (Tarman, 2019; Thanarajah et al., 2019; Wang et al., 2004).

Withdrawal generally includes cravings and a drive to repeat addictive behavior. Studies using fMRI brain scans showed greater activation of brain reward and motivation centers in obese individuals compared to lean individuals, which means they are more likely to struggle with cravings and uncontrolled eating (Becetti et al., 2023). In a study using the *Highly Processed Food Withdrawal Scale (ProWS)*, researchers found that withdrawal from highly processed foods (such as pizza, chocolate, pretzels, and gummy candy) paralleled the course of drug withdrawal, with the most intense symptoms between days two and five during an attempt to cut down on processed foods (Schulte et al., 2018).

ANIMAL MODELS OF FOOD ADDICTION

Animal studies of food addiction have been an important piece of the puzzle because they remove human risk factors such as self-esteem, media, and culture as drivers of eating behavior. Research on rodents (rats and mice) reveals changes to the neuron function in the brain and microbiome that indicate withdrawal symptoms in response to certain foods in ways that are similar to changes seen with drug addiction (Becetti et al., 2023; Brownell & Gold, 2012). These changes in neuron function are thought to contribute to binge-eating behavior due to the addictive properties of certain foods such as sugar (Avena & Hoebel, 2012; Laque et al., 2022). For example, a study of sugar addiction performed with rats found that, after a month of intermittent bingeing on sugar, the rats showed neurological and behavior changes similar to the effects of drugs of abuse (Avena et al., 2008).

FOOD ADDICTION AND EATING DISORDERS

The line between describing a person as having a food addiction and diagnosing someone with BED is an area of debate. A food addiction implies there are triggering foods that lead to over-consumption and bingeing behavior that should be removed from the diet. Whereas treatment for BED is generally in alignment with the eating approach recommended by the Academy of Nutrition and Dietetics, "All foods can fit within this pattern [of healthy eating] if consumed in moderation with appropriate portion size and combined with physical activity" (Freeland-Graves & Nitzke, 2013, p. 1). For example, it is fine to eat a cookie once or twice a week, but it may be a problem if one is eating ten cookies in a sitting or if eating cookies every day instead of vegetables. The concern is that being overly restrictive and entirely cutting out certain foods can cause feelings of deprivation that will drive someone to overeat the next time that food is available (Costin & Grabb, 2011).

The food addiction field has a different perspective. They argue that certain foods are very triggering for some people and cause an addictive response similar to drugs of abuse (Sheppard, 2024; Thompson, 2024). For these people, a diet focused on moderation that includes triggering foods is unlikely to be effective because when they ingest the triggering food, it is likely to stimulate cravings and binge-eating behavior. From that perspective, abstinence from triggering foods is the best option to manage the addictive power of these foods. Similar to alcohol addiction, many alcoholics report that the only way to stay sober is to completely avoid drinking any alcohol. Of course, we cannot abstain from all food in the same way we can from all alcohol, however, we can identify which foods are triggering for us and avoid consuming those triggering foods.

Recovery from food addiction also similarly requires awareness and vigilance around environmental triggers (Treasure et al., 2018). For the alcoholic, it might be important to avoid going to a bar as a likely trigger to want to drink alcohol. For the food addict, it might be important to avoid going to a donut shop for the same reason, that it is likely to trigger them to eat a food that would initiate a binge response. This is the approach used in the food addiction field and promoted in 12-step addiction recovery groups such as Overeaters Anonymous (OA), Food Addicts Anonymous (FAA), and Food Addicts in Recovery Anonymous (FA), which follow a similar 12-step program as promoted in Alcoholics Anonymous (AA).

Food Acceptance

There is a risk in vilifying certain foods as "bad," "unhealthy," or "junk" foods. Restrictive eating disorders such as anorexia and orthorexia include anxiety associated with food (Steinglass et al., 2012). Labeling a group of foods as bad can increase anxiety around food. In the book *8 Keys to Recovery from an Eating Disorder*, they state, "If you binge or binge and purge, abstaining from certain foods, such as sugar and white flour, can elevate their status in your mind and make you want them even more, contributing to a later binge" (Costin & Grabb, 2011, p. 66). The concern is that the abstinence model found in the 12-step recovery programs is too rigid when applied to food and may not be an appropriate fit for eating disorder clients who often struggle with perfectionism and obsessive thinking.

Eating disorder treatment often focuses on acceptance of a wide range of foods, including "junk" foods, as being safe and appropriate in moderation. It is therefore imperative that we are cautious in our use of the term food addiction, and recognize that, as with all addiction, it is not black and white. People fall along a spectrum of responses to triggering foods, where the same foods are not an issue for some and cause great activation leading to distress for others. Similar to the spectrum of response to alcohol where some people can drink in moderation with no problems, some binge on alcohol occasionally with few consequences, and others consume alcohol in a compulsive, out-of-control way that causes impairment and distress (Mills, 2022). We must each evaluate for ourselves where we fall on the spectrum of food addiction.

DIFFERENTIATING FOOD ADDICTION FROM AN EATING DISORDER

Within the eating disorder treatment community, there are concerns that food addiction research does not appropriately consider how a person with an eating disorder may respond differently to the questions on the YFAS. These differences can skew the results and lead to false positives showing higher rates of food addiction associated with eating disorders than actually exist (Wiss & Brewerton, 2020). For example, the YFAS asks if you feel a perceived loss of control over food. A client with AN might perceive a loss of control over food in a very different way than someone without that disorder since AN tends to include extreme efforts at controlling any form of food consumption. Some of the greatest controversy around food addiction has focused on concerns for clients with clinically significant eating disorders that may attach stigma, fear, and guilt to the idea of being addicted to certain foods, which can exacerbate disordered eating patterns, especially those related to food restriction.

Some of the traits that describe food addiction (e.g., feeling out of control) are similar to diagnostic criteria for eating disorders, especially BED, but they do not completely overlap. This suggests there may be key differences that need to be examined and elucidated (Hauck et al., 2020). It is important to understand which aspects of addictive eating behaviors are due to learned and habitual cues, and which are due to substance dependence, to provide the best treatment approach (di Giacomo et al., 2022; Ratković et al., 2023).

EXORPHINS

We recognize at face value that some foods are more addictive than others. Most people do not crave broccoli the same way they crave chocolate. The powerful drive toward consuming caffeine and sugar even when we are trying to cut back is a familiar wrestling match. However, we are often unaware of the addictive properties of seemingly "normal" or average foods. Many would be surprised to hear that bread and cheese also promote addictive reactions in our brains. These foods contain proteins termed *exorphins* that, in people with genetic susceptibility, can interact with opioid receptors like other addictive substances. If we are sensitive to this type of exorphin, then when we eat bread and cheese, our opioid receptors light up, which leads to a dopamine release and feelings of pleasure similar to other addictive substances. If we eat them regularly and then stop, we may experience cravings and withdrawal symptoms, such as feeling tired and sad (Brogan & Marriott, 2019).

CASOMORPHIN IN DAIRY

For those who crave dairy, it is essential to understand the role of casein (pronounced kay-seen). Casein is a family of proteins found in milk. Casein contains *casomorphins*, a compound that stimulates the opioid receptors in the brain that contribute to feeling pleasure and satisfaction associated with eating dairy products. It keeps people eating dairy products like cheese and milk even if they recognize that their bodies do not handle them well (e.g., they have diarrhea, feel gassy, or have itchy skin after they eat dairy). Recent research shows us that, for a subset of the population, eating dairy foods may be contributing to significant mental health issues such as psychosis, Schizophrenia, bipolar disorder, depression, and autism (Hockey et al., 2020; Severance et al., 2010; Thiruvengadam et al., 2021). Therefore, it may be important to explore removing dairy products from a person's diet for three weeks (as suggested in the Elimination Diet mentioned in Chapter 8) to see if there are any changes and improvements in mental health symptoms that may have been exacerbated by frequent dairy consumption.

GLIADORPHIN IN GLUTEN

Gluten can also be problematic and addictive for people. Gluten is a protein found in wheat and other grains. We often hear about the connection between gluten and celiac (coeliac) disease, an autoimmune disorder diagnosed with a lab test. When people with celiac disease eat gluten, they experience an immune response in the small intestine that, over time, damages the small intestine's lining and causes malabsorption (difficulty absorbing some nutrients). Symptoms can include diarrhea, fatigue, weight loss, rashes, bloating, and anemia (Mayo Clinic, 2022).

However, even those who do not have celiac disease may unknowingly struggle with gluten's negative impact on their overall health. The doctor may confirm the lack of celiac disease, yet negative symptoms may persist when gluten is consumed. This is known as *non-celiac gluten sensitivity (NCGS)*. A growing body of research has linked gluten to various inflammatory disorders in people with NCGS, with symptoms including diarrhea, constipation, headache, joint and muscle pain and numbness, chronic fatigue, brain fog, and depression. Practitioners diagnose NCGS by tracking what happens when someone eats gluten. Symptoms usually occur after they eat gluten-containing foods, disappear when they remove gluten from the diet, and relapse when they return to eating gluten (Czaja-Bulsa, 2015). Gluten sensitivity can even have an impact on major mental health disorders. Dating back to the 1950s, several studies linked NCGS with schizophrenia and autism spectrum disorder (ASD), with reported improvement in psychiatric symptoms after implementing a gluten-free diet (Ji, 2018).

Like dairy, gluten can impact the brain in ways that are similar to other addictive substances. Gluten contains an exorphin called *gliadorphin* peptides that can act on opioid receptors. Like casomorphins, for the portion of the population sensitive to these gliadorphin peptide proteins, when these people eat food with gluten, the body releases these peptides into the bloodstream. It stimulates opioid receptors in the body to release dopamine. As a result, they will feel a wave of pleasure when they eat gluten, and if they eat gluten for a considerable time and then stop, they will have unpleasant withdrawal symptoms similar to any drug withdrawal. At the same time, those sensitive to gluten will show other signs of irritation due to long-term gluten consumption, including gut dysbiosis, which increases intestinal permeability and allows more gliadorphin peptides from the intestines into the bloodstream. More gliadorphins means an increased opioid pleasure/pain cycle associated with gluten consumption. Like any addictive process, this dopamine rollercoaster takes a toll on a person's mental health while keeping them hooked on gluten-eating behavior due to cravings and discomfort (Woodford, 2021).

CASE STUDY: GLUTEN AND PSYCHOSIS

A 37-year-old woman with no history of mental illness began having psychotic, paranoid delusions focused on believing that friends and family were talking about her and part of a conspiracy to manipulate her. These symptoms worsened when her apartment was burglarized and vandalized. In her paranoia, she was convinced her family was involved and began making threats against family members. She was admitted to an inpatient psychiatric facility and diagnosed with paranoid schizophrenia. Her evaluation noted significant iron deficiency, vitamin deficiencies (especially vitamins B12 and D2), and a history of unintentional weight loss and hair thinning. After a one-month inpatient stay, the patient was discharged with a recommendation to continue taking psychiatric medications and iron and vitamin supplements.

Six weeks after discharge, her primary care physician evaluated her and found her to be excessively thin. Psychiatric conditions generally develop during early adulthood, so it was unusual for a client to have her first psychotic break in her late 30s. With this late onset of psychotic symptoms and no family history of psychiatric disorders, her physician thought a diagnosis of an underlying medical condition rather than a primary psychiatric disorder better explained her symptoms. Ultimately, the client was diagnosed with celiac disease and Hashimoto's thyroiditis (an autoimmune thyroid disorder). Although she had no stomach or gut symptoms, her weight loss and nutrient deficiencies were likely due to the impaired absorption of micronutrients commonly associated with celiac disease.

After six months of taking her prescribed medication, she was still having psychiatric symptoms, including paranoia. Her response to receiving the diagnosis of celiac disease was that she thought her doctors were trying to trick her and refused a gluten-free diet. Her paranoia persisted and she eventually lost her job, became homeless, attempted suicide, and her family took out a restraining order against her.

The client was rehospitalized at a psychiatric facility and placed on a gluten-free diet. After three months at the psychiatric facility, her delusions wholly resolved, and negative lab tests revealed that her celiac disease was in remission. She tapered down and then stopped taking the psychiatric medication and remained symptom-free for several months.

Sadly, after the patient inadvertently ingested gluten, she became delusional and was again hospitalized. Her labs indicated that her celiac disease was again active, and her iron deficiency had returned. At the publication of the case study, the patient refused to follow a gluten-free diet due to a delusion that the celiac disease diagnosis was incorrect.

This case study was adapted from Delichatsios, H., & Fasano, A. Case 14-2016: A woman with a thyroid nodule and psychosis. New England Journal of Medicine, 375(9), e20. https://doi.org/10.1056/NEJMc1607733. Copyright © (2016) Massachusetts Medical Society. Reprinted with permission from Massachusetts Medical Society.

CAFFEINE AND SUGAR ADDICTION

CAFFEINE

Any discussion of food addiction must include the impact of caffeine on a person's brain. *Caffeine* is a stimulant in coffee, tea, soda, and chocolate, and is included in the DSM-5 under substance-related and addictive disorders because some caffeine users "display symptoms consistent with problematic use" (American Psychiatric Association, 2013). While not at the same level as alcohol, which is more often categorized as a drug or substance of abuse than food, caffeine has clear hallmarks of the addictive process, including tolerance (needing more and more caffeine to experience the same positive feeling) and physiological withdrawal symptoms such as "caffeine headaches." It is habit-forming with feelings of emotional and psychological dependence and denial of its negative impact on overall health. So, despite our national love affair with caffeinated drinks and chocolate, it is important to pause and consider the possible negative impacts this substance may be having on our mental health. At this point, many readers may stop feeling interested in this topic and internally think, "Do not take away my caffeine!" It's okay, we understand.

In his book *Caffeine* (Pollan, 2020), Michael Pollan states that caffeine is so widely consumed worldwide that, for most of us, the altered state of being caffeinated feels like our standard state of consciousness. It has such a huge consumption rate that it makes caffeine the most widely used psychoactive substance and the only one we routinely give to children in the form of chocolate and soda. According to Pollan, its popularity has raised it to the level of normality, if not necessity, for many people, and we have become blind to the impact of this powerful and addictive substance.

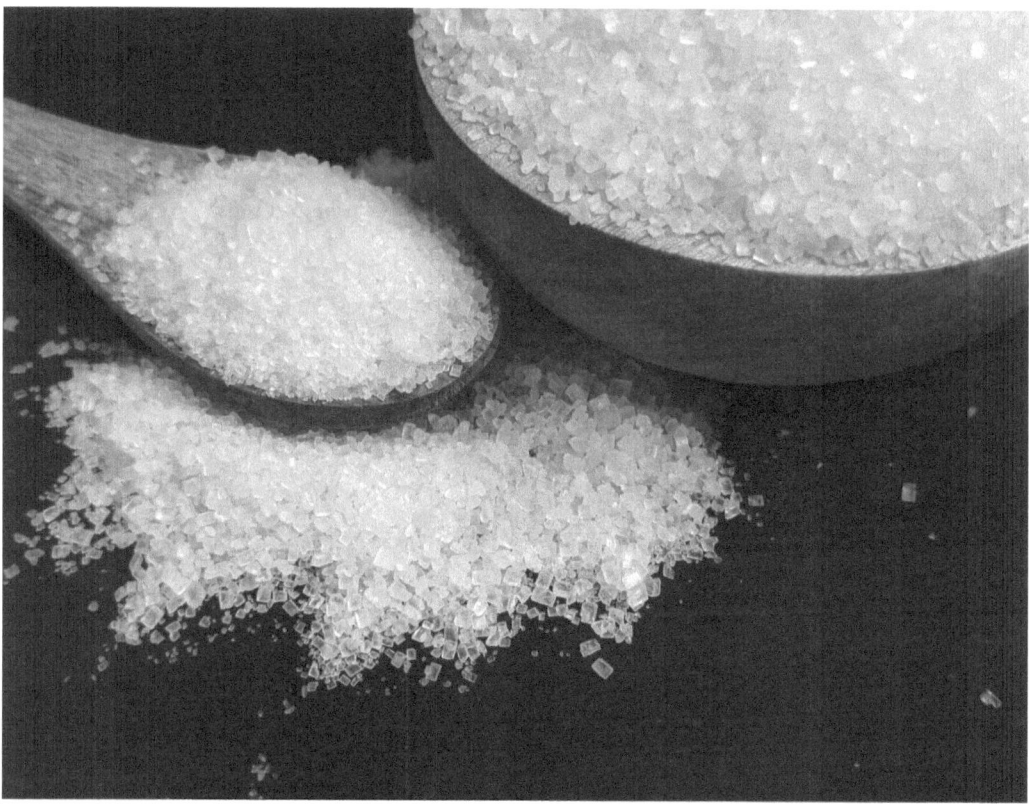

FIGURE 13.2   Granulated sugar, another highly addictive substance. (Shutterstock).

SUGAR

While there is still controversy about whether or not sugar is truly addictive, sugar has the second highest score for food addiction on the YFAS after caffeine. It has been identified in the food addiction field as the first food to be eliminated to recover from cravings and compulsive eating (Tarman, 2019). It is clearly problematic for some people, yet most people see it as an accepted and essential part of the food system. In research on drug abuse, we accept that a substance is addictive if it causes certain addictive symptoms, such as cravings, bingeing, tolerance, and withdrawal. We see all these addictive symptoms associated with the consumption of sugar, which shows that sugar is indeed addictive (Lenoir et al., 2007).

Going back to Pavlov's dogs, we can learn to pair images and smells with anticipating eating foods that will make us feel good. We react both to real food and images of food with *cue-induced cravings* that can be associated with overeating. For someone vulnerable to sugar addiction, being in an environment where there are many sugary environmental cues (e.g., vending machine, cookies in the break room, a bowl of candy on a desk) can lead to intense sugar cravings and addictive-like eating behaviors (Joyner et al., 2015; Massicotte et al., 2019; Sun & Kober, 2020). The good news is a conditioned response can be reconditioned and will fade over time when triggering foods are avoided and replaced with healthy alternatives (Meule, 2020).

In his book *Metabolical* (Lustig, 2021), Robert Lustig argues that, in many ways, sugar is more like a drug of abuse than it is a food. It is similar to alcohol in that it is not essential for animal life, causes damage to the body in chronically high doses, and a sizable percentage of the population is addicted. Like alcohol, not everyone exposed to sugar gets addicted, but enough do get addicted to sugar and suffer the effect of their addiction to warrant public health interventions.

The manufacturing that results in table sugar and high-fructose corn syrup requires an intensive refinement process to create the form of sugar added to nearly every package of processed foods that is quite different from the sugar found in nature. It is the refinement of sugar that adds to its addictive properties and causes it to behave like drugs of abuse. For example, in nature, sugar cane has a fibrous stalk that protects the sucrose from being easily eaten by mammals, so historically, humans could only consume it in small quantities. Modern agriculture quickly strips away the fibrous stalk and transforms the sucrose into a food we can now eat in very large doses that our brain is not designed to handle (Tarman, 2019).

The very small and quickly digested sugar particles release opioids and dopamine in the brain, creating pleasure sensations. They also set off a chemical process that delays the release of acetylcholine (a neurotransmitter), which increases tolerance to sugar so that we must eat more sugar to experience the same level of pleasure. When people stop eating sugar, they often experience withdrawal symptoms, including increased cravings and compulsive eating (DiNicolantonio et al., 2018). We end up eating more and more sugar as part of our daily diet, craving its effects, and are often unaware that it is the primary driver behind our choosing to eat tasty, processed foods that make us feel good in the short term and terrible in the long term.

ARTIFICIAL SWEETENERS

Artificial sweeteners are a popular alternative for consumers who do not want to eat sugar. Many people choose foods with artificial sweeteners such as aspartame, sucralose, and stevia to avoid sugar-related problems, especially calories. However, there are concerns that artificial sweeteners might be problematic for some people. For example, research suggests that artificial sweeteners trick the brain into thinking that sugar is coming, stimulating appetite and insulin release, and increasing cravings for sugar and processed carbohydrates (Lenoir et al., 2007; Pepino et al., 2013). So, just experiencing the sweetness of artificial sweeteners can stimulate the sugar addiction process in the body. There is also evidence that some artificial sweeteners can leave you feeling more hungry after you consume them compared to when you consume sugar (Egan, 2024; Perlmutter, 2022; van Opstal et al., 2019). In addition, there is growing evidence that artificial sweeteners are associated with our increasing rates of chronic disease. Recent correlative studies argue that artificially sweetened beverages can be associated with an increased risk of obesity, diabetes, cardiovascular disease, depression, and dementia (Avena et al., 2008; Azad et al., 2017; Guo et al., 2014; Lustig, 2021; Ruanpeng et al., 2017). So even artificial sweeteners do not offer an easy way out of the well-entrenched sugar addiction that grips the U.S.

FOOD FOR THOUGHT: OBESITY AND FOOD ADDICTION

There is a tendency to blame someone who is obese that it is their fault because they are lazy and undisciplined. However, new research is showing that there appear to be many factors that lead to obesity and make some people at higher risk than others. This model of food addiction argues that some people are more susceptible to developing unhealthy eating patterns (like binge eating) when they regularly consume highly processed foods due to how their body responds to those substances.

Many people point to a person's genetic makeup as the cause of obesity. There is certainly evidence in the form of twin studies that demonstrate a solid inherited component to a person's BMI, which means that some people are genetically vulnerable to becoming obese (Kim et al., 2022). For many, this casts a hopeless gloom that being obese is inevitable and that they are at the mercy of their genes and helpless to make any changes that would help them to lose weight. However, being genetically vulnerable does not make it a foregone conclusion that a person will become obese, since we must also look at the impact of the environment on that vulnerability.

We are still struggling to understand the depth of how genetics impact obesity. One hypothesis is a genetic mutation that decreases the production of the enzyme uricase, which amplifies the effect of fructose (now available in large quantities due to high fructose corn syrup) to promote fat storage and insulin resistance (Johnson et al., 2022). Anybody with that genetic mutation living in an environment filled with foods that contain high fructose corn syrup would be vulnerable to weight gain if they eat those foods.

Genetics research has found a significant association between a specific gene, the dopamine receptor gene (DRD2 A1+), and addiction to alcohol, cocaine, nicotine, and opioids (Brownell & Gold, 2012; Le Foll et al., 2009), as well as to obesity (Noble et al., 1994). People with this gene also have fewer D_2 dopamine receptors, which interferes with the dopamine reward system and makes it harder to feel good. Substances that produce a strong dopamine reaction (like alcohol and ultra-processed foods) that can provide more stimulation for their limited dopamine receptors would naturally drive increased cravings and addictive behavior for a person with that dopamine receptor gene.

The field of *epigenetics* argues that, in addition to whether a person carries a specific gene, we must also acknowledge the impact of the environment on whether or not that gene is activated so that it produces a specific effect in the body. Therefore, specific genes may make us genetically vulnerable to obesity if they interact with an environment that preys upon that vulnerability and causes the genes to be activated so that a person struggles with weight gain and increased adiposity (higher body fat).

In addition to having certain genes activated by the environment that influence eating behavior, there is also evidence that once a person has begun to gain weight, a cycle begins that perpetuates weight gain as well as inflammation and disease states. In his book *Always Hungry*, David Ludwig argues that we should think about obesity as a disorder where there has been a change in our fat cells that causes them to act upon our metabolism in a way that increases cravings and a constant feeling of hunger. "Overeating doesn't make us fat. The process of becoming fat makes us overeat" (Ludwig, 2016, p. 9).

Body fat is a complex metabolic tissue that influences our appetite, how we burn calories, and how our body regulates our weight. When fat (adipose) tissue reaches its capacity to store fat, the fat cells hit a critical threshold and begin to send distress signals to the immune system, resulting in chronic inflammation (Zatterale et al., 2022). This inflammation worsens insulin resistance, which causes the fat cells to resist releasing any fat to be used as energy (i.e., weight loss) and increases hunger and overeating.

Once in this inflamed state, highly processed foods will exacerbate the issue as the body attempts to store energy from those foods in the fat cells. Yet we keep eating highly processed foods due to their addictive nature, so the inflammation grows and continues. Obesity is then more likely to develop in those who are sensitive to addictive foods and is maintained by the cycle of never-ending hunger and cravings that result from inflammation and insulin resistance. Eating healthy food and avoiding addictive foods becomes increasingly difficult when you are always hungry and craving, and so the weight gain creeps in day-by-day while the person suffers from the constant struggle to feel satiated. As with many genetic vulnerabilities, a look at lifestyle can give meaning to breaking dysfunctional cycles through tools that can impact genetic destiny.

REFERENCES

American Psychiatric Association. (2013). *Diagnostic and statistical manual of mental disorders: DSM-5* (5th ed.). American Psychiatric Association. http://dsm.psychiatryonline.org/doi/book/10.1176/appi.books.9780890425596

Avena, N. M., Bocarsly, M. E., Rada, P., Kim, A., & Hoebel, B. G. (2008). After daily bingeing on a sucrose solution, food deprivation induces anxiety and accumbens dopamine/acetylcholine imbalance. *Physiology & Behavior, 94*(3), 309–315.

Avena, N. M., & Hoebel, B. G. (2012). Bingeing, withdrawal, and craving: An animal model of sugar addiction. In K. D. Brownell & M. S. Gold (Eds.), *Food and addiction: A comprehensive handbook* (1st ed., pp. 206–213). Oxford University Press.

Avena, N. M., Rada, P., & Hoebel, B. G. (2008). Evidence for sugar addiction: Behavioral and neurochemical effects of intermittent, excessive sugar intake. *Neuroscience & Biobehavioral Reviews, 32*(1), 20–39.

Azad, M. B., Abou-Setta, A. M., Chauhan, B. F., Rabbani, R., Lys, J., Copstein, L., Mann, A., Jeyaraman, M. M., Reid, A. E., & Fiander, M. (2017). Nonnutritive sweeteners and cardiometabolic health: A systematic review and meta-analysis of randomized controlled trials and prospective cohort studies. *CMAJ, 189*(28), E929–E939.

Bartoshuk, L. (2011). Addicted to food: An interview with Bart Hoebel. In *APS observer* (Vol. 22): Association for Psychological Science.

Becetti, I., Bwenyi, E. L., de Araujo, I. E., Ard, J., Cryan, J. F., Farooqi, I. S., Ferrario, C. R., Gluck, M. E., Holsen, L. M., Kenny, P. J., Lawson, E. A., Lowell, B. B., Schur, E. A., Stanley, T. L., Tavakkoli, A., Grinspoon, S. K., & Singhal, V. (2023). The neurobiology of eating behavior in obesity: Mechanisms and therapeutic targets: A report from the 23rd Annual Harvard Nutrition Obesity Symposium. *The American Journal of Clinical Nutrition, 118*(1), 314–328. https://doi.org/10.1016/j.ajcnut.2023.05.003

Brogan, K., & Marriott, N. (2019). *Own your self: The surprising path beyond depression, anxiety, and fatigue to reclaiming your authenticity, vitality, and freedom* (1st ed.). Hay House, Inc.

Brownell, K. D., & Gold, M. S. (2012). *Food and addiction: A comprehensive handbook* (1st ed.). Oxford University Press.

Costin, C., & Grabb, G. S. (2011). *8 keys to recovery from an eating disorder: Effective strategies from therapeutic practice and personal experience (8 keys to mental health)*. WW Norton & Company.

Czaja-Bulsa, G. (2015). Non coeliac gluten sensitivity - A new disease with gluten intolerance. *Clinical Nutrition, 34*(2), 189–194. https://doi.org/10.1016/j.clnu.2014.08.012

Delichatsios, H., & Fasano, A. (2016). Case 14-2016: A woman with a thyroid nodule and psychosis. *New England Journal of Medicine, 375*(9), e20. https://doi.org/10.1056/NEJMc1607733

Di Chiara, G., & Imperato, A. (1988). Drugs abused by humans preferentially increase synaptic dopamine concentrations in the mesolimbic system of freely moving rats. *Proceedings of the National Academy of Sciences, 85*(14), 5274–5278.

di Giacomo, E., Aliberti, F., Pescatore, F., Santorelli, M., Pessina, R., Placenti, V., Colmegna, F., & Clerici, M. (2022). Disentangling binge eating disorder and food addiction: A systematic review and meta-analysis. *Eating and Weight Disorders - Studies on Anorexia, Bulimia and Obesity, 27*(6), 1963–1970. https://doi.org/10.1007/s40519-021-01354-7

DiNicolantonio, J. J., O'Keefe, J. H., & Wilson, W. L. (2018). Sugar addiction: Is it real? A narrative review. *British Journal of Sports Medicine, 52*(14), 910–913.

Dufty, W. (1975). *Sugar blues* (1st ed.). Chilton Book Co.

Egan, J. M. (2024). Physiological integration of taste and metabolism. *New England Journal of Medicine, 390*(18), 1699–1710. https://doi.org/doi:10.1056/NEJMra2304578

Epel, E. S., Tomiyama, A. J., Mason, A. E., Laraia, B. A., Hartman, W., Ready, K., Acree, M., Adam, T. C., St Jeor, S., & Kessler, D. (2014). The reward-based eating drive scale: A self-report index of reward-based eating. *PLoS One, 9*(6), e101350. https://doi.org/10.1371/journal.pone.0101350

Examine.com. (2024). *What are the 11 diagnostic criteria in the Yale Food Addiction Scale?* https://examine.com/conditions/food-addiction/faq/what-are-the-11-diagnostic-criteria-in-the-yale-food-addiction-scale/

Freeland-Graves, J. H., & Nitzke, S. (2013). Position of the academy of nutrition and dietetics: Total diet approach to healthy eating. *Journal of the Academy of Nutrition and Dietetics, 113*(2), 307–317. https://doi.org/10.1016/j.jand.2012.12.013

Gearhardt, A. N., & Corbin, W. R. (2012). Food addiction and diagnostic criteria for dependence. In K. D. Brownell & M. S. Gold (Eds.), *Food and addiction: A comprehensive handbook* (1st ed.). Oxford University Press.

Gearhardt, A. N., Corbin, W. R., & Brownell, K. D. (2009). Preliminary validation of the Yale Food Addiction Scale. *Appetite, 52*(2), 430–436. https://doi.org/10.1016/j.appet.2008.12.003

Gearhardt, A. N., Corbin, W. R., & Brownell, K. D. (2016). Development of the Yale Food Addiction Scale Version 2.0. *Psychology of Addictive Behaviors, 30*(1), 113–121. https://doi.org/10.1037/adb0000136

Gordon, E. L., Ariel-Donges, A. H., Bauman, V., & Merlo, L. J. (2018). What is the evidence for "Food addiction?" A systematic review. *Nutrients, 10*(4), 477. https://www.mdpi.com/2072-6643/10/4/477

Guo, X., Park, Y., Freedman, N. D., Sinha, R., Hollenbeck, A. R., Blair, A., & Chen, H. (2014). Sweetened beverages, coffee, and tea and depression risk among older US adults. *PLoS One, 9*(4), e94715. https://doi.org/10.1371/journal.pone.0094715

Hauck, C., Cook, B., & Ellrott, T. (2020). Food addiction, eating addiction and eating disorders. *Proceedings of the Nutrition Society, 79*(1), 103–112. https://doi.org/10.1017/S0029665119001162

Hockey, M., McGuinness, A. J., Marx, W., Rocks, T., Jacka, F. N., & Ruusunen, A. (2020). Is dairy consumption associated with depressive symptoms or disorders in adults? A systematic review of observational studies. *Critical Reviews in Food Science and Nutrition*, *60*(21), 3653–3668. https://doi.org/10.1080/10 408398.2019.1703641

Hollis, J. (1985). *Fat is a family affair*. Hazelden.

Ifland, J., Sheppard, K., & Wright, T. (2012). From the front lines: The impact of refined food addiction on well-being. In K. D. Brownell & M. S. Gold (Eds.), *Food and addiction: A comprehensive handbook* (1st ed., pp. 349–353). Oxford University Press.

Ji, S. (2018). *60 years of research links gluten grains to schizophrenia*. https://greenmedinfo.com/ blog/60-years-research-links-gluten-grains-schizophrenia

Johnson, P. M., & Kenny, P. J. (2010). Addiction-like reward dysfunction and compulsive eating in obese rats: Role for dopamine D2 receptors. *Nature Neuroscience*, *13*(5), 635–641. https://doi.org/10.1038/nn.2519

Johnson, R. J., Sánchez-Lozada, L. G., Nakagawa, T., Rodriguez-Iturbe, B., Tolan, D., Gaucher, E. A., Andrews, P., & Lanaspa, M. A. (2022). Do thrifty genes exist? Revisiting uricase. *Obesity*, *30*(10), 1917–1926. https://doi.org/10.1002/oby.23540

Joyner, M. A., Gearhardt, A. N., & White, M. A. (2015). Food craving as a mediator between addictive-like eating and problematic eating outcomes. *Eating Behaviors*, *19*, 98–101.

Kenny, P. J. (2013). The food addiction. *Scientific American*, *309*(3), 44–49. http://www.jstor.org/stable/26017984

Kessler, D. A. (2009). *The end of overeating: Taking control of the insatiable American appetite*. Rodale Books.

Kim, S. Y., Yoo, D. M., Kwon, M. J., Kim, J. H., Kim, J. H., Bang, W. J., & Choi, H. G. (2022). Differences in nutritional intake, total body fat, and BMI score between twins. *Nutrients*, *14*(17). https://doi. org/10.3390/nu14173655

Laque, A., Wagner, G. E., Matzeu, A., De Ness, G. L., Kerr, T. M., Carroll, A. M., de Guglielmo, G., Nedelescu, H., Buczynski, M. W., Gregus, A. M., Jhou, T. C., Zorrilla, E. P., Martin-Fardon, R., Koya, E., Ritter, R. C., Weiss, F., & Suto, N. (2022). Linking drug and food addiction via compulsive appetite. *British Journal of Pharmacology*, *179*(11), 2589–2609. https://doi.org/10.1111/bph.15797

Le Foll, B., Gallo, A., Le Strat, Y., Lu, L., & Gorwood, P. (2009). Genetics of dopamine receptors and drug addiction: A comprehensive review. *Behavioural Pharmacology*. *20*(1), 1–17. https://doi.org/10.1097/ FBP.0b013e3283242f05

Lembke, A. (2021). *Dopamine nation: finding balance in the age of indulgence*. Dutton.

Lenoir, M., Serre, F., Cantin, L., & Ahmed, S. H. (2007). Intense sweetness surpasses cocaine reward. *PLoS One*, *2*(8), e698. https://doi.org/10.1371/journal.pone.0000698

Ludwig, D. (2016). *Always hungry?: conquer cravings, retrain your fat cells, and lose weight permanently* (1st ed.). Grand Central Life & Style.

Lustig, R. H. (2021). *Metabolical: the lure and the lies of processed food, nutrition, and modern medicine*. HarperWave.

Massicotte, E., Deschênes, S. M., & Jackson, P. L. (2019). Food craving predicts the consumption of highly palatable food but not bland food. *Eating and Weight Disorders-Studies on Anorexia, Bulimia and Obesity*, *24*, 693–704.

Mayo Clinic. (2022). *Celiac disease*. Mayo Clinic. https://www.mayoclinic.org/diseases-conditions/celiac-disease/symptoms-causes/syc-20352220?p=1

Meule, A. (2015). Back by popular demand: A narrative review on the history of food addiction research. *Yale Journal of Biology and Medicine*, *88*(3), 295–302.

Meule, A. (2020). The psychology of food cravings: The role of food deprivation. *Current Nutrition Reports*, *9*(3), 251–257. https://doi.org/10.1007/s13668-020-00326-0

Mills, K. (2022). Speaking of psychology. In *Can you be addicted to food? With Ashley Gearhardt, PhD*. https://www.apa.org/news/podcasts/speaking-of-psychology/food-addiction

Minirth, F. B. (1990). *Love hunger*. T. Nelson.

Noble, E. P., Noble, R. E., Ritchie, T., Syndulko, K., Bohlman, M. C., Noble, L. A., Zhang, Y., Sparkes, R. S., & Grandy, D. K. (1994). D2 dopamine receptor gene and obesity. *International Journal of Eating Disorders*, *15*(3), 205–217. 10.1002/1098-108x(199404)15:3<205::aid-eat2260150303>3.0.co;2-p

Pepino, M. Y., Tiemann, C. D., Patterson, B. W., Wice, B. M., & Klein, S. (2013). Sucralose affects glycemic and hormonal responses to an oral glucose load. *Diabetes Care*, *36*(9), 2530–2535.

Perlmutter, D. (2022). *Drop acid: The surprising new science of uric acid – The key to losing weight, controlling blood sugar and achieving extraordinary health*. Little, Brown Spark.

Pollan, M. (2020). *Caffeine: How caffeine created the modern world*. Audible Originals.

Praxedes, D. R. S., Silva-Junior, A. E., Macena, M. L., Oliveira, A. D., Cardoso, K. S., Nunes, L. O., Monteiro, M. B., Melo, I. S. V., Gearhardt, A. N., & Bueno, N. B. (2022). Prevalence of food addiction determined by the Yale Food Addiction Scale and associated factors: A systematic review with meta-analysis. *European Eating Disorders Review*, *30*(2), 85–95. https://doi.org/10.1002/erv.2878

Praxedes, D. R. S., Silva-Júnior, A. E., Macena, M. L., Oliveira, A. D., Cardoso, K. S., Nunes, L. O., Monteiro, M. B., Melo, I. S. V., Gearhardt, A. N., & Bueno, N. B. (2024). Correction to 'Prevalence of food addiction determined by the Yale Food Addiction Scale and associated factors: A systematic review with meta-analysis. *European Eating Disorders Review, 32*(3), 610–611. https://doi.org/10.1002/erv.3078

Pursey, K. M., Stanwell, P., Gearhardt, A. N., Collins, C. E., & Burrows, T. L. (2014). The prevalence of food addiction as assessed by the Yale Food Addiction Scale: A systematic review. *Nutrients, 6*(10), 4552–4590.

Randolph, T. G. (1956). The descriptive features of food addiction. Addictive eating and drinking. *Quarterly Journal of Studies on Alcohol, 17*(2), 198–224. https://doi.org/10.15288/qjsa.1956.17.198

Ratković, D., Knežević, V., Dickov, A., Fedrigolli, E., & Čomić, M. (2023). Comparison of binge-eating disorder and food addiction. *Journal of International Medical Research, 51*(4), 03000605231171016. https://doi.org/10.1177/03000605231171016

Ruanpeng, D., Thongprayoon, C., Cheungpasitporn, W., & Harindhanavudhi, T. (2017). Sugar and artificially sweetened beverages linked to obesity: A systematic review and meta-analysis. *QJM: An International Journal of Medicine, 110*(8), 513–520. https://doi.org/10.1093/qjmed/hcx068

SAMHSA. (2023). *SAMHSA announces National Survey on Drug Use and Health (NSDUH) results detailing mental illness and substance use levels in 2021.* https://www.hhs.gov/about/news/2023/01/04/samhsa-announces-national-survey-drug-use-health-results-detailing-mental-illness-substance-use-levels-2021.html

Schulte, E. M., & Gearhardt, A. N. (2018). Associations of food addiction in a sample recruited to be nationally representative of the United States. *European Eating Disorders Review, 26*(2), 112–119. https://doi.org/10.1002/erv.2575

Schulte, E. M., Smeal, J. K., Lewis, J., & Gearhardt, A. N. (2018). Development of the highly processed food withdrawal scale, *Appetite, 131*, 148–154. https://doi.org/10.1016/j.appet.2018.09.013

Severance, E. G., Dickerson, F. B., Halling, M., Krivogorsky, B., Haile, L., Yang, S., Stallings, C. R., Origoni, A. E., Bossis, I., Xiao, J., Dupont, D., Haasnoot, W., & Yolken, R. H. (2010). Subunit and whole molecule specificity of the anti-bovine casein immune response in recent onset psychosis and schizophrenia. *Schizophrenia Research, 118*(1–3), 240–247. https://doi.org/10.1016/j.schres.2009.12.030

Sheppard, K. (1989). *Food addiction: The body knows.* Health Communications.

Sheppard, K. (2024). *The Kay Sheppard plan: A program for freedom from food addiction.* https://kaysheppard.com/

SHiFT. (n.d.). *SHiFT recovery by Acorn.* Sobriety, Hope, Freedom, and Transformation (SHiFT). https://foodaddiction.com/

Steinglass, J., Albano, A. M., Simpson, H. B., Carpenter, K., Schebendach, J., & Attia, E. (2012). Fear of food as a treatment target: Exposure and response prevention for anorexia nervosa in an open series. *International Journal of Eating Disorders, 45*(4), 615–621.

Sun, W., & Kober, H. (2020). Regulating food craving: From mechanisms to interventions, *Physiology & Behavior, 222*, 112878. https://doi.org/10.1016/j.physbeh.2020.112878

Sussman, S., & Sussman, A. N. (2011). Considering the definition of addiction. *International Journal of Environmental Research and Public Health, 8*(10), 4025–4038. https://www.mdpi.com/1660-4601/8/10/4025

Tarman, V. (2019). *Food junkies: Recovery from food addiction.* Dundurn.

Thanarajah, S. E., Backes, H., DiFeliceantonio, A. G., Albus, K., Cremer, A. L., Hanssen, R., Lippert, R. N., Cornely, O. A., Small, D. M., & Brüning, J. C. (2019). Food intake recruits orosensory and post-ingestive dopaminergic circuits to affect eating desire in humans. *Cell Metabolism, 29*(3), 695–706.e4.

Thiruvengadam, M., Venkidasamy, B., Thirupathi, P., Chung, I. M., & Subramanian, U. (2021). β-Casomorphin: A complete health perspective. *Food Chemistry, 337*, 127765. https://doi.org/10.1016/j.foodchem.2020.127765

Thompson, S. P. (2024). *Bright line eating.* https://www.brightlineeating.com/

Treasure, J., Leslie, M., Chami, R., & Fernández-Aranda, F. (2018). Are trans diagnostic models of eating disorders fit for purpose? A consideration of the evidence for food addiction. *European Eating Disorders Review, 26*(2), 83–91. https://doi.org/10.1002/erv.2578

van Opstal, A. M., Kaal, I., van den Berg-Huysmans, A. A., Hoeksma, M., Blonk, C., Pijl, H., Rombouts, S. A. R. B., & van der Grond, J. (2019). Dietary sugars and non-caloric sweeteners elicit different homeostatic and hedonic responses in the brain. *Nutrition, 60*, 80–86. https://doi.org/10.1016/j.nut.2018.09.004

Volkow, N. D., Fowler, J. S., & Wang, G. J. (2002). Role of dopamine in drug reinforcement and addiction in humans: Results from imaging studies. *Behavioural Pharmacology, 13*(5–6), 355–366. https://doi.org/10.1097/00008877-200209000-00008

Wang, G.-J., Volkow, N. D., Thanos, P. K., & Fowler, J. S. (2004). Similarity between obesity and drug addiction as assessed by neurofunctional imaging: A concept review. *Journal of Addictive Diseases, 23*(3), 39–53.

Wiss, D., & Brewerton, T. (2020). Separating the signal from the noise: How psychiatric diagnoses can help discern food addiction from dietary restraint. *Nutrients, 12*(10), 2937.

Woodford, K. B. (2021). Casomorphins and gliadorphins have diverse systemic effects spanning gut, brain and internal organs. *International Journal of Environmental Research and Public Health, 18*(15), 7911. https://doi.org/10.3390/ijerph18157911

Zatterale, F., Raciti, G. A., Prevenzano, I., Leone, A., Campitelli, M., De Rosa, V., Beguinot, F., & Parrillo, L. (2022). Epigenetic reprogramming of the inflammatory response in obesity and type 2 diabetes. *Biomolecules, 12*(7). https://doi.org/10.3390/biom12070982

Section VI

Where Do We Go from Here?

14 The Politics of Food

Why do some people have plenty of good food while others barely have enough to eat? This is a complex issue that touches many lives in many ways. In the U.S., the United States Department of Agriculture (USDA) is responsible for monitoring the food system. These responsibilities include tracking the quality of food production, distribution, and consumption, in other words, the wellbeing of livestock, pesticides in the fields, transporting of goods to food manufacturers and grocery stores, all the way to becoming the foods that people purchase and eat.

Recognizing that food security is an issue for many U.S. families, the USDA created a Community Food Security Assessment Toolkit to be used in a series of focus groups to gather data on access to food (Cohen et al., 2002). The following questions from their toolkit can be informative when working to better understand food security in the U.S.

1. Do you think that many households in the community have a problem with food security?
2. What is the extent of the problem?
3. Why do you think that household food security is a problem? (That is, how do you see the problem manifest itself?)
4. How do people cope with the problem of food insecurity?
5. What are the contributing factors?

FOOD INSECURITY

To understand food insecurity, we must first define food security. The USDA defines *food security* as "access by all people at all times to enough food for an active, healthy life." Food security means a household has the ability to acquire the quantity and quality of needed food, that they have the means to travel to the store, the money to pay for the food that is being sold, and the time and ability to cook and store the food (USDA, 2023). The USDA estimates that almost 90 percent of U.S. households were food secure in 2022, which looks good on paper but the real story is more nuanced.

The USDA defines *food insecurity (FI)* as households that are "uncertain of having, or unable to acquire, at some time during the year, enough food to meet the needs of all their members because they had insufficient money or other resources for food." A household with FI experiences an ongoing struggle to obtain food for a variety of reasons, worries about their ability to obtain food, and may experience periods of hunger and discomfort due to a lack of food. Frequently, part of the challenge of acquiring not just food, but healthy food, is the unfortunate reality that many people reside in neighborhoods known as food deserts or food swamps, where there is either minimal food available or the only convenient food is fast food or highly processed packaged foods (see more on this later in the chapter).

People who experience FI regularly face challenges such as insufficient food quantity, poor food quality, limited nutritional diversity, and compromised food safety. One example of FI is a family of four where the children only eat breakfast and lunch on the days they go to school because the family cannot afford more than one simple meal per day at home each evening. Another example is a college student who skips meals to pay rent and buy books.

As though being hungry wasn't bad enough, sometimes people must engage in behaviors that they find humiliating and demeaning to acquire enough food for themselves and their families (Whittle et al., 2015). People participate in socially unacceptable methods of obtaining food, including scrounging from family and friends, begging from strangers, relying on charity, exchanging sex for food, dumpster diving, foraging street garbage cans, and stealing food. Even within the social safety net systems, customers of food pantries, soup kitchens, and community development programs often feel stigmatized and demeaned for accessing and taking part in those programs

DOI: 10.1201/9781032647647-20

(Lindberg et al., 2023). Struggling to obtain food can become a source of shame and can influence a lifetime of fear-based thoughts and behaviors around food and eating.

STATISTICS ON FOOD INSECURITY

So how many people does FI affect and which segments of the population are at higher risk of FI? The U.S. government began measuring household FI in 1995 and releases an annual *Household Food Security* report that details national trends in population FI. In 2023, the average number of households in the U.S. that reported FI was 13.5 percent of the population, which equals 18 million households. This means more than 1 out of 10 people did not have the ability to acquire adequate nutritious food for their household (Rabbitt et al., 2023).

Looking historically, 13.5 percent of hungry Americans is a lot. The *Household Food Security* data over the last 24 years shows that the current rate of FI and very low food security is higher than averages in the past, and moving toward the high rates of FI during the recession years from 2008 to 2014, when large portions of the population were struggling financially (see Figure 14.1). In a separate 2023 study that examined FI in the first year of the novel coronavirus (COVID-19) pandemic when jobs were lost and food supply chains were disrupted, the researchers reported an increased risk of FI among lower-income racial minority families, young women, and college students (Ellakany et al., 2022; Kim-Mozeleski et al., 2023). However, these figures often do not account for the quality of the food consumed or the socially stigmatizing situations involved in obtaining the food such as begging or stealing. This broader view of FI leads to a discussion about *nutrition equity* and how access to quality food is impacted by social, political, and environmental influences.

One area of FI that has been gaining attention is the high rate of FI among college students. Numerous studies report higher than average rates of FI on college campuses, at both the undergraduate and graduate levels. A 2020 systematic review of 51 studies of U.S. colleges, universities,

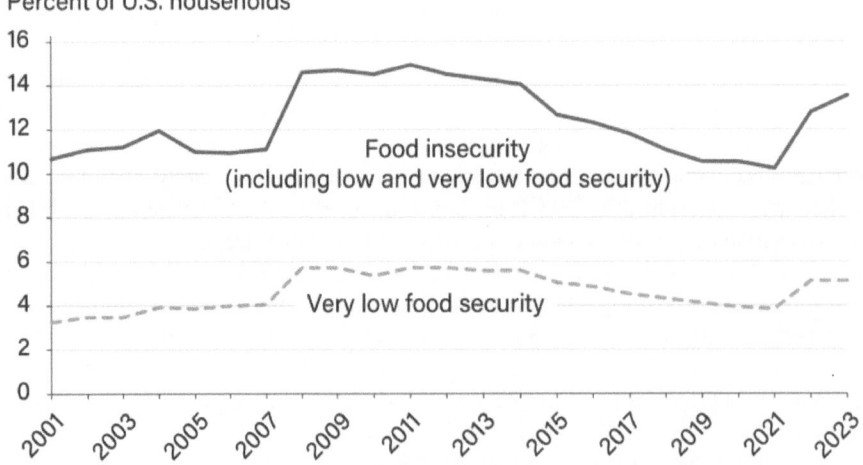

Trends in the prevalence of food insecurity and very low food security in U.S. households, 2001–23

Percent of U.S. households

Source: USDA, Economic Research Service using data from U.S. Department of Commerce, Bureau of the Census, Current Population Survey Food Security Supplements.

FIGURE 14.1 Trends in prevalence rates of food insecurity and very low food security in U.S. households, 2001–23 *Household Food Security* report (USDA, 2023). (Courtesy of the United States Department of Agriculture.)

and community colleges by Nikolaus et al. estimated that an average of 41 percent of college students struggle with FI (2020). The issue is exacerbated at historically black colleges and universities where as many as 73 percent of college students experience some level of FI (Duke et al., 2023). Qualitative studies highlighted the hidden nature of the problem, as college students reported not notifying family members because they did not want to worry them or lying to friends that they had already eaten (Meza et al., 2019). College students at higher risk include those who are from lower-income households, first-generation college students, non-traditionally aged, those with a reported disability, a member of a racial/ethnic minority, transgender, and non-binary gender identifying (Hagedorn-Hatfield et al., 2022; Olfert et al., 2023). Other risk factors include never having cooked for themselves and having busy schedules with little time for food shopping and cooking. We will discuss strategies for maintaining a healthy diet during the college years in Chapter 15.

RACE AND ETHNICITY

When we examine FI by race and ethnicity, it is clear that the rate is much higher for people of color. In the 2023 USDA report titled *Food Security Status of U.S. Households in 2022* (USDA, 2023), race and ethnicity are divided into four categories: Black (non-Hispanic), White (non-Hispanic), Hispanic, and Other (non-Hispanic). The Other (non-Hispanic) group includes people who identify as multiple races, American Indian, Alaskan Native, Asian, Hawaiian, or Pacific Islander. Examining the trend over the last 20 years, it is clear that those who identify as Black (non-Hispanic) and Hispanic reported significantly higher levels of FI than the other two groups and the average of all households (see Figure 14.2).

THE IMPACT OF FOOD INSECURITY ON HEALTH

FI focuses not only on insufficient quantities of food but also includes eating poor-quality food that contributes to chronic health disorders both physical and mental. Long-term consumption of poor-quality food has clear associations with many types of chronic diseases like type 2 diabetes,

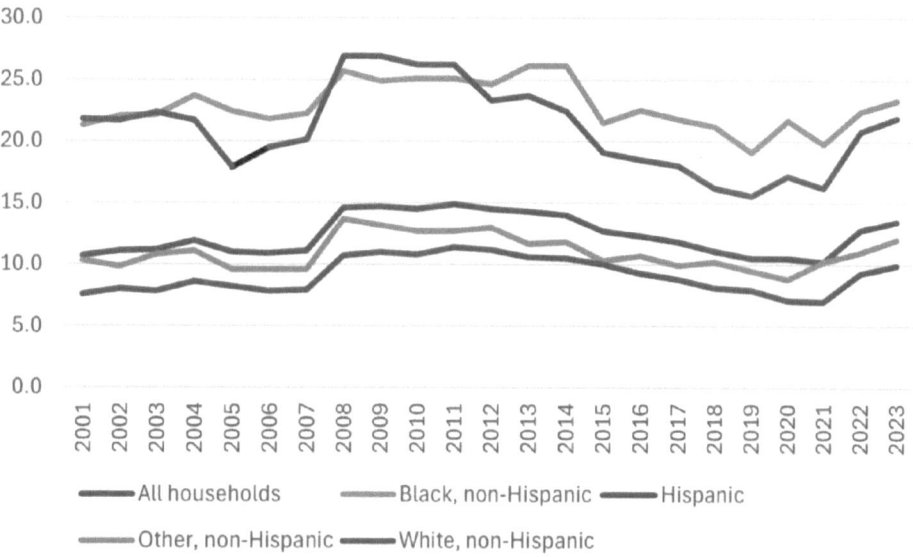

FIGURE 14.2 Trends in food insecurity by race and ethnicity, 2001–23 (USDA, 2023). (Adapted from *Trends in Food Insecurity by Race and Ethnicity, 2001–23*, Food Security in the U.S., United States Department of Agriculture.)

asthma, heart disease, and Crohn's disease. It is common to see co-morbid illnesses where a person has both a physical disease and a mental health disorder, and both are impacted by poor food quality (Anema et al., 2011).

FI is a major risk factor for both developing depression and increasing pre-existing depressive symptoms. As has been discussed in previous chapters, physical health and mental health are intricately intertwined, and food has the power to impact the entire body. In the case of FI, mental illness such as depression can be both the outcome of FI as well as the cause of it. In other words, being food insecure makes it more likely that you will be depressed, and being depressed makes it more likely that you will be food insecure (Pourmotabbed et al., 2020). For example, it is easy to imagine a parent who is distressed about not being able to provide food for their children having feelings of sadness, hopelessness, and guilt, then finally giving up, pulling the covers over their head, and avoiding the whole issue of trying to provide for their family. The research also tells us that depression is often a predictor of FI where someone who is depressed has a difficult time gathering up the energy and organization required to acquire, cook, and store food (Gundersen & Ziliak, 2015). This is corroborated by a large study of 14,000 children which found that mothers who were moderately to severely depressed had a 79 percent higher risk of household FI (Noonan et al., 2016). As you can imagine, in a community with widespread poor access to food, the risk of a negative spiral into debilitating depression is even worse.

It is interesting to note that the level of distress around FI is intensified in wealthy countries where the expectation is that everybody has access to plenty of healthy food. Often called *relative FI*, there is increased secrecy and shame if yours is the household without enough food while others in the same community are food secure and often unaware of the difference in circumstances. Even households that have not previously experienced FI can be thrown into an unstable state (even if temporary) when a key provider becomes ill or loses their job. Suddenly FI looms as a new and difficult challenge with an immediate ripple effect. A family may unexpectedly need to rely on food pantries, apply for financial aid, or skip meals, which can lead to feeling needy and embarrassed. The feelings of shame around FI are amplified in a wealthy country where it is easy to negatively compare yourself to more affluent neighbors, which implies anybody who is not food secure is somehow failing to fulfill social expectations. The additional stress of having to work to acquire food can drain a person's strength and resources and cause them to fail in other responsibilities like going to work or completing a writing assignment, which is especially difficult when you are comparing yourself to neighbors who are currently more stable around food. Elgar and colleagues close their article on relative FI with the statement, "Indeed, the surest way to *feel* food insecure is to be continually reminded of how little food you have when others have plenty" (2021, p. 7).

The impact of FI sometimes looks different in children. Children with persistent FI are at greater risk of experiencing mood and behavioral challenges. These can show up as increased emotional symptoms, including feeling low, irritable, or nervous. Since children often act on their distressed moods with dysfunctional behavior changes, a child who is food insecure is more likely to develop both internalizing and externalizing behaviors. When under the stress of deep hunger, the child may hurt themselves (internalizing) with behaviors such as cutting or developing an eating disorder or hurting others (externalizing) with behaviors such as tantrums, bullying, and breaking things. They are more likely to show symptoms of mood disorders like depression and anxiety and to have behavioral challenges like inattention and hyperactivity (Althoff et al., 2016). In Chapter 2, we covered more detailed information about childhood mental health disorders and how distress is sometimes displayed differently in children compared to adults.

THE COST OF FOOD INSECURITY

As a wealthy society, FI is expensive and avoidable. FI comes with tremendous financial costs to our national budget. There are clear connections between FI and preventable illnesses in adults such as type 2 diabetes. There is also a link between lack of food or quality food to lost productivity at work or school, and behavioral and developmental issues in children, such as increased moodiness and conduct problems (e.g., rule breaking) in children with ADHD (Booth & Pollard, 2020; Hatsu et al., 2022). The magnitude of the cost to us as a society was detailed in a study performed by Shepard et al. who estimated that FI costs our nation at least $167 billion due to the combination of "lost economic productivity per year, more expensive public education because of the rising costs of poor education outcomes, avoidable healthcare costs, and the cost of charity to keep families fed." This cost does not include the *Supplemental Nutrition Assistance Program (SNAP)* or other key federal nutrition programs (Shepard et al., 2011).

Luckily, the rapidly growing body of research about the deleterious impact of FI has put pressure on national leaders to take action. In March of 2023, the Biden administration launched the *White House Challenge to End Hunger and Build Healthy Communities* (Stephenson, 2022). This legislation dedicated $8 billion in new commitments to focus on five key pillars of the food system:

Pillar 1 – Improve Food Access and Affordability
Pillar 2 – Integrate Nutrition and Health
Pillar 3 – Empower Consumers to Make and Have Access to Healthy Choices
Pillar 4 – Support Physical Activity for All
Pillar 5 – Enhance Nutrition and Food Security Research

VIOLENCE AND FOOD

With so many committed people concerned about access to both sufficient quantity and quality of food, you may wonder how people become food insecure. What environmental pressures put some people more at risk for FI than others? Are there invisible structures in the U.S. food system that make it more difficult for some communities to maintain a healthy diet? What does violence have to do with not having enough food to eat?

Pairing violence with food is not an obvious combination for most people, other than perhaps in the infamous scene from the movie Animal House where one student yells, "Food fight!" in the cafeteria, and an all-out food war takes place. However, when looking at our national food systems, it is clear that some people have access to high-quality foods and others do not. Some neighborhoods have grocery stores and other neighborhoods require that their residents drive 10 miles for a head of lettuce. If these differences are based on ethnic and socioeconomic communities, then are they a form of social repression? Are our leaders in government making decisions that prioritize corporate interests over individual needs and is that a form of violence?

TYPES OF VIOLENCE

Johan Galtung, a peace scholar and Norwegian theorist, was one of the first to identify different types of violence: direct violence, structural violence, and then later added cultural violence (1969, 1990). According to Galtung, what usually comes to mind when we think about violence is called direct violence. *Direct violence* is when a person intentionally inflicts physical harm on another human. Of course, the most pressing examples of direct violence might be a mass shooting where people are killed or maimed, bullying on a school playground, sexual assault, or any form of physical abuse. This is the violence we often read about in the news and see in the video games that our children play. The examples are endless and all too familiar in our society. While we all recognize the damage caused by direct violence, the often invisible structural and cultural forms of violence can be just as damaging because they are the beliefs and systemic structures that are used to deny or justify direct violence.

Structural violence describes a form of violence where social structures or social institutions harm people by preventing them from attaining their basic needs (Lee, 2016), where there is harm to humans as a result of injustices in our societies (Empowering Nonviolence, 2023). These social injustices are embedded and normalized in our political, economic, and cultural systems, which masks the harm they inflict on individuals and groups by limiting access to resources of segments of the population which restricts their ability to reach their full potential (Lindberg et al., 2023). For example, many people of color in lower socioeconomic groups struggle to afford healthcare services because insurance premiums and costs for care continue to go up largely due to ongoing pressure from corporations that maintain huge profits with the current healthcare system.

Cultural violence is how people justify direct and structural violence by sending the message that the people who are the target of the violence are less important and somehow deserve the injuries that they received. These ideas are passed along in the form of stories, songs, language use, aspects of religions or traditions, science, assumptions, and stereotypes (Galtung, 1990). For example, one of the historic forms of cultural violence is the belief that Africans are primitive and intellectually inferior to Caucasians, which gave sanction to the African slave trade.

A more current example is bullying on a school playground. Bullying is minimized in a school with a zero-tolerance policy, where teachers and staff have been trained to identify and immediately act when they see bullying, with a clear structure for how the school will work with the parents and discipline a child for bullying behavior. In contrast, bullying thrives in schools where overwhelmed teachers turn a blind eye because they feel it is not their job to parent someone else's child, they are just there to teach. In the first example, the school as a system is working to create a safe environment. In the second example, the school creates an environment that is unsafe by not providing the necessary staffing and procedures to keep the kids safe (a form of structural violence). Often this lack of school bullying policy is justified by promoting the belief that the fault lies with the parents and not the teachers or the school and is therefore the parents' responsibility and they are to blame (a form of cultural violence).

With this example, we could also take another step back and say that structural and cultural violence are part of a bigger picture. Structural violence includes government policies that perpetuate schools to be underfunded in certain neighborhoods, which creates overwhelmed teachers and staff with less bandwidth to recognize and deal with bullying. The belief system or cultural violence that justifies the lack of state funding for the school may focus on the school being in a poor neighborhood, so it is perceived as the fault of the neighborhood that the kids are not safe rather than an indication that our school funding policies are not working very well for a lot of families.

VIOLENCE IN THE FOOD SYSTEM

So, what do these forms of violence have to do with food? All three forms of violence are possible with food, so let's review some examples. We will begin with direct violence. Remember that direct violence is when someone intentionally causes harm to another. Direct violence could occur if someone intentionally poisoned someone else's food or allowed food to be sold that was known to be unsafe. Luckily, this form of food violence is rare compared to the other forms of violence with food.

Structural violence looks at systems that are in place, such as government policies, that end up harming people by how they implement the rules and laws. An example of structural violence in the U.S. food system is farm subsidies that make high-quality fresh produce and meat less available and more expensive than less nutrient-dense foods (see more in the *Food for Thought* section below). Policymakers are aware that low-income communities have fewer options and less money to spend on high-quality food, and as a result generally have poorer health. Therefore, the policies that maintain these food price inequities are inflicting structural violence on the communities that have worse health due to their diet and are thereby harmed by these policies.

Cultural violence associated with food exists in the form of blaming people who are overweight or unhealthy for eating poor-quality food. We shame people in families, social media, and the healthcare system for their lack of discipline to make good food choices which results in them being fat and sick. We often ignore that there are many factors that influence what we eat, including cost, misinformation, and availability of healthy foods. The fact that we allow food corporate interests to influence our food research and policies speaks to the structural violence that keeps people confused about what to eat. Food decisions are made in different environments, some that support high consumption of fresh fruits and vegetables, others that offer mostly convenience foods as the only viable option (see Food Apartheid below). It is a form of cultural violence when we judge people for eating ultra-processed foods while at the same time making it the only food available.

Of Note ... DIET MISINFORMATION AND THE LOW-FAT MOVEMENT

One of the biggest areas of deception that influenced our understanding of healthy and unhealthy foods for decades was the idea that too much saturated fat in the diet was the primary driver of poor health and the number one killer of adults in the U.S. by causing obesity and heart disease. "Eating fat makes you fat" or so the theory goes and causes you to have a heart attack or a stroke. So where did we get this idea that eating fat is bad for you? Credit is generally given to Ancel Keys and his 1957 publication of the *Seven Countries Study*. In this study, Keys sought to understand the link between specific dietary patterns and heart disease by studying people from different regions around the world (Aboul-Enein et al., 2020). The study findings were that people who had high blood cholesterol (serum lipid) levels and high blood pressure (hypertension) were at higher risk of dying from a heart attack or stroke and that replacing dietary saturated fat from animal products with unsaturated fat from vegetable oils would lower cholesterol and decrease the risk of a heart attack or stroke. This is known as the *diet-heart* hypothesis. By the 1980s, Keys' theories received international recognition and were the basis of health education, public health policy, and nutritional science for decades. Thus, was born the crusade for the low-fat, low-cholesterol, low-calorie diet. The intense focus on a low-fat diet to avoid heart disease still lingers almost 70 years later, especially related to calorie counting and the diet industry.

Through his book *Good Calories, Bad Calories*, Gary Taubes (2007) became a leading voice in the controversy over dietary fat. Taubes persuasively argued that the real dietary driver of heart disease is refined carbohydrates due to their dramatic effect on insulin, and that there is no compelling scientific evidence that dietary saturated fat and cholesterol cause obesity and heart disease. He concluded that the key to good health is the *kind* of calories we take in, not the number of calories, especially when it is in the form of ultra-processed foods.

Sadly, evidence that the diet-heart hypothesis was incorrect was available in the 1970s but was never published. Beginning in 2013, unpublished data from two large studies were recovered and analyzed to understand the research that had been performed to test the diet-heart hypothesis. The Sydney Diet Heart Study (1966–1973) and the Minnesota Coronary Experience (1968–1973) were both very large and rigorous studies whose participants replaced saturated fat (e.g., butter and lard) with unsaturated fat (e.g., corn oil) for up to four years. Both studies showed that eating unsaturated fat did effectively lower serum (blood) cholesterol levels; however, those lowered levels did not prevent death due to heart disease, which contradicts the core of the diet-heart hypothesis (Ramsden et al., 2016). Since then, numerous researchers have demonstrated significant flaws in Ancel Keys' research, and multiple reviews of the data on saturated fat and heart disease have found no clear link (Astrup et al., 2020; Olszewski, 2020; Teicholz, 2014). The evidence is clear. Eating saturated fat like that found in butter and bacon does *not* increase your risk of having a heart attack.

WELCOME TO THE NEIGHBORHOOD

The study of *nutrition equity* examines systemic factors that influence the food system and access to healthy food in our communities. In a study of nutrition equity in urban neighborhoods, Freedman et al. argued that FI is tied to racial oppression in that the current food system makes access to food difficult in many of these neighborhoods. Many African American and Hispanic neighborhoods have a reduced access to healthy foods, often described as food deserts, food swamps, and food apartheid. This reduced access to healthy foods results in communities eating higher quantities of low-quality food due to their availability, which then creates diet-related racial inequities resulting in poorer health (Freedman et al., 2022).

Food Deserts

Food desert is a term used to describe communities with minimal access to food. The term "food desert" was originally coined by the Scottish Nutrition Task Force in 1995 and later popularized in 2010 as part of Michelle Obama's *Let's Move!* campaign. It describes communities that lack grocery stores or require considerable travel to have access to anything other than packaged food, especially prevalent in low-income communities (Karpyn et al., 2019). These are communities where more than a third of the population lives more than a mile (for urban areas) or 10 miles (for rural areas) from the nearest supermarket, supercenter, or large grocery store. Research has identified over 6500 food deserts in the U.S. that impact an estimated 11.5 million people in low-income communities (Vinella-Brusher, 2023).

While poverty is always a major factor with food deserts, the characteristics are different between urban and rural communities. In urban areas, food deserts include a larger minority population, compared to small town and rural areas with limited food access where the defining characteristic was lack of transportation to grocery stores. Consumers in both communities often shop at the closest convenience store where they pay higher prices for a limited range of foods, especially with few choices for fresh fruits and vegetables, compared to the supply and variety offered at a supermarket or large grocery store.

Food Swamps

The term *food swamp* has been used to describe areas that have a high density of fast-food restaurants and convenience stores but lack grocery stores that sell healthier, less processed foods. A quick drive in a food swamp and you will see block after block of common fast-food names like McDonalds and Burger King, as well as convenience stores like 7-Eleven and Quik Mart, but no sign of a grocery store. In food swamps, food is available to consumers but there is undue pressure to eat energy-dense snack foods and deep-fried poor-quality fast foods. The unhealthy food sources inundate consumers and make it less likely for them to make healthy food choices, which increases their risk for obesity and obesity-related diseases (Bevel et al., 2023; Cooksey-Stowers et al., 2017; Rose et al., 2009; Yang et al., 2020).

For example, a study of food swamps in Baltimore City, Maryland examined associations between food availability and dietary behaviors among urban adolescent girls (Hager et al., 2017). The study evaluated the consumption of fruits, vegetables, snacks, and desserts for 634 predominantly African American girls in sixth and seventh grades from 22 urban schools. Communities were mapped and categorized as food swamps based on a total of the number of convenience and small grocery corner stores that primarily sold processed foods within a quarter mile of homes. The results demonstrated that the girls whose homes were included in the food swamp geography ate more snacks and desserts than the girls who were not in the food swamps.

Food Apartheid

The term *food apartheid* emphasizes that racism underlies many of the decisions made by those in power to build food systems that make it difficult to access healthy food, especially in communities of color in urban cities (Hochedez, 2021). These communities of primarily poor minorities lack healthy food and have an overabundance of fast-food outlets and convenience stores. Food apartheid is a more recent food equity concept coined by food justice activist Karen Washington (BUGs, n.d.)

in response to the argument that the term "food desert" implies a naturally occurring phenomenon, but the social inequity in our food system is not natural. Food apartheid better describes the perspective that specific groups of people have been more negatively impacted by the current food system, largely based on decreased access to healthy foods, and acknowledges that human decisions and actions that have been happening for decades such as city planning that contributes to the availability of food and policies that impact the cost of food created and maintain this inequitable food system (University of Minnesota Duluth, April 6, 2021). Luckily, there is increasing awareness of this issue, which is being met by city planning projects in major U.S. cities, including Philadelphia, PA (Gripper et al., 2022), Salt Lake City, UT (Joyner et al., 2022), Grand Rapids, MI (O'Brien et al., 2023), and New Haven, CT (Corcoran, 2021).

Food Systems Planning is an emerging field of study for U.S. urban planners, which has created increased awareness and activity to build healthier communities (Vinella-Brusher, 2023). Food activists recommend that policy makers, funding agencies, and community stakeholders can improve the health disparities caused by food apartheid by establishing sustainable improved access to healthier food, such as renovating public areas to create walkable neighborhoods with produce stands, farmers markets, and community gardens (Bevel et al., 2023; Gripper et al., 2022). Numerous food systems projects have sprouted up (pun intended) in different cities. For example, in Washington, DC, the city began waiving taxes and fees for grocery stores located in neighborhoods lacking access to groceries and fresh food (DC Office of the Deputy Mayor for Planning and Economic Development, n.d.). Another example is Boston's 2013 zoning code update to facilitate urban agriculture by supporting food production activities such as small-scale farms, rooftop greenhouses, backyard honeybees, and raising chicken and fish in their urban neighborhoods (Boston Planning & Development Agency, 2014; Vinella-Brusher, 2023).

CONCERNS ABOUT THE U.S. DIETARY GUIDELINES

We have been discussing the powerful topic of how our eating decisions are influenced by our environment. We have looked at local influences like city planning to determine what foods are easily accessible in our community, and both obvious and subtle forms of marketing that enter our homes and our minds through a multitude of media. Now let us take a look at how the federal government influences our understanding of what constitutes a healthy diet through the publication of the *U.S. Dietary Guidelines.*

As discussed in Chapter 4, the Dietary Guidelines were originally to be based only on nutrition science. Over time, it has not been the nutrition scientists who have the final say in what is included in the Dietary Guidelines. Lobbyists from the food industry and politicians are heavily involved in the development process by influencing the USDA and Health and Human Services (HHS) leadership, which of course impacts the final recommendations (Hyman, 2020; Kristal et al., 2005; Zeraatkar et al., 2019).

One of the concerns about the Dietary Guidelines is that the USDA has a conflict of interest in how to approach recommended foods. The USDA is tasked with looking out for the needs of farmers (i.e., making sure the farmers are making enough money) as well as assuring a healthy food supply for the American people. However, what is good for the financial wellbeing of the farmers is not always what is best for the health and wellbeing of the consumers of their products (Wendel et al., 2011). In an interview with *Time Magazine* (Heid, 2016), Dr. Marion Nestle, author of *Food Politics*, stated that when she served as one of the experts hired to design the 1992 Dietary Guidelines, "I was told we could never say 'eat less meat' because USDA would not allow it." The meat and dairy industry successfully put pressure on the USDA so that more of their products would be recommended by the Dietary Guidelines. Since then, the debate has raged on about how much meat, if any, is best to consume for your health.

The 1992 *Food Guide Pyramid* Dietary Guidelines followed the trend at the time and advised a low-fat high-carbohydrate diet even though that did not match the good scientific evidence of the time. The tip of the pyramid recommended consuming fats and oils sparingly with no distinction

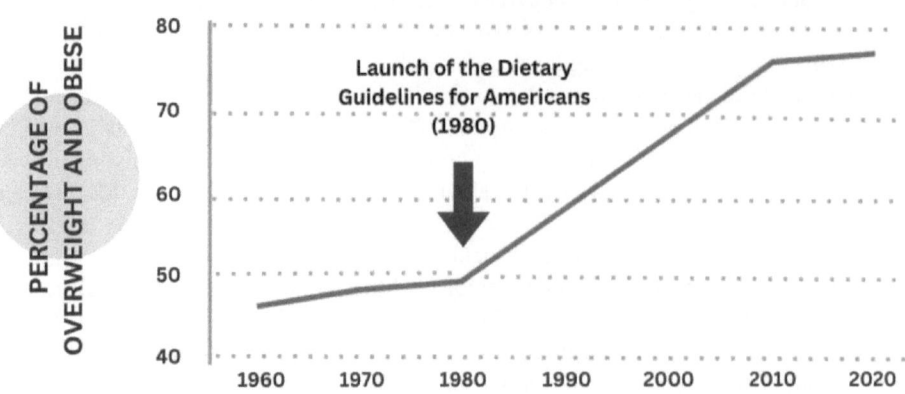

FIGURE 14.3 U.S. Dietary Guidelines for Americans and Obesity (Nutrition Coalition, 2023). (Courtesy of the Nutrition Coalition.)

about the type of fat. Even when it was written, the science for 30 or 40 years indicated that the type of fat made a big difference in how it impacted overall health. The body processes the healthy fat in an avocado very differently than the unhealthy fat in French fries.

One of the key concerns about the food pyramid was that it over-emphasized eating more processed carbohydrates (bread, cereal, pasta, and crackers), which for many people ended up contributing to weight gain. In fact, when we look at the trend of weight gain and obesity since the first Dietary Guidelines in 1980, we see an increase in the percentage of overweight and obese individuals in the U.S. population from 1980 to 2020 (see Figure 14.3) (Nutrition Coalition, 2023).

When the *MyPlate* Dietary Guidelines came out in 2011, the government advised people to eat a half plate of fruits and veggies at each meal. Ironically, at the same time they stacked the deck against consumers by making junk food cheaper and easier to buy than fresh produce through government farm subsidies and other policies (more on this in the *Food for Thought* section of this chapter).

In 2015, Congress mandated the first-ever outside peer review of the Dietary Guidelines by the National Academy of Sciences, Engineering, and Medicine. The results of the review concluded that the process of deciding what to include in the Dietary Guidelines needed to be restructured to increase the "scientific rigor" in how they reviewed the research literature to better match current scientific standards so that the final product would be more evidence-based. They reported that in setting new standards for the process of writing the Dietary Guidelines, there also needed to be increased efforts to minimize the bias and conflicts of interest that continued to exist for guidelines developers and consultants who influence what is included in the final versions of the Dietary Guidelines. "As part of following these standards, it will be important to review the potential biases and conflicts of interest for writing team members, and ensure external reviewers represent a diverse set of viewpoints" (National Academies of Sciences, Engineering, and Medicine, 2017, p. 68).

By 2020, the Dietary Guidelines removed the upper limits on dietary fat and dietary cholesterol and increased portions of daily fruits and vegetables, which are seen as improvements. Unfortunately, there was still no inclusion of research on the health risks and negative environmental consequences associated with ultra-processed foods and conventional factory-farmed meat (more on organic vs. conventional farming practices in Chapter 15). Nutrition activist groups such as the Nutrition Coalition are taking action to address these issues in the 2025 Dietary Guidelines.

Many consumers are impacted by the Dietary Guidelines without their awareness in the form of federally funded food programs in schools, public hospitals, government offices, and prisons with policies that mandate all food served must follow the guidelines. For example, students in school meal programs that follow U.S. Dietary Guidelines are offered and often eat higher quantities of vegetables and dairy products at school than they do at home (Finkelstein et al., 2004). All public schools are supposed to offer meals based on the guidelines, which are generally lower in added sugars and sodium and higher in whole grains (Wang et al., 2023). Unfortunately, a high percentage of schools do not meet the current Dietary Guidelines for school meals, so there is still work to be done around how best to implement the guidelines in public institutions.

CASE STUDY: OPPOSITIONAL DEFIANT DISORDER

Dr. Champion began work with a young boy, age five, who had been diagnosed with oppositional defiant disorder (ODD). The young client had also been tested for autism spectrum disorder, which was ruled negative by the family's psychiatrist.

The client routinely lashed out at his mother, nanny, and teachers, both verbally and physically. His outbursts would often leave him exhausted afterward. The client's mother reported that she and the nanny had tried everything they could think of to control or redirect his behavior. When he had an incident-free day at school, he would come home and attack his little brother (age three), mother, and nanny by throwing toys, biting, hitting, screaming, and then locking himself in his room. The angry outbursts were increasing in frequency and the irritability was unbearable. When the mother or nanny would try to console him, he would push them away, often hitting and biting as well. The family had learned to walk on eggshells to avoid conflict and worsening his symptoms.

At the time of the initial intake, the mother was at her wit's end and reported having tried everything she could think of. She was resistant to their doctor's recommendation to put him on medication and sought out natural treatments and dietary changes before using the medication as a last resort.

During the intake, Dr. Champion noticed that most of the time, the client's symptoms presented after times of higher stimulation and shortly after meals or snacks. The child ate a cleaner version of the Standard American Diet for kids, consisting of organic macaroni and cheese, organic chicken nuggets or hot dogs, and organic pizza. Dr. Champion asked the mother to keep a log of the foods the child ate for seven days and note any changes in behavior alongside the food intake.

To be expected, the boy ate the same foods repeatedly despite being offered new foods to try at most meals. The mother reported that he did not like to try new foods, and it was often a struggle to get him to eat what the family was having. Many times when a new food was placed on his plate, he would fling himself to the ground in a fit, yell, and then stomp off to his room, leaving the mother in tears from the stress.

From the food and mood tracking, Dr. Champion noted a strong connection between three foods and the boy's outbursts – gluten, dairy, and sugar. These are very common gut disruptors but especially so for young children with mood dysregulation. To avoid increasing family conflict, the first nutritional swap was gluten. Whole wheat pasta and macaroni and cheese were replaced with gluten-free options, using brown rice pasta. This food conversion process took about 30 days as the mother replaced everything in the house with gluten-free options. (The mother also noted a reduction in her own gastrointestinal symptoms!)

After the gluten-free options were introduced, we began to work on dairy. The dairy replacement was a much more challenging aspect since the casein in dairy is addictive. The child initially threw fits when not served his macaroni and cheese. The non-dairy options did not work well. However, the family persisted and decided to give up dairy and show the young boy that no one in the family was eating any dairy. This process continued for 30 days until the boy finally quit asking for cheese and milk. Again, his symptoms improved and now were hardly noticeable except when he would have sugar. Dr. Champion worked with the mother to make delicious fruit-based swaps for his favorite desserts and moved to use monk fruit, stevia, and honey (which the boy could tolerate) when they wanted a treat.

From intake to complete symptom remediation, this process took approximately 90 days. At the final session, the mother reported feeling like she had her little boy back and no medication was necessary for this young boy. When he has an outburst, the mother gently reminds her son about the sugar he consumed (e.g., classroom birthday parties), and he goes outside to play, run, and jump to burn the sugar off. Typically, he is fine within about 2 hours after burning off the excess energy.

THE LABELING OF FOOD ADDITIVES

Food ingredient lists often include a long list of ingredients most people do not recognize or understand. Many of these ingredients fall under the heading of food additives. A *food additive* is "any substance used in the production, processing, treatment, packaging, transportation or storage of food" (U.S. Department of Health and Human Services, 2014).

GRAS FOODS

We have all read food labels with a long list of ingredients that we can barely pronounce much less know what they are. These ingredients are often a group of chemicals or substances added to food that, according to the Food and Drug Administration (FDA), are considered safe by experts. Most additives are listed by the FDA as *Generally Recognized As Safe (GRAS)*. The GRAS list began in 1958 with 700 substances. It was initially created to cover ingredients that were widely known to be safe, such as vegetable oil. The current GRAS list contains over 1100 ingredients or food substances that are often included as part of "natural ingredients" on a food ingredient list (U.S. Food and Drug Administration, 2022; FEMA, 2024).

Food watchdog groups have expressed concern about potential health risks associated with GRAS ingredients due to a lack of sufficient evidence that they are safe for long-term human consumption. In 2017, the Center for Science in the Public Interest (CSPI) and other public-interest groups filed a lawsuit challenging that the FDA had too weak of a policy for allowing food manufacturers to add food substances to the GRAS list without sufficient evidence of their safety. While the final ruling did not change the GRAS approval policy, it did acknowledge concerns about the current FDA practice around GRAS ingredients (CSPI, 2021). CSPI continues to publish information about potential risks associated with food additives, and maintains a list on their webpage titled *Chemical Cuisine Ratings* which ranks food additives from "safe" to "avoid" for those interested in better understanding the potential impact of the food additives that they consume (CSPI, 2023).

THE STORY OF TRANS FATS

An example of a GRAS substance is trans fats. Industrial *trans fats* are created through hydrogenation of plant-based oils to create products like shortening and margarine. This takes the liquid vegetable oils and makes them into a solid substance that is often used in commercial baked goods because they are cheaper than animal fats like butter and lard, do not turn rancid, and can withstand higher heat without breaking down which increases shelf life for the products, and decreases saturated fats which makes them more marketable.

Before the 1990s, trans fats were in thousands of foods but were not required to be listed in the top part of their Nutrition Facts labels and could only be found listed in the ingredients as partially hydrogenated oil and vegetable shortening. Fortunately, in the 1990s, a large body of research sounded the alarm that trans fats increase the risk for heart disease, stroke, and diabetes, and may promote obesity and insulin resistance. In response, trans fats were added to the top of Nutrition Facts labels in 2006, and a series of national policy changes led to the near elimination of trans fats in the U.S. food supply by 2018 (The Nutrition Source, 2023). However, while we have been effective at decreasing the trans fats in the U.S., outside the U.S. there is still more work to be done since consumption of trans fats remains high. In 2018, the World Health Organization (WHO) began a campaign to remove trans fats from global food supplies, potentially saving approximately ten million lives (Jacobs, 2018). Since 2018, 43 countries have adopted new regulations to limit trans fats in the food supply. New incentives and policies, as well as mechanisms to create more accountability by food manufacturers, are in place to continue the push to restrict the use of trans fats in processed food products worldwide (Steele et al., 2024).

FOOD FOR THOUGHT: FARM AND FOOD SUBSIDIES

Cost is an important influence on access to food and food selection behavior. Fast food and ultra-processed foods are generally convenient and inexpensive, which makes them an easy choice. In contrast, fresh fruits and vegetables, especially organic produce, can be expensive, and high-quality fat like coconut oil and organic eggs and meat are generally very pricey. There is a political component to this aspect of the fund industry as well.

Farm subsidies are a key government process that influences the cost of food to consumers. Farm subsidies are funding and insurance programs for farmers that are budgeted for and managed through the Farm Bill, a federal law that governs agricultural and food programs. The Farm Bill is renewed by Congress every five years, with input and influence from many sources, including food manufacturers who lobby to keep the prices for their processed foods low compared to unprocessed whole foods.

Currently our federal tax dollars go toward farm subsidies that support staple *food commodities* – corn, soybeans, wheat, cotton, rice, peanuts, dairy, and sugar (CRS, 2024). These farm subsidies allow farmers to sell these products at much lower prices and still make a profit. Ultra-processed foods generally include many of these subsidized foods in their products, often in unrecognizable forms like ascorbic acid and maltodextrin, which are both made from corn or rice. While U.S. Dietary Guidelines recommend limiting the consumption of saturated fats, sugar, salt, and refined grains, the funding through the Farm Bill actually encourages people to eat more of these ingredients by making these foods less expensive.

In the end, a large proportion of farm subsidies go to support the production of food commodities (e.g., soy, corn, and dairy) that are often converted into high fat, highly refined foods and soft drinks sweetened with corn syrup (McCarthy, 2016). By using inexpensive ingredients made from food products that are subsidized, food manufacturers can sell ultra-processed products at low prices compared to the cost of many whole foods, making ultra-processed foods cheap and abundant. In reality, those foods are expensive. In addition to paying the purchase price, we pay for them with our tax dollars in our farm subsidies, in our environmental cleanup dollars due to damaging farming practices, as well as our healthcare dollars due to the negative health impact associated with eating large quantities of ultra-processed foods (The Editors, 2012).

There is evidence that one avenue to improve population health in the U.S. is to change our farm subsidy programs. Among U.S. adults, increased consumption of subsidized foods is associated with a higher risk of cardiovascular disease due to higher rates of obesity, elevated cholesterol, and other risk factors that result from eating large amounts of ultra-processed foods (Siegel et al., 2016). Changes in farm subsidy policies can improve population dietary behaviors by leveling the playing field between whole foods and ultra-processed foods, which would make whole foods comparatively more affordable and thereby increase consumption of healthier foods and decrease consumption of foods high in unhealthy fats, sodium, sugar, and food additives (Niebylski et al., 2015).

In spite of the low-cost of ultra-processed foods due to farm subsidies, the overall cost of food has continued to rise. While there has been a slow and steady rise in the cost of food over the last 50 years, the recent spike in food prices since 2020 has placed a tremendous burden on U.S. families (see Figure 14.4). This has increased the need for another type of subsidy in the form of federal food assistance.

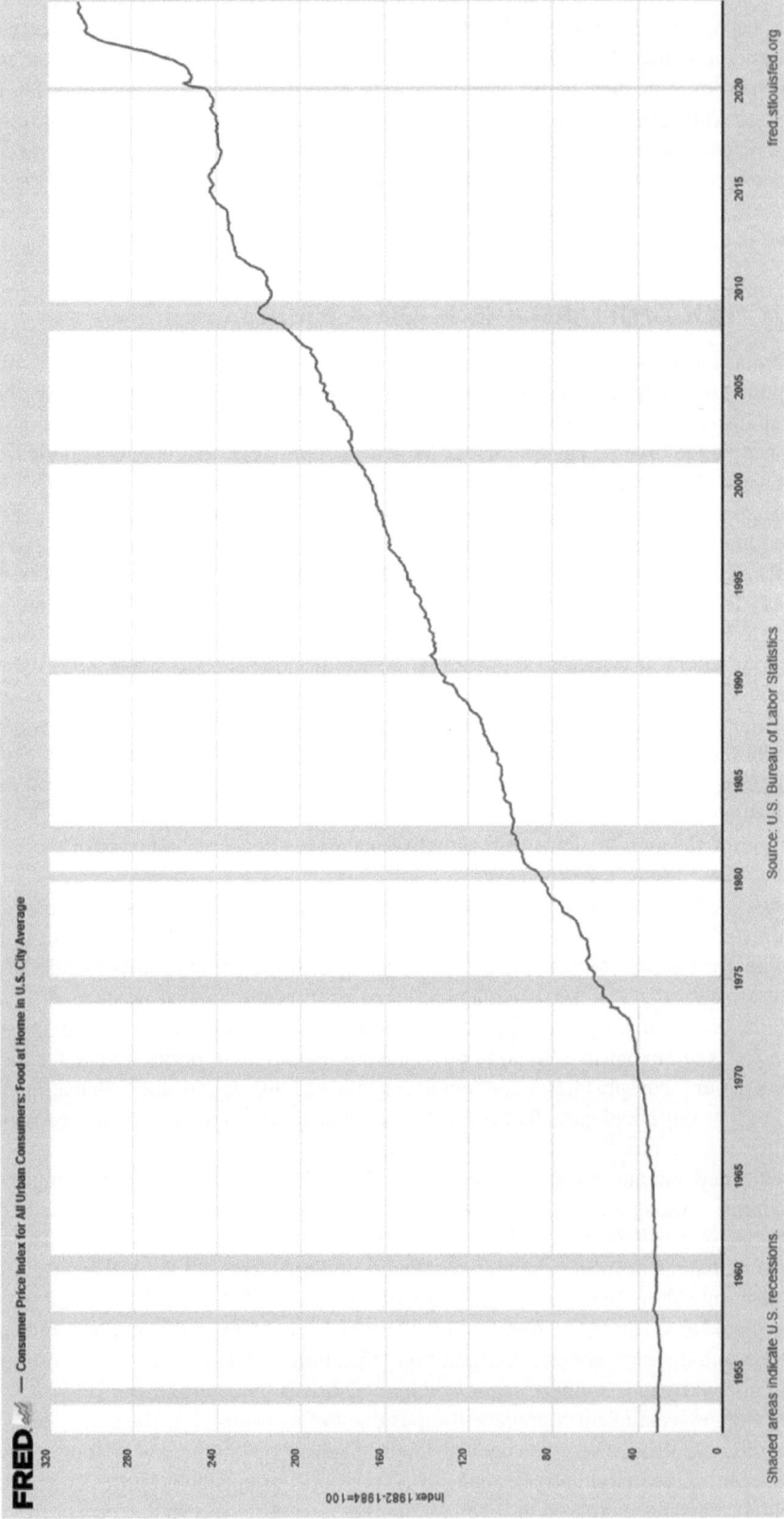

FIGURE 14.4 Average cost of food in U.S. cities (U.S. Bureau of Labor Statistics, 2024). (Courtesy of the U.S. Bureau of Labor Statistics.)

The federal USDA *Supplemental Nutrition Assistance Program (SNAP)* is the country's largest *food subsidy* program and has been an effective means of using tax dollars to put food within reach for those in need. It has been a crucial safety net that helps put food on tables to avoid hunger and FI. This food subsidy program reduces poverty and FI for the over 40 million Americans it serves. Most of the people who participate in SNAP are children, elderly adults, and people with a disability (USDA, 2024).

Similar to farm subsidies, there is room for improvement in SNAP that could make a big difference in what people are eating. While SNAP has succeeded in providing food security, it has failed to protect its participants from the damage associated with obesity and diet-related diseases. In fact, SNAP recipients have lower-quality diets than income eligible (e.g., low-income) participants who do not participate in SNAP (Zhang et al., 2018). Unfortunately, even when whole foods are available, SNAP recipients often end up consuming large quantities of sugar-sweetened beverages and processed meats for a number of reasons, including preference, habit, convenience, marketing, and to stretch the limited dollars that they receive when processed foods are less expensive (Leung et al., 2013).

An argument has been made that limiting the amount of ultra-processed foods and sugar-sweetened beverages that is allowed to be purchased with SNAP funds would help improve the quality of the diets and thereby the health of some of our most vulnerable population (Hyman, 2020). Others feel this approach is too restrictive and controlling. A study published in *JAMA Internal Medicine* in 2016 provided evidence that a combination approach would work best. The study authors recommended that SNAP recipients have both processed food restrictions as well as incentives to buy healthy foods, which was the most effective approach to decrease consumption of less healthy foods and increase consumption of fruits and vegetables (Harnack et al., 2016). Other successful programs have allowed participants to use SNAP funds at farmers markets and have given extra SNAP money for every dollar spent on local fruits and vegetables. These steps to reform SNAP can help improve the physical and mental health of millions of Americans.

REFERENCES

Aboul-Enein, B. H., Puddy, W. C., & Bernstein, J. (2020). Ancel Benjamin Keys (1904–2004): His early works and the legacy of the modern Mediterranean diet. *Journal of Medical Biography, 28*(3), 139–147.

Althoff, R. R., Ametti, M., & Bertmann, F. (2016). The role of food insecurity in developmental psychopathology. *Preventive Medicine, 92*, 106–109. https://doi.org/10.1016/j.ypmed.2016.08.012

Anema, A., Weiser, S. D., Fernandes, K. A., Ding, E., Brandson, E. K., Palmer, A., Montaner, J. S. G., & Hogg, R. S. (2011). High prevalence of food insecurity among HIV-infected individuals receiving HAART in a resource-rich setting. *AIDS Care, 23*(2), 221–230. https://doi.org/10.1080/09540121.2010.498908

Astrup, A., Magkos, F., Bier, D. M., Brenna, J. T., de Oliveira Otto, M. C., Hill, J. O., King, J. C., Mente, A., Ordovas, J. M., & Volek, J. S. (2020). Saturated fats and health: A reassessment and proposal for food-based recommendations: JACC state-of-the-art review. *Journal of the American College of Cardiology, 76*(7), 844–857. https://www.jacc.org/doi/abs/10.1016/j.jacc.2020.05.077

Bevel, M. S., Tsai, M.-H., Parham, A., Andrzejak, S. E., Jones, S., & Moore, J. X. (2023). Association of food deserts and food swamps with obesity-related cancer mortality in the US. *JAMA Oncology, 9*(7), 909–916. https://doi.org/10.1001/jamaoncol.2023.0634

Booth, S., & Pollard, C. M. (2020). Food insecurity, food crimes and structural violence: An Australian perspective. *Australian and New Zealand Journal of Public Health, 44*(2), 87–88. https://doi.org/10.1111/1753-6405.12977

Boston Planning & Development Agency. (2014). *Urban Agriculture Rezoning Initiative.* https://archive.org/details/Urban_Agriculture_Rezoning_Initiative_Neighborhood_Meeting

BUGs. (n.d.). *Co-Founder Karen Washington, Rise & Root Farm, Chester, NY.* Black Farmers & Urban Gardners (BUGs). https://www.blackurbangrowers.org/about

Cohen, B., Andrews, M., & Kantor, L. S. (2002). *Community food security assessment toolkit.* Economic Research Service. https://www.ers.usda.gov/publications/pub-details/?pubid=43179

Cooksey-Stowers, K., Schwartz, M. B., & Brownell, K. D. (2017). Food swamps predict obesity rates better than food deserts in the United States. *International Journal of Environmental Research and Public Health, 14*(11), 1366. https://www.mdpi.com/1660-4601/14/11/1366

Corcoran, M. P. (2021). Beyond 'food apartheid': Civil society and the politicization of hunger in new haven, Connecticut. *Urban Agriculture & Regional Food Systems*, *6*(1), e20013.

CRS. (2024). *Farm bill primer: What is the Farm Bill?* Congressional Research Service. https://crsreports. congress.gov/product/pdf/IF/IF12047

CSPI. (2021). *Secret GRAS rule*. Center for Science in the Public Interest. https://www.cspinet.org/case/ secret-gras-rule

CSPI. (2023). *Chemical Cuisine ratings*. https://www.cspinet.org/page/chemical-cuisine-ratings

DC Office of the Deputy Mayor for Planning and Economic Development. (n.d.). *Supermarket tax incentives*. https://dmped.dc.gov/page/supermarket-tax-incentives

Duke, N. N., Campbell, S. D., Sauls, D. L., Stout, R., Story, M. T., Austin, T., Bosworth, H. B., Skinner, A. C., & Vilme, H. (2023). Prevalence of food insecurity among students attending four Historically Black Colleges and Universities. *Journal of American College Health*, *71*(1), 87–93.

Elgar, F. J., Pickett, W., Pförtner, T.-K., Gariépy, G., Gordon, D., Georgiades, K., Davison, C., Hammami, N., MacNeil, A. H., Azevedo Da Silva, M., & Melgar-Quiñonez, H. R. (2021). Relative food insecurity, mental health and wellbeing in 160 countries. *Social Science & Medicine*, *268*, 113556. https://doi. org/10.1016/j.socscimed.2020.113556

Ellakany, P., Zuñiga, R. A. A., El Tantawi, M., Brown, B., Aly, N. M., Ezechi, O., Uzochukwu, B., Abeldaño, G. F., Ara, E., & Ayanore, M. A. (2022). Impact of the COVID-19 pandemic on student' sleep patterns, sexual activity, screen use, and food intake: A global survey. *PLoS One*, *17*(1), e0262617.

Empowering Nonviolence. (2023). *Violence*. https://www.nonviolence.wri-irg.org/en/print/pdf/node/40497

FEMA. (2024). *About FEMA GRAS Program*. Flavor & Extract Manufacturers Association. https://www. femaflavor.org/gras

Finkelstein, E., French, S., Variyam, J. N., & Haines, P. S. (2004). Pros and cons of proposed interventions to promote healthy eating. *American Journal of Preventive Medicine*, *27*(3), 163–171.

Freedman, D. A., Clark, J. K., Lounsbury, D. W., Boswell, L., Burns, M., Jackson, M. B., Mikelbank, K., Donley, G., Worley-Bell, L. Q., Mitchell, J., Ciesielski, T. H., Embaye, M., Lee, E. K., Roche, A., Gill, I., & Yamoah, O. (2022). Food system dynamics structuring nutrition equity in racialized urban neighborhoods. *The American Journal of Clinical Nutrition*, *115*(4), 1027–1038. https://doi.org/10.1093/ajcn/ nqab380

Galtung, J. (1969). Violence, peace, and peace research. *Journal of Peace Research*, *6*(3), 167–191. https://doi. org/10.1177/002234336900600301

Galtung, J. (1990). Cultural violence. *Journal of Peace Research*, *27*(3), 291–305.

Gripper, A. B., Nethery, R., Cowger, T. L., White, M., Kawachi, I., & Adamkiewicz, G. (2022). Community solutions to food apartheid: A spatial analysis of community food-growing spaces and neighborhood demographics in Philadelphia. *Social Science & Medicine*, *310*, 115221, https://doi.org/10.1016/ j.socscimed.2022.115221

Gundersen, C., & Ziliak, J. P. (2015). Food insecurity and health outcomes. *Health Affairs*, *34*(11), 1830–1839.

Hagedorn-Hatfield, R. L., Hood, L. B., & Hege, A. (2022). A decade of college student hunger: What we know and where we need to go. *Frontiers in Public Health*, *10*, 837724.

Hager, E. R., Cockerham, A., O'Reilly, N., Harrington, D., Harding, J., Hurley, K. M., & Black, M. M. (2017). Food swamps and food deserts in Baltimore City, MD, USA: Associations with dietary behaviours among urban adolescent girls. *Public Health Nutrition*, *20*(14), 2598–2607. https://doi.org/10.1017/ S1368980016002123

Harnack, L., Oakes, J. M., Elbel, B., Beatty, T., Rydell, S., & French, S. (2016). Effects of subsidies and prohibitions on nutrition in a food benefit program: A randomized clinical trial. *JAMA Internal Medicine*, *176*(11), 1610–1618. https://doi.org/10.1001/jamainternmed.2016.5633

Hatsu, I. E., Eiterman, L., Stern, M., Lu, S., Johnstone, J. M., Leung, B. M. Y., Srikanth, P., Robinette, L., Tost, G., Odei, J. B., Gracious, B. L., & Arnold, L. E. (2022). Household food insecurity is associated with symptoms of emotional dysregulation in children with attention deficit hyperactivity disorder: The MADDY study. *Nutrients*, *14*(6), 1306. https://www.mdpi.com/2072-6643/14/6/1306

Heid, M. (January 8, 2016). Experts say lobbying skewed the U.S. dietary guidelines. *Time Magazine, Health – Diet & Nutrition*. https://time.com/4130043/lobbying-politics-dietary-guidelines/

Hochedez, C. (2021). *Food justice: A conceptual framework and a category of action. Perspectives from the Latin American context (HAL Id: halshs-03017065)*. HAL SHS sciences humaines et sociales. https:// shs.hal.science/halshs-03017065

Hyman, M. (2020). *Food fix: How to save our health, our economy, our communities and our planet–one bite at a time*. Hachette.

Jacobs, A. (May 14, 2018). Trans Fats Should be Eliminated Worldwide by 2023, W.H.O. Says. *The New York Times*. https://www.nytimes.com/2018/05/14/health/trans-fats-who-ban.html

Joyner, L., Yagüe, B., Cachelin, A., & Rose, J. (2022). Farms and gardens everywhere but not a bite to eat? A critical geographic approach to food apartheid in Salt Lake City. *Journal of Agriculture, Food Systems, and Community Development, 11*(2), 67–88.

Karpyn, A. E., Riser, D., Tracy, T., Wang, R., & Shen, Y. (2019). The changing landscape of food deserts. *UNSCN Nutrition, 44*, 46.

Kim-Mozeleski, J. E., Pike Moore, S. N., Trapl, E. S., Perzynski, A. T., Tsoh, J. Y., & Gunzler, D. D. (2023). Food insecurity trajectories in the US during the first year of the COVID-19 pandemic. *Preventing Chronic Disease, 20*, E03. https://doi.org/10.5888/pcd20.220212

Kristal, A. R., Peters, U., & Potter, J. D. (2005). Is it time to abandon the food frequency questionnaire? *Cancer Epidemiology, Biomarkers & Prevention, 14*(12), 2826–2828.

Lee, B. X. (2016). Causes and cures VII: Structural violence. *Aggression and Violent Behavior, 28*, 109–114. https://doi.org/10.1016/j.avb.2016.05.003

Leung, C. W., Blumenthal, S. J., Hoffnagle, E. E., Jensen, H. H., Foerster, S. B., Nestle, M., Cheung, L. W., Mozaffarian, D., & Willett, W. C. (2013). Associations of food stamp participation with dietary quality and obesity in children. *Pediatrics, 131*(3), 463–472.

Lindberg, R., McKenzie, H., Haines, B., & McKay, F. H. (2023). An investigation of structural violence in the lived experience of food insecurity. *Critical Public Health, 33*(2), 185–196. https://doi.org/10.1080/09581596.2021.2019680

McCarthy, M. (2016). US food subsidies fuel obesity, study finds. *BMJ: British Medical Journal, 354*. https://www.jstor.org/stable/26946165

Meza, A., Altman, E., Martinez, S., & Leung, C. W. (2019). "It's a feeling that one is not worth food": A qualitative study exploring the psychosocial experience and academic consequences of food insecurity among college students. *Journal of the Academy of Nutrition and Dietetics, 119*(10), 1713–1721.e1. https://doi.org/10.1016/j.jand.2018.09.006

National Academies of Sciences, Engineering, and Medicine. (2017). *Redesigning the process for establishing the Dietary Guidelines for Americans*. The National Academies Press. https://doi.org/10.17226/24883

Niebylski, M. L., Redburn, K. A., Duhaney, T., & Campbell, N. R. (2015). Healthy food subsidies and unhealthy food taxation: A systematic review of the evidence. *Nutrition, 31*(6), 787–795. https://doi.org/10.1016/j.nut.2014.12.010

Nikolaus, C. J., An, R., Ellison, B., & Nickols-Richardson, S. M. (2020). Food insecurity among college students in the United States: A scoping review. *Advances in Nutrition, 11*(2), 327–348.

Noonan, K., Corman, H., & Reichman, N. E. (2016). Effects of maternal depression on family food insecurity. *Economics & Human Biology, 22*, 201–215.

Nutrition Coalition. (2023). *US Dietary Guidelines for Americans—101*. https://www.nutritioncoalition.us/dietary-guidelines-for-americans-dga-introduction

O'Brien, J., Patrell-Fazio, E., & Steere, J. (2023). *Developing food justice policy solutions and educational resources to address food apartheid in Grand Rapids, MI*. School for Environment and Sustainability, University of Michigan. https://dx.doi.org/10.7302/7156

Olfert, M. D., Hagedorn-Hatfield, R. L., Houghtaling, B., Esquivel, M. K., Hood, L. B., MacNell, L., Soldavini, J., Berner, M., Savoie Roskos, M. R., Hingle, M. D., Mann, G. R., Waity, J. F., Knol, L. L., Walsh, J., Kern-Lyons, V., Paul, C., Pearson, K., Goetz, J. R., Spence, M., … Coleman, P. (2023). Struggling with the basics: Food and housing insecurity among college students across twenty-two colleges and universities. *Journal of American College Health, 71*(8), 2518–2529. https://doi.org/10.1080/07448481.2021.1978456

Olszewski, T. M. (2020). Diet-heart debates: Past, present and future. *Clinical Handbook of Coronary Artery Disease, 308*.

Pourmotabbed, A., Moradi, S., Babaei, A., Ghavami, A., Mohammadi, H., Jalili, C., Symonds, M. E., & Miraghajani, M. (2020). Food insecurity and mental health: A systematic review and meta-analysis. *Public Health Nutrition, 23*(10), 1778–1790. https://doi.org/10.1017/S136898001900435X

Rabbitt, M. P., Hales, L. J., Burke, M. P., & Coleman-Jensen, A. (2023). *Household food security in the United States in 2022*. Economic Research Service, U.S. Department of Agriculture.

Ramsden, C. E., Zamora, D., Majchrzak-Hong, S., Faurot, K. R., Broste, S. K., Frantz, R. P., Davis, J. M., Ringel, A., Suchindran, C. M., & Hibbeln, J. R. (2016). Re-evaluation of the traditional diet-heart hypothesis: Analysis of recovered data from Minnesota coronary experiment (1968–73). *BMJ, 353*, i1246. https://doi.org/10.1136/bmj.i1246

Rose, D., Bodor, J. N., Swalm, C. M., Rice, J. C., Farley, T. A., & Hutchinson, P. L. (2009). Deserts in New Orleans? Illustrations of urban food access and implications for policy. University of Michigan National Poverty Center/USDA Economic Research Service Research, Ann Arbor, MI.

Shepard, D. S., Setren, E., & Cooper, D. (2011). *Hunger in America: Suffering we all pay for*. https://www.americanprogress.org/article/hunger-in-america/

Siegel, K. R., Bullard, K. M., Imperatore, G., Kahn, H. S., Stein, A. D., Ali, M. K., & Narayan, K. (2016). Association of higher consumption of foods derived from subsidized commodities with adverse cardio-metabolic risk among US adults. *JAMA Internal Medicine, 176*(8), 1124–1132.

Steele, L., Drummond, E., Nishida, C., Yamamoto, R., Branca, F., Perez, C. P., Allemandi, L., Arnanz, L., Schoj, V., Khanchandani, H. S., Bhardwaj, S., Garg, R., Frieden, T. R., & Cobb, L. K. (2024). Ending trans fat—the first-ever global elimination program for a noncommunicable disease risk factor. *Journal of the American College of Cardiology, 84*(7), 663–674. https://doi.org/doi:10.1016/j.jacc.2024.04.067

Stephenson, J. (2022, October). White house releases strategy to address hunger, nutrition, and health in the US. *JAMA Health Forum, 3*, e224293–e224293. American Medical Association.

Taubes, G. (2007). *Good calories, bad calories: challenging the conventional wisdom on diet, weight control, and disease* (1st ed.). Knopf.

Teicholz, N. (2014). *The big fat surprise: Why butter, meat and cheese belong in a healthy diet.* Simon and Schuster.

The Editors. (2012). For a healthier country, overhaul farm subsidies. *Scientific American.* https://www.scientific american.com/article/fresh-fruit-hold-the-insulin/

The Nutrition Source. (2023). *Shining the spotlight on trans fats.* Harvard T.H. Chan School of Public Health. https://www.hsph.harvard.edu/nutritionsource/what-should-you-eat/fats-and-cholesterol/types-of-fat/transfats/

University of Minnesota Duluth. (April 6, 2021). *Food Apartheid.* https://sustainability.d.umn.edu/food-apartheid

U.S. Bureau of Labor Statistics. (2024). *Consumer Price Index for All Urban Consumers: Food at Home in U.S. City Average [CUSR0000SAF11].* FRED, Federal Reserve Bank of St. Louis. https://fred.stlouisfed.org/series/CUSR0000SAF11

U.S. Department of Health and Human Services. (2014). *What is a food additive?* https://www.hhs.gov/answers/public-health-and-safety/what-is-a-food-addititve/index.html

U.S. Food and Drug Administration. (2022). *Generally Recognized as Safe (GRAS).* https://www.fda.gov/food/food-ingredients-packaging/generally-recognized-safe-gras

USDA. (2023). *Food security status of U.S. households in 2023: Trends in prevalence.* USDA. https://www.ers.usda.gov/topics/food-nutrition-assistance/food-security-in-the-u-s/key-statistics-graphics/

USDA. (2024). *SNAP in Action Dashboard.* USDA Food and Nutrition Service. https://www.fns.usda.gov/data-research/data-visualization/snap/action

Vinella-Brusher, E. (2023). *Reckoning with food apartheid: Lessons from US cities and counties.* Gillings School of Global Public Health, University of North Carolina at Chapel Hill. https://doi.org/10.17615/vyfr-8y52

Wang, L., Cohen, J. F. W., Maroney, M., Cudhea, F., Hill, A., Schwartz, C., Lurie, P., & Mozaffarian, D. (2023). Evaluation of health and economic effects of United States school meal standards consistent with the 2020–2025 dietary guidelines for Americans. *The American Journal of Clinical Nutrition, 118*(3), 605–613. https://doi.org/10.1016/j.ajcnut.2023.05.031

Wendel, B., Corry, J., & Boon, A. (2011). *Forks over Knives documentary.* https://www.forksoverknives.com/the-film/

Whittle, H. J., Palar, K., Hufstedler, L. L., Seligman, H. K., Frongillo, E. A., & Weiser, S. D. (2015). Food insecurity, chronic illness, and gentrification in the San Francisco Bay Area: An example of structural violence in United States public policy. *Social Science & Medicine, 143*, 154–161. https://doi.org/10.1016/j.socscimed.2015.08.027

Yang, M., Wang, H., & Qiu, F. (2020). Neighbourhood food environments revisited: When food deserts meet food swamps. *The Canadian Geographer/Le Géographe Canadien, 64*(1), 135–154.

Zeraatkar, D., Johnston, B. C., & Guyatt, G. (2019). Evidence collection and evaluation for the development of dietary guidelines and public policy on nutrition. *Annual Review of Nutrition, 39*, 227–247.

Zhang, F. F., Liu, J., Rehm, C. D., Wilde, P., Mande, J. R., & Mozaffarian, D. (2018). Trends and disparities in diet quality among US adults by supplemental nutrition assistance program participation status. *JAMA Network Open, 1*(2), e180237. https://doi.org/10.1001/jamanetworkopen.2018.0237

15 Making Food Decisions

Choosing what, when, and how to eat food can involve some complicated decision-making. There are a lot of factors to consider as we journey into better understanding what works best for our body at any given time. This chapter explores ways to prioritize making nutrition changes that best suit your needs, as well as to address some common challenges and strategies associated with changing how we eat.

CHANGE CAN BE HARD

Changing what and how we eat food can be very difficult and confusing. Often, we get clear about wanting to make a change (e.g., eat less sugar, limit daily calories), which we feel resolute about and can sometimes manage for a few days or even a few weeks, and then stress rushes in, our time becomes limited, or a schedule change that keeps us from cooking or grocery shopping. The reality of change is that it takes place within the context of real life – not some ideal world. We may ask ourselves, "Why can't I do better?"

The topic of *willpower* often arises and can easily get cast as the villain in our story of eating better. Lack of willpower is a common concern associated with feeling out of control with our eating. The idea that someone has a lack of willpower implies a judgment that they have poor discipline and a weak character, which can contribute to guilt and low self-esteem around eating. This raises the question, "Is lack of willpower a character flaw or is there more to consider?" Some interesting research shows that willpower is less about *will* and more about learning new skills such as delayed gratification to feel we are in alignment with and committed to our true goals and values.

Delayed Gratification

The landmark Marshmallow Test performed at Stanford University in 1970, led by psychologist Walter Mischel, examined willpower and self-control associated with delaying the reward of eating fun food (Mischel & Ebbesen, 1970). In the study, researchers offered four-year-old students at the Bing research nursery school a marshmallow and gave them a choice: Eat this one now or wait 15 minutes and then enjoy two marshmallows. The researchers then video-recorded the children's responses. The children who were able to sit in the room alone with their marshmallow and wait the (what seemed like forever) 15 minutes without eating the marshmallow were rewarded by the researchers with the promised second marshmallow. The children who ate their marshmallow during the 15 minutes were not given a second marshmallow. The children who were able to wait and delay gratification used some interesting techniques to stop themselves from eating the first marshmallow, including distracting themselves with singing and hopping and putting the marshmallow under the napkin so that they did not have to look at it while they were waiting.

The study then followed these children over the years to see if there was a difference between the group of children who were able to wait for the second marshmallow and the group who did not. The researchers concluded that the ability to delay immediate gratification was a learned skill that predicted success in their adult life (Mischel, 2014). The skill that the children demonstrated was how to strategically focus their attention away from the enticing object (in this case the marshmallow) to decrease its power over them. Redirecting one's attention onto higher-value thoughts or activities helps decrease obsessing thoughts that often heighten feelings of agitation and powerlessness. For example, if you decided to experiment with removing gluten from your diet for a couple of weeks to see if it improved your frequent bouts of constipation, initially you are likely to experience

DOI: 10.1201/9781032647647-21

strong cravings. Obsessing thoughts might sound like, "I really want that piece of bread. Just one more piece and then I will quit. It would just taste so good. I can't stand not eating that bread right now." These thoughts are likely to make you feel agitated and deprived. If instead you could shift your attention to more helpful thoughts it might sound like, "I am a little uncomfortable right now, but it is worth it to see if this will help me feel better. Rather than stand here in the kitchen staring at the bread, I am going to go outside and play with my dog."

Urge Surfing

Another strategy for dealing with cravings is *urge surfing*. This mindfulness technique originated in psychotherapy working with clients poised to quit smoking tobacco (Marlatt & Gordon, 1985). Like an ocean wave, urges gradually intensify, peak, and fade away. The first waves are some of the most difficult to ride. Rather than giving in to an urge, a person trains themselves to ride it out, like a surfer riding a wave. After a short time, the urge will pass on its own. When urges go unfed, future urges gradually become weaker (Therapist Aid, 2021).

Keeping this image of waves cresting and falling when applied to urges or cravings when we feel pulled into emotional eating can increase feeling empowered to ride the wave of the craving. It allows us to notice and accept sad or frustrated emotions and then choose activities other than eating in that moment of heightened emotions that can coast us on to something else away from eating (Bowen & Marlatt, 2009). If the urge to eat is due to emotions and not hunger, the strongest urges often only last a short time and then fade. If we can redirect ourselves for that initial period, we can survive the urge wave without giving in to undesirable behavior, for example, eating foods that make us feel bad. We might negotiate with ourselves that we can still have the desired food later when we are not so drawn to it to reduce intensification of the craving that can result from overly rigid food restriction. Recognizing that the urges will quickly subside if we do not act on them is very affirming and can help us feel calmer and more deliberate about our eating behavior. Focusing on the thought, "I can push through this short wave," can help to counteract the misleading feeling that this level of discomfort will continue until you give in to the urge.

Willpower as a Limited Fuel Source

Urge surfing requires some willpower and is a good strategy for short bursts of discipline, but it does not work well if it is your only strategy for making dietary changes. Willpower, as a conscious effort to regulate behaviors, is a limited resource. Short-term, willpower can be an effective way to "muscle through" completing difficult tasks. However, over time willpower fades for all of us, where we just cannot sustain that determined mindset to keep pushing ourselves to do something that feels really uncomfortable.

A 1998 experiment conducted by psychologist Roy Baumeister investigated the effectiveness of willpower as a resource for influencing human behavior. The experiment measured two aspects of willpower: self-control and persistence. The experimental participants were asked to control themselves and not eat freshly baked chocolate chip cookies while sitting in a room for 15 minutes. Immediately afterward they were asked to solve a puzzle that was impossible to solve, as the researchers measured how long the participant would persevere and keep trying to solve the puzzle. The control groups, who were either offered no food at all or who were told not to eat radishes (rather than cookies, which was not very difficult for them), were also asked to solve the same unsolvable puzzles.

The results were clear. The control groups spent more than twice the amount of time on the unsolvable puzzles than the experimental group that resisted eating the chocolate chip cookies before attempting to solve the puzzles. Resisting eating the cookies left the participants with less energy and drive to do something difficult and uncomfortable. They had used up their supply of willpower and no longer cared enough to keep trying to solve the puzzles. These results provided the initial support for the concept of *ego depletion*, which suggests we become depleted when using willpower and then have less energy to devote to a new task. "Resisting temptation seems to have produced a psychic cost, in the sense that afterward participants were more inclined to give up easily in the face of frustration" (Baumeister, 2018, p. 23).

This experiment demonstrated that willpower only takes us so far. We can count on willpower for short periods of focused exertion but cannot rely on it for long-term change. The act of changing our eating practices does not work as a short-term change or we will quickly revert back to our old style of eating. We can only resist the ice cream in the freezer for a while before we give in to its beckoning call and eat it. To create lasting change, we will need to look beyond willpower to other sources of information and motivation to guide our eating decisions, like paying attention to body cues and environmental pressures, and intentionally focusing our thoughts on what we hope to accomplish rather than on what we are giving up. The helpful reality check is we may not be able to keep the ice cream in the house if we only want to eat it on special occasions. Creating systems and a supportive environment facilitates consciously choosing what to eat as part of a healthy eating plan that is aligned with our desired results.

The Downside of Willpower

For people with a history of an eating disorder or who are at greater risk for developing disordered eating, willpower can be a dangerous narrative to follow when considering nutritional needs. Willpower can become elevated to a measure of one's self-worth when embedded in unhealthy ideas that maintain disordered eating. A drive for perfection may turn into, "I have the willpower to do things others can't do." A desire to be special or unique may become, "I get a lot of attention for my willpower over food" and "Being thin and not eating are signs of true willpower and success" (Costin & Grabb, 2011, pp. 84, 127).

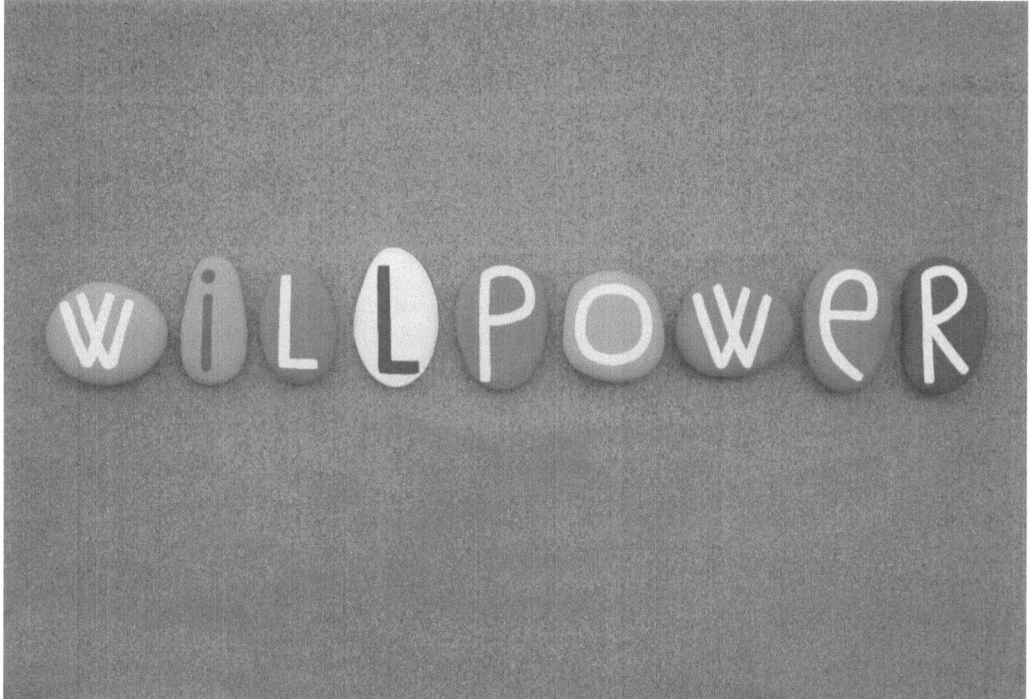

FIGURE 15.1   Willpower alone does not sustain long-term change. Credit: yournameonstones (Shutterstock).

The positive attention given in response to demonstrating willpower to resist eating food can exacerbate overly restrictive eating behavior and inadvertently support unhealthy attitudes around food. Willpower can mask an unhealthy relationship with food and an urgent need for control, which can invoke guilt, shame, and a desire for even more willpower until food becomes all-consuming, which is a losing game. Willpower can become about restraining yourself rather than having a mindful, trusting, and intuitive relationship with your food decisions.

One of the biggest risks of utilizing willpower to avoid eating food is that it encourages following external beliefs for eating (e.g., 2000 calories per day is correct for all people) with little priority given to staying attuned to internal cues. It can become a problem if we develop a habit of using will-power to ignore hunger and fullness cues, as well as our need for comfort, rest, and affection. The field of Intuitive Eating was developed to reacquaint people with these internal cues around food.

MANAGING HUNGER AND THIRST

Recognizing and honoring your body's hunger and fullness cues supports a healthy relationship between food and body. Diet culture centers around over-riding hunger cues (e.g., growling stomach) to follow an eating plan that may or may not be a good fit for your body on that day. Understanding different nutritional plans can provide good information about different eating options, but the only real test of success is how that eating program feels in your body. Eating is very personal and the only way to know what works best for us is to go on a journey of discovery. Intuitive eating can help with that journey by providing some guidelines for areas to explore that can offer important information about what works for you.

INTUITIVE EATING

Intuitive Eating (IE) is an approach to nutrition focused on awareness of bodily sensations, thoughts, and feelings. An intuitive eater is attentive to their body signals and plans their eating to maintain comfortable levels of hunger and fullness to prevent feeling anxious and desperate to eat food or guilty and overfull from eating too much. IE also focuses attention on our thoughts and feelings around food that often drive our eating behavior, especially the ways we are critical of our desire to eat and feel guilt and shame around food and our body. Emotional eating is recognized in IE as an attempt to ease or change our emotions by eating food, and we are encouraged to pause to notice and accept our emotions and then decide if eating is the best way to satisfy our needs in that moment (Tribole & Resch, 2020). Research investigating the effectiveness of IE indicates that this approach to nutrition decreases disordered eating and promotes greater body appreciation (Babbott et al., 2023; Bruce & Ricciardelli, 2016).

An important IE concept is the *forbidden fruit* effect. This concept argues that when desirable foods are forbidden (i.e., avoided or excluded from the diet), the human brain increases its focus and desire for that food. This can develop into a preoccupation or obsession with certain foods and can make them more desirable because they are not allowed. Sometimes this leads to the *Last Supper* phenomenon where a diet is preceded by consuming forbidden foods that will "never be eaten again" once the diet begins. Almost a "farewell-to-food party" that begins the next restrictive dieting cycle (Tribole & Resch, 2020). To avoid this affect, it can be helpful to intentionally include forbidden foods as part of your normal diet to alleviate any building tension around those foods. If we eat small amounts frequently, they lose a lot of their power and specialness and become just another part of our multi-faceted diet. This often helps decrease bingeing behavior and keeps us in the driver's seat for what we choose to eat.

An important part of learning to eat intuitively is the development of greater *interoception*, which is the ability to perceive physical sensations that arise from within the body such as hunger, fatigue, muscle tension, and bodily functions like the need to urinate. By paying better attention to our bodily sensations, we are better able to pick up on cues such as hunger and satiety before they

TABLE 15.1

Hunger and Fullness Scale

Level 1	Famished, lightheaded, urgent
Level 2	Very hungry, irritable, distracted
Level 3	**Ready to eat, interested, stomach growling**
Level 4	**Starting to think about food, noticing any nearby food**
Level 5	**Almost done eating, just a few bites more**
Level 6	**Comfortably full, satiated, content**
Level 7	Over full, uncomfortable, slightly unpleasant
Level 8	Stuffed, distended belly, nauseous

Source: Created by Andrea Cook.

intensify to a level that causes distress. Feeling desperately hungry increases anxiety, agitation, and irritability, sometimes called being "hangry." Increased interoception helps us regulate emotions by enhancing our ability to recognize and respond to bodily sensations connected to different feelings, such as a clenched fist linked to anger or a quivering lower lip in response to sadness (Price & Hooven, 2018). When we are more sensitive to noticing that we are starting to get upset, either because we are hungry or for another reason, we can more quickly act to resolve the situation. Here again mindfulness and eating behavior are intricately woven into our self-regulation system and are carefully tied to how we manage our emotional wellbeing.

A method to improve interoception associated with eating is to increase familiarity with your different levels of hunger and fullness. This can be accomplished by checking in and rating those sensations throughout the day using the following Hunger and Fullness Scale (see Table 15.1). The goal is to start and stop eating at levels 3 through 6, before you feel desperately hungry or overly full.

Of Note . . . HARA HACHI BU

Hara hachi bu is a 2500-year-old Japanese Confucian mantra said before meals to remind yourself to stop eating when you are mostly full rather than over full (Buettner & Skemp, 2016). Hara hachi bu translates to "eat until only mostly full" or "eat until 80% full." Similar to the Hunger and Fullness Scale, hara hachi bu, incorporates mindfulness to stay attentive to hunger and fullness cues while eating. This practice has contributed to the Japanese people thriving into old age as the country with the oldest population (Shirai & Tsushita, 2024).

To explore this pattern of eating, we invite you to make a note when you are starting to feel full during a meal. Slow down and pay attention to how you are feeling, "Hmm, I am starting to feel full. I think two or three more bites would feel good, then I am probably done. Let's see how it feels after two or three more bites."

HYDRATION

Perhaps you have been told to consider the possibility of thirst rather than hunger as the need your body is attempting to communicate. Just as our bodies need nutrients from a variety of food sources for fuel, *hydration* is also imperative for our physical and mental wellbeing. Among its many functions, hydration assists in transporting nutrients to cells and removing waste from them via the blood. It also plays a role in protecting the joints and organs as a key part of synovial fluid and it helps regulate body temperature and electrolyte balance for minerals like potassium, magnesium, and sodium.

The human brain primarily consists of water. Thus, when the brain is dehydrated, it is unable to function properly and you may experience lethargy and cognitive impairment related to concentration, memory, and critical thinking (Kranz, 2024; Riebl & Davy, 2013). It is also possible to be over-hydrated, which can be associated with patterns of disordered eating where a person is attempting to control their hunger by drinking a lot of fluids (Walsh, n.d.).

Something to keep in mind when it comes to thirst is that symptoms of diabetes include increased thirst (polydipsia), dry mouth, and frequent urination (Cleveland Clinic, n.d.). Many people with polydipsia who are pre-diabetic or diabetic have a difficult time feeling hydrated and feel constantly thirsty, so their body cues may be giving them misinformation about their hydration needs.

CREATING A PERSONAL FOOD PLAN

Limited free time, exhaustion, and periods of stress can lead to overwhelm and interfere with maintaining new lifestyle changes. Planning for access to nutrient-rich regular feedings through meals and snacks is essential to equip yourself with enough energy to tackle a full day of responsibilities. For example, college students' schedules are often jam-packed with tasks and activities. Your day may look like running to early morning classes, then studying at the library immediately after, and then returning home to complete assignments due later that evening. College life can pose a challenge to maintain consistent fuel from food. Thus, planning, by either packing easy and on-the-go meals and snacks or setting aside time to purchase food can be essential for many students. A busy schedule is not a good rationale for going without food since it is counter-productive to studying and attending class when you are hungry and struggling to concentrate. The goal is to create a food plan where you have access to good food and the opportunity to eat before you are so hungry that you wolf down your food and then feel overfull.

The incorporation of snacks can be an important part of daily dietary intake (Enriquez & Gollub, 2023). Focus on snack foods that both feel good in your body and satisfy your hunger. Sometimes you may need to be creative to both honor a craving and keep yourself satiated, such as opting for the cookie because it's what you really want and adding nut butter so that it keeps you full longer. As long as your body can handle them, nuts and seeds make easy to-go snacks that fit easily in a backpack or jacket pocket and which offer protein and fats that help with satiety and stabilizing blood glucose. It can be helpful to add them any time you are eating a simple carbohydrate like bread or crackers to help slow down the absorption, smooth out your blood glucose, and keep you feeling full for longer. Throw in some fruit for complex carbohydrates that provide fiber and micronutrients, which help you feel full and provide essential vitamins and minerals for mental well-being.

MALNUTRITION AND ACADEMIC PERFORMANCE

Research indicates that nutrition has an immense impact on academic performance. Malnutrition is linked to mental health conditions including diminished brain function, changes in mood and behavior, and problems with learning and memory (Khalil, 2022). Poor nutrition leaves you feeling depleted, with poor concentration and increased anxiety and depressive symptoms, which can negatively influence social behaviors as well as academic motivation (Keck et al., 2020). Malnutrition's association with a decline in cognition and concentration, energy, and the body's ability to perform day-to-day tasks clearly has an impact on academic performance. For example, college students in the U.S. whose eating habits include daily breakfast consumption and a wider variety of macronutrients and micronutrients in their diet report greater academic success (higher GPA averages) compared to students who do not eat breakfast or receive enough dietary nutrients (e.g. a lack of variety and nutritional density) (Reuter et al., 2021).

Malnutrition in college students happens for a number of reasons. Sometimes it is due to a busy schedule or loss of appetite due to stress, anxiety, or depression. Other times it is due to a lack of access to food. A large percentage of college students face food insecurity while attending school.

There is clear evidence that food insecurity is linked to lower academic performance and overall wellbeing for college students (Loofbourrow & Scherr, 2023; Weaver et al., 2020). Students who do not receive enough nutrients face negative consequences associated with cognitive function, including concentration and memory. Lack of nourishment also results in more rapid energy depletion, which can hinder the ability to focus or maintain motivation related to academic tasks or group socializing. Additionally, the stress of uncertainty about obtaining future meals can interfere with focus on academics as the body is innately inclined to dedicate greater focus on nutritional necessity and survival.

PREPARING FOR STRESSFUL TIMES

College student populations can face immense periods of stress. The sheer intensity of going through a life transition to begin navigating life independently as a young adult, plus the social pressures and culture shock of campus life combined with academic commitments and performance exams, can place tremendous pressure on college students. This compounds the significance of consuming adequate nourishment to manage daily life tasks and to protect oneself from the consequences of poor nutrition and stress.

Preparing for extra-busy schedules and increased pressures during exam periods can be an essential part of a college student's nutrition plan. Think of yourself as an athlete in training for a "big game" like a final exam. Eating foods with a variety of macronutrients and micronutrients will ensure a higher likelihood of your body receiving the vital energy it needs. Energy-dense foods, carbohydrates, and mindful caffeine intake can also support a healthy body dedicated to academics (MacDonald, 2019). Importantly, planning by meal-prepping and thoughtful food shopping before your schedule becomes too overwhelming or time sensitive can make incorporating mealtimes much quicker and easier in the moment.

LATE-NIGHT EATING

On those busy days, sometimes we fly through the day rushing to get everything done, and then collapse and finally eat some food at night. Recent research has explored whether the time of day when we eat our meals has an impact, especially late-night eating, which is very common. It turns out that the timing of your meals impacts your body, including hormone-driven hunger levels, energy, and body composition.

A 2022 study conducted at Harvard Medical School, explored the effect of college student meal schedules on appetite and the body's rate of energy consumption (Vujovic et al., 2022). Study participants were divided into two groups: the early mealtime group and the later mealtime group. The results reported that, in comparison to the early mealtime group, students in the late mealtime group woke up hungrier and had lower leptin levels, the hormone that manages the body's cues for feeling satiated. The late mealtime group participants also woke up with less energy and showed an increase in lipid (body fat) storage. This demonstrated that eating later in the day increases daytime hunger and fat storage and decreases available energy.

There is evidence that focusing your meals to earlier in the day has health benefits including reductions in fasting glucose, insulin resistance, and inflammation (Currenti et al., 2021). When research looked at the impact of restricting eating to early in the day (between 8:00 am and 2:00 pm) compared to the control group eating schedule (between 8:00 am and 8:00 pm), they found that having your last meal of the day at 2:00 pm decreased fasting glucose and insulin levels, and improved insulin sensitivity. In previous chapters, we discussed the negative implications of high glucose and insulin levels on mental health and focused primarily on the glycemic load of foods to help prevent glucose spikes caused by simple carbohydrates. This research reminds us that it is not just what you eat, but also when you eat it, that impacts how it is digested and absorbed into the bloodstream. If you have concerns about chronically high morning glucose levels associated with pre-diabetes and diabetes and its correlated depression, then eating earlier in the day (perhaps finish your last meal by 6:00 or 7:00 pm) may be another tool in your toolkit for managing your glucose levels and your depressive symptoms.

THE IMPACT OF FASTING

Thus far in this book we have focused on what and how to eat. Now let us consider what happens if we do not eat. *Fasting* has recently experienced a resurgence and has become a popular topic of discussion, and not just for weight loss. It is being used as a tool to optimize metabolism, boost mental clarity, and enhance vitality. Yet fasting is nothing new. Fasting has been part of human culture for thousands of years in various religious and spiritual traditions, healing practices, and social movements. It has long been touted for its healing benefits, including improved energy, focus, mood, sleep, and digestive health (Bland, 2019). Yet when we hear of fasting, many of us cringe and think, "I could never go a day without food" and wonder, "Why would I do that on purpose?"

The term fasting covers a broad range of behaviors. Fasts can last anywhere from 12 hours to 3 days or more. The most popular style of fasting is *intermittent fasting* (also known as time-restricted eating), where a person goes 14 to 18 hours without food on most days, shortening their eating window to a specific limited range. A common time-restricted eating schedule is the 16:8 method, where you fast for 16 hours and then have an 8-hour eating window, such as starting your first meal of the day at 11:00 am and ending your last meal of the day by 7:00 pm (Myers & Goldhamer, 2024). Another popular intermittent fasting approach is the 5:2 plan, where you eat normally for five days of the week, and then fast or eat minimal calories on the other two days (Naidoo, 2023). The range of fasting includes anything from a period of having no food of any kind and drinking only water (known as a water fast) to a period of highly reduced calorie or minimal food intake, such as a bone broth fast. Prolonged or multi-day fasting has additional healing benefits for some but is also more difficult and comes with greater risks.

CONTRAINDICATIONS FOR FASTING

Fasting is not recommended for people with disordered eating or a history of or current eating disorder. The highly restrictive nature of fasting can exacerbate the unhealthy pattern of rigid food restriction associated with eating disorders like anorexia and avoidant restrictive food intake disorder (ARFID). Fasting is also not advisable for people who are underweight, pregnant or lactating, or children under 12 years of age, as they have changing and sensitive nutritional needs (Varady et al., 2022). Also, all medications will respond differently when you fast since it changes how it is digested and absorbed when there is no food in the system, so it is important to involve your doctor in your fasting decisions if you are taking medication, especially thyroid and diabetes medications (Pelz, 2022).

FROM STARVATION TO AGRICULTURE

Proponents of fasting remind us that our bodies are designed to go through periods without food. During our hunting and gathering years, evolution designed us to live through periods of food abundance and periods of food scarcity. Our bodies developed the ability to store fat during times of abundance and to utilize that fat later to avoid starvation. Mind you, that is the first distinction that needs to be made. Fasting is voluntary and done for positive health, spiritual, and social benefits, while starvation is not.

Large scale food scarcity and starvation were primary concerns for survival until only very recently. About 12,000 years ago, a revolutionary event occurred. Humans developed agriculture. This newfound ability to produce a more stable and abundant food supply dramatically reduced the constant threat of starvation. The Industrial Age brought about the mass production of food, with increasing rates of highly processed and preserved foods that stabilized the food supply by providing foods with a long shelf life that could be transported and stored for long periods without refrigeration. Unfortunately, it also changed the nature of many of these foods so that our bodies were digesting something different and new compared to the foods we ate before that period in history.

METABOLIC SYNDROME

If the entire history of human evolution was represented as a 24-hour clock, these massive changes in our food occurred within only the last 0.1 millisecond! Our species' dietary habits drastically changed, but our genetics did not (The Galen Foundation, 1999). Our ancient survival programming to eat as much as possible and store fat has become a serious problem. These recent changes to our food supply bring new, life-threatening chronic food-related health threats, especially *metabolic syndrome (MetS)* which is associated with obesity, especially when it includes visceral adiposity (belly fat). MetS is diagnosed when someone has at least 3 out of 5 health conditions that increase their risk of cardiovascular disease, stroke, and type 2 diabetes: high blood glucose (i.e., pre-diabetes and insulin resistance), high cholesterol or high triglycerides in the blood (i.e., dyslipidemia or dyslipidaemia), high blood pressure (i.e., hypertension), and a large waist circumference (i.e., abdominal obesity) (see Figure 15.2) (AHA, 2023).

Recently we have expanded our understanding of the negative impact of MetS to include mental illness. Mental health issues including depression, anxiety, Alzheimer's disease, schizophrenia, ADHD, bipolar disorder, and autism spectrum disorder have been linked with MetS (Kouvari et al., 2022; Moradi et al., 2021; Nousen et al., 2013; Tahmi et al., 2021; Tang et al., 2017; Zuin et al., 2021). There is a bi-directional relationship between mental illness and MetS, since MetS increases your risk of developing a psychiatric disorder and because mental health symptoms make it harder to maintain good self-care habits and increase the risk of adopting unhealthy behaviors like poor diet,

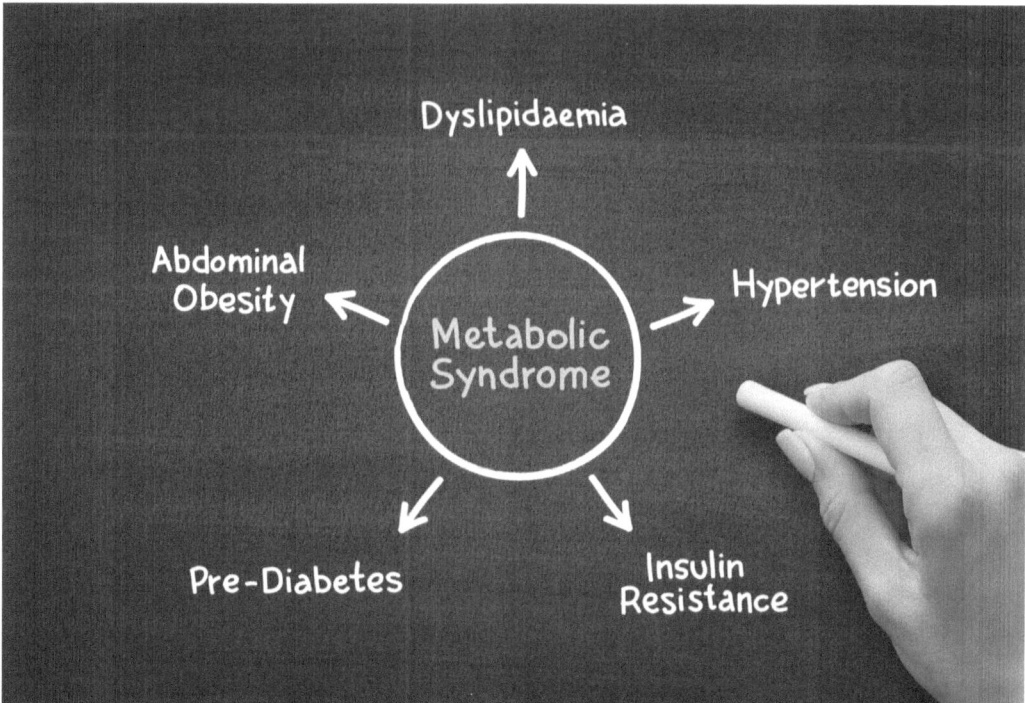

FIGURE 15.2 Health conditions associated with metabolic syndrome that increase risk of disease. Credit: dizain (Shutterstock).

smoking, alcohol use, and a sedentary lifestyle that contribute to developing MetS (Richard et al., 2023). Unfortunately, another risk factor among the mentally ill is the common side effect of weight gain associated with many of the medications prescribed for psychiatric disorders, which increases the risk of developing MetS (Brunero & Lamont, 2009).

FASTING BENEFITS

As discussed previously, the field of Metabolic Psychiatry has focused on the connection between metabolic health and mental health. Much of the research in that field has focused on the ketogenic diet, which shares many of the benefits of fasting, including reducing the chronically high glucose levels that are a primary driver of MetS. When carbohydrate consumption is significantly limited (keto) or removed (fasting), the body will use up its available stores of glucose and then turn to burning fat in the form of ketone bodies as its primary fuel source (Phinney et al., 2011). While there is controversy over the recommended levels of carbohydrate restriction and fasting, there is robust clinical evidence of the beneficial effects of well-constructed ketogenic diets and fasting plans to improve metabolic health and reverse symptoms of MetS (Cabo & Mattson, 2019; Chaix et al., 2019; Kunduraci & Ozbek, 2020; Li et al., 2017; Volek et al., 2024).

By reducing carbohydrate intake and glucose levels, the body can be conditioned to use fat (both dietary fat as well as fat stored in the body) as the primary energy source, while still using glucose as needed, a state often referred to as "fat adapted" or having achieved "metabolic flexibility" (Berg, 2024). In this state, many people find their cravings and intense hunger calm down, sleep and satiety improve, and they are more easily and comfortably able to go for longer periods without food.

A few words of caution. If you drink alcohol while reducing food carbohydrate intake, your body will burn the carbohydrates in the alcohol for energy and will resist shifting to metabolic flexibility. So, if your priority is to become fat-adapted, you may need to stop drinking alcohol for a while. Also, when your body is transitioning to using fat as the primary energy source, you may experience increased cravings for carbohydrates for the first week or two and then a decrease in cravings. Remember in the chapter about the microbiome, we discussed that the makeup of the gut bacteria is heavily influenced by diet. A diet high in carbohydrates supports different gut bacteria than a diet low in carbohydrates. These gut bacteria influence cravings to motivate you to eat food that helps them thrive. Fasting and low carbohydrate diets kill unhelpful gut bacteria and allow your beneficial bacteria to thrive, which initially can be an uncomfortable process during the "bad" bacteria die-off period. "Those bad bacteria will shout at you as they are dying off, often triggering cravings for chocolate, carbohydrates, or sugars" (Pelz, 2022, p. 174). It is important to remember that this is a short-term feeling while your gut is healing, and that the cravings die down when they are not fed.

FASTING AND MENTAL HEALTH

Two key mechanisms that underlie the connection between MetS and psychiatric disorders are *inflammation* and *BDNF (brain-derived neurotrophic factor)*. In both rodent and human studies, MetS was associated with increased cytokine levels (a marker for inflammation in the body) and decreased levels of BDNF (a protein that promotes neuron growth and connections in the brain) (Nousen et al., 2013). Fasting can help.

There is a growing body of research demonstrating the benefits of different types of fasting for improving mental health. Research has shown improved depression, anxiety, focus, memory, alertness, and a sense of tranquility associated with fasting (Currenti et al., 2021; Fond et al., 2013; Sharifi et al., 2024). Two of the beneficial mechanisms that result from fasting are decreased inflammation and increased production of BDNF, which has demonstrated benefits to relieving symptoms of both MetS and mental illness (Aksungar et al., 2007; Mattson et al., 2017; McAllister et al., 2020; Patterson & Sears, 2017; Seidler & Barrow, 2022; Sharifi et al., 2024).

If you are interested in trying fasting and are currently eating a diet high in carbohydrates, especially through ultra-processed foods, it may be advisable to prepare for fasting with a period of reduced carbohydrate intake to make the fasting process more comfortable. For example, a keto-genic diet (as discussed in Chapter 8) adds dietary fat to keep you satiated and decreases carbohydrates from 200–350 grams per day in the average American diet to 20–50 grams per day. It is important to start slowly to allow your body and mind to adapt to this new approach to eating. It is often helpful to start with intermittent fasting before attempting a multi-day water fast, which generally makes for a more positive experience (Pelz, n.d.). While intermittent fasting is generally well tolerated, multi-day water fasts come with risks and should only be attempted with proper supervision.

FOOD FOR THOUGHT: HEALTHY EATING ON A BUDGET

Eating a variety of food that is loaded with energy-dense nutrients and enjoyment makes for a well-rounded and nutritious diet. However, the increased cost of high-quality food can make the food shopping feel daunting. Therefore, doing some planning ahead of time can help you feel more relaxed about healthy food shopping without breaking the bank.

Food shopping trips can become expensive quickly. Focusing on whole food ingredients for meal prepping for regular meals and snacks offers food diversity (e.g., making a variety of meals with the same purchase) with financial practicality. Whole foods are nutrient-packed food sources that often cost the same or less than processed foods. Fruits and vegetables, whole grains like quinoa and brown rice, nuts and seeds, legumes such as lentils and soybeans, and meat and animal products like chicken, fish, beef, eggs, and dairy are categorized under the whole foods umbrella. Including on-the-go foods like frozen meals and protein bars can be a viable option for especially busy days but may not always be the most cost-effective choice on a daily basis.

The conversation around whether to purchase organic versus conventional (non-organic) foods remains complex and nuanced. *Organic* products are grown without synthetic pesticides or fertilizers and without the routine use of antibiotics or growth hormones for animal products. One of the challenging factors is that there is a lot of variation in farming practices and regulatory codes used in both organic and conventional farming.

Development of U.S. national organic standards started in the 1980s. The primary differentiation between organic and conventional farming focuses on the types of inputs (e.g., fertilizers and pesticides) used during the growing process, with organic pushing for more natural inputs (e.g., cow manure as fertilizer) instead of chemically processed synthetic inputs. Organic animal ranching for meat, dairy, or eggs has regulations that protect animal welfare by requiring that the animals are treated humanely with specifications such as adequate space for natural movement, company with other animals, natural light, and ventilation (Seufert et al., 2017).

Organic farming in its original conceptualization, also focused on differences in farming practices described as *sustainable agriculture* that are more environmentally sensitive and work to improve the quality of the soil and the agricultural water systems. There have long been concerns that regulatory agencies do not mandate sustainable agriculture practices, especially for farms with large-scale organic production. Farming practices like cover crops to replenish nutrients back into the soil and water conservation systems, while still encouraged and recommended, are generally not as well codified into organic certification requirements (Guthman, 2004). A recent addition to sustainable agriculture is the term *regenerative farming* which focuses on farming practices that improve soil health, increase biodiversity (the variety of species of plants and animals), and protect watersheds (Koman et al., 2021; White, 2020).

Not everyone agrees that there is sufficient evidence of the benefits of organic products to justify their higher cost (Paarlberg, 2023). For example, there is debate over what constitutes an acceptable exposure to pesticides, considering both initial pesticide levels upon consumption as well as the potential for pesticide levels in the body to build up over time (Damalas & Eleftherohorinos,

2011). A systematic review of the nutrient and contaminant levels in food explored if organic food has a significantly higher density of micronutrients and a significantly lower level of contaminants (such as pesticides) when compared to conventional foods. The study concluded that there was a lack of strong evidence that organic foods are significantly more nutritious than conventional foods, but there was evidence that consuming organic foods may reduce exposure to pesticide residues in fruits and vegetables and antibiotic-resistant bacteria in chicken and pork (Smith-Spangler et al., 2012).

A *pesticide* is any substance used to prevent, destroy, or repel pests such as insects, mice, and weeds. "Pesticides are toxic substances, and exposure to them can cause acute or chronic adverse health effects" (Namulanda, 2016, p. 6). According to the World Health Organization (WHO), pesticides play a significant role in food production to protect crops against insects, weeds, fungi, and other pests. Pesticides can have negative health effects on humans depending on the quantity and ways in which a person is exposed. Those working in agriculture who are directly exposed to pesticides are at the highest risk for high exposure which can lead to pesticide poisoning (WHO, 2022).

Recent research has been examining the association between pesticide exposure and psychiatric illness, especially depression and anxiety. There is evidence of the association between pesticide poisoning and depression (Freire & Koifman, 2013; Frengidou et al., 2024) likely due to disruptions in brain neurochemistry that cause psychiatric symptoms (Stallones & Beseler, 2016). That has raised questions about the mental health impact of long-term low-level exposure to pesticides from eating foods that have pesticide residue levels considered normal and acceptable within the conventional food industry standards.

The toxic effect of low doses of pesticides on human health is largely unknown, although there are growing concerns about their safety. Evidence is mounting that long-term exposure to low doses of pesticides may lead to an array of negative health consequences, including cancer, neurodegenerative diseases, reproductive and developmental issues, and respiratory problems (Hernández et al., 2013). To examine this issue, it was important to look at pesticide levels in people who did not work in the agricultural industry nor were exposed to high levels of pesticides in an acute pesticide exposure event. Meaning their primary exposure to pesticides was in the food and water they consumed. A recent large study measured urinary concentrations of six widely used pesticides in over 5000 participants not associated with the agricultural industry and compared them to survey data about nutrition habits and mental health. The results found evidence that increased exposure to pesticides significantly increased the risk of depressive symptoms (Wu et al., 2023).

Even if you are concerned about the impact of pesticides from the foods you consume, for many it is just too expensive to eat organic foods every day. To help you get the biggest bang for your buck and prioritize which foods make the most difference to buy organic, the Environmental Working Group (EWG) provides a guide for buying fresh produce based on the level of pesticide residue commonly found on those foods. Each year the EWG publishes two lists at www.ewg.org to help with food purchase decisions: the *Dirty Dozen* and the *Clean Fifteen*. The Dirty Dozen lists the 12 fruits and vegetables found to have the most pesticide residue, while the Clean Fifteen lists the produce with the least pesticide residue.

For those who struggle with mental illness, learning to buy and prepare whole foods can be especially important. The SMILES diet study analyzed the cost of a diet high in whole nutrient-dense foods for people diagnosed with a mental illness. The experimental group whole foods diet was found to be more financially friendly on average than the control group diet which included more prepared foods (Chatterton et al., 2018). When the study also included the reduction in expenditures from psychiatric medication, treatment services, and lost wages due to improved mental health from an improved diet, the cost-effectiveness of this approach became even more apparent.

To help with the cost of food, many students are eligible for the SNAP program (Supplemental Nutrition Assistance Program), also known as food stamps, which is a federal financial support system for grocery shopping needs. In addition to using SNAP funds at grocery stores, many farmer's markets accept SNAP funds to make fresh local produce more affordable. Other resources include community gardens that offer reduced-price goods and campus-partnered food programs, like food pantries, which offer more cost-effective and fresh food options for students on a budget. Although high-quality cuts of meat and fresh fruits and vegetables may be preferable, incorporating canned and frozen whole foods can be an important way to decrease costs and improve convenience.

Knowing your budget and getting support through local resources may be a first step toward maximizing your purchase power. Other options may include making a shopping list before you enter the shopping area. Grocery shopping can feel formidable. When sticking to a grocery budget, planning ahead by jotting down your list of "wants" and "needs" for your upcoming snacks and meals can support effective spending and avoid succumbing to enticing food advertisements while walking down the aisles. Focus your shopping on the perimeter of the grocery store, which is filled with whole foods like fresh produce and meat, while the center aisles of the store focus more on processed foods which can be more expensive.

When preparing meals, keep things simple! Complex recipes can become overwhelming and interfere with your motivation to nourish yourself. If you feel overwhelmed and frustrated, you are more likely to give up and search for quick food sources. Storing food properly decreases food spoilage and food waste. Utilize freezer space to preserve portions of prepared meals for later to create a quick meal option when you are in a hurry.

It is important to be gentle with yourself and realistic about your schedule. You may not have the bandwidth for extravagant home-cooked meals, and that is okay! Selecting time-efficient, less-intensive options can still support you to eat a high-quality diet while decreasing the likelihood of overwhelm. You might even find out that cooking for yourself is fun!

REFERENCES

AHA. (2023). *What is metabolic syndrome?* American Heart Association. https://www.heart.org/en/health-topics/metabolic-syndrome/about-metabolic-syndrome

Aksungar, F. B., Topkaya, A. E., & Akyildiz, M. (2007). Interleukin-6, c-reactive protein and biochemical parameters during prolonged intermittent fasting. *Annals of Nutrition and Metabolism*, *51*(1), 88–95. https://doi.org/10.1159/000100954

Babbott, K. M., Cavadino, A., Brenton-Peters, J., Consedine, N. S., & Roberts, M. (2023). Outcomes of intuitive eating interventions: A systematic review and meta-analysis. *Eating Disorders*, *31*(1), 33–63.

Baumeister, R. F. (2018). *Self-regulation and self-control: Selected works of Roy Baumeister*. Routledge.

Berg, E. (2024). *How to Really Become Fat Adapted*. https://www.drberg.com/blog/how-to-really-become-fat-adapted

Berkeley University Health Services. (2018). *Finals week nutrition tips*. UC Berkeley. https://uhs.berkeley.edu/news/finals-week-nutrition-tips

Bland, J. S. (2019). Fasting physiology and therapeutic diets: A look back to the future. *Integrative Medicine*, *18*(1), 16–21.

Bowen, S., & Marlatt, A. (2009). Surfing the urge: Brief mindfulness-based intervention for college student smokers. *Psychology of Addictive Behaviors*, *23*(4), 666–671. https://doi.org/10.1037/a0017127

Bruce, L. J., & Ricciardelli, L. A. (2016). A systematic review of the psychosocial correlates of intuitive eating among adult women, *Appetite*, *96*, 454–472, https://doi.org/10.1016/j.appet.2015.10.012

Brunero, S., & Lamont, S. (2009). Systematic screening for metabolic syndrome in consumers with severe mental illness. *International Journal of Mental Health Nursing*, *18*(2), 144–150. https://doi.org/10.1111/j.1447-0349.2009.00595.x

Buettner, D., & Skemp, S. (2016). Blue zones: Lessons from the world's longest lived. *American Journal of Lifestyle Medicine*, *10*(5), 318–321.

Cabo, R., & Mattson, M. P. (2019). Effects of intermittent fasting on health, aging, and disease. *New England Journal of Medicine*, *381*(26), 2541–2551. https://doi.org/doi:10.1056/NEJMra1905136

Chaix, A., Lin, T., Le, H. D., Chang, M. W., & Panda, S. (2019). Time-restricted feeding prevents obesity and metabolic syndrome in mice lacking a circadian clock. *Cell Metabolism*, *29*(2), 303–319. e304. https://doi.org/10.1016/j.cmet.2018.08.004

Chatterton, M. L., Mihalopoulos, C., O'Neil, A., Itsiopoulos, C., Opie, R., Castle, D., Dash, S., Brazionis, L., Berk, M., & Jacka, F. (2018). Economic evaluation of a dietary intervention for adults with major depression (the "SMILES" trial). *BMC Public Health*, *18*(1), 11.

Cleveland Clinic. (n.d.). *Diabetes.* https://my.clevelandclinic.org/health/diseases/7104-diabetes

Costin, C., & Grabb, G. S. (2011). *8 keys to recovery from an eating disorder: Effective strategies from therapeutic practice and personal experience (8 keys to mental health).* WW Norton & Company.

Currenti, W., Godos, J., Castellano, S., Caruso, G., Ferri, R., Caraci, F., Grosso, G., & Galvano, F. (2021). Association between time restricted feeding and cognitive status in older Italian adults. *Nutrients, 13*(1), 191. https://www.mdpi.com/2072-6643/13/1/191

Damalas, C. A., & Eleftherohorinos, I. G. (2011). Pesticide exposure, safety issues, and risk assessment indicators. *International Journal of Environmental Research and Public Health, 8*(5), 1402–1419. https://www.mdpi.com/1660-4601/8/5/1402

Enriquez, J. P., & Gollub, E. (2023). Snacking consumption among adults in the United States: A scoping review. *Nutrients, 15*(7). https://doi.org/10.3390/nu15071596

Fond, G., Macgregor, A., Leboyer, M., & Michalsen, A. (2013). Fasting in mood disorders: Neurobiology and effectiveness. A review of the literature. *Psychiatry Research, 209*(3), 253–258. https://doi.org/10.1016/j.psychres.2012.12.018

Freire, C., & Koifman, S. (2013). Pesticides, depression and suicide: A systematic review of the epidemiological evidence. *International Journal of Hygiene and Environmental Health, 216*(4), 445–460.

Frengidou, E., Galanis, P., & Malesios, C. (2024). Pesticide exposure or pesticide poisoning and the risk of depression in agricultural populations: A systematic review and meta-analysis. *Journal of Agromedicine, 29*(1), 91–105.

Guthman, J. (2004). The trouble with 'Organic Lite' in California: A rejoinder to the 'Conventionalisation' debate. *Sociologia Ruralis, 44*(3), 301–316. https://doi.org/10.1111/j.1467-9523.2004.00277.x

Hernández, A. F., Parrón, T., Tsatsakis, A. M., Requena, M., Alarcón, R., & López-Guarnido, O. (2013). Toxic effects of pesticide mixtures at a molecular level: Their relevance to human health, *Toxicology, 307*, 136–145, https://doi.org/10.1016/j.tox.2012.06.009

Keck, M. M., Vivier, H., Cassisi, J. E., Dvorak, R. D., Dunn, M. E., Neer, S. M., & Ross, E. J. (2020). Examining the role of anxiety and depression in dietary choices among college students. *Nutrients, 12*(7), 2061. https://www.mdpi.com/2072-6643/12/7/2061

Khalil, N. A. (2022). Malnutrition of micronutrients and brain disorders. In W. Mohamed & T. Yamashita (Eds.), *Role of micronutrients in brain health* (pp. 167–182). Springer Singapore. https://doi.org/10.1007/978-981-16-6467-0_10

Koman, E., Laurilliard, E., Moore, A., & Ruiz-Uribe, N. (2021). Restoration through regeneration: A scientific and political lens into regenerative agriculture in the United States. *Journal of Science Policy & Governance, 19*, 1–28.

Kouvari, M., D'Cunha, N. M., Travica, N., Sergi, D., Zec, M., Marx, W., & Naumovski, N. (2022). Metabolic syndrome, cognitive impairment and the role of diet: A narrative review. *Nutrients, 14*(2), 333. https://www.mdpi.com/2072-6643/14/2/333

Kranz, R. (2024). *Symptoms of dehydration: What they are and what to do if you experience them.* https://www.health.harvard.edu/staying-healthy/symptoms-of-dehydration-what-they-are-and-what-to-do-if-you-experience-them

Kunduraci, Y. E., & Ozbek, H. (2020). Does the energy restriction intermittent fasting diet alleviate metabolic syndrome biomarkers? A randomized controlled trial. *Nutrients, 12*(10), 3213. https://www.mdpi.com/2072-6643/12/10/3213

Li, C., Sadraie, B., Steckhan, N., Kessler, C., Stange, R., Jeitler, M., & Michalsen, A. (2017). Effects of a one-week fasting therapy in patients with type-2 diabetes mellitus and metabolic syndrome–A randomized controlled explorative study. *Experimental and Clinical Endocrinology & Diabetes, 125*(09), 618–624.

Loofbourrow, B. M., & Scherr, R. E. (2023). Food insecurity in higher education: A contemporary review of impacts and explorations of solutions International Journal of Environmental Research and Public Health, *20*(10). https://doi.org/10.3390/ijerph20105884

MacDonald, L. (2019). *Exam time- eating strategies.* NutriNews, The University of Arizona. https://nutrition.arizona.edu/news/2019/12/exam-time-eating-strategies

Marlatt, G. A., & Gordon, J. R. (1985). *Relapse prevention: Maintenance strategies in the treatment of addictive behaviors.* Guilford Press.

Mattson, M. P., Longo, V. D., & Harvie, M. (2017). Impact of intermittent fasting on health and disease processes. *Ageing Research Reviews, 39*, 46–58, https://doi.org/10.1016/j.arr.2016.10.005

McAllister, M. J., Pigg, B. L., Renteria, L. I., & Waldman, H. S. (2020). Time-restricted feeding improves markers of cardiometabolic health in physically active college-age men: A 4-week randomized pre-post pilot study. *Nutrition Research, 75*, 32–43, https://doi.org/10.1016/j.nutres.2019.12.001

Mischel, W. (2014). *The marshmallow test: Mastering self-control* (1st ed.). Little, Brown and Company.

Mischel, W., & Ebbesen, E. B. (1970). Attention in delay of gratification. *Journal of Personality and Social Psychology, 16*(2), 329–337. https://doi.org/10.1037/h0029815

Moradi, Y., Albatineh, A. N., Mahmoodi, H., & Gheshlagh, R. G. (2021). The relationship between depression and risk of metabolic syndrome: A meta-analysis of observational studies. *Clinical Diabetes and Endocrinology, 7*(1), 4. https://doi.org/10.1186/s40842-021-00117-8

Myers, T., & Goldhamer, A. (2024). *Can fasting save your life?* Book Publishing Company.

Naidoo, U. (2023). *Calm your mind with food: A revolutionary guide to controlling your anxiety* (1st ed.). Little, Brown Spark.

Namulanda, G. (2016). Acute nonoccupational pesticide-related illness and injury—United States, 2007–2011. *MMWR. Morbidity and Mortality Weekly Report, 63*(55). National Center for Environmental Health, CDC. https://www.cdc.gov/mmwr/volumes/63/wr/mm6355a2.htm.

Nousen, E. K., Franco, J. G., & Sullivan, E. L. (2013). Unraveling the mechanisms responsible for the comorbidity between metabolic syndrome and mental health disorders. *Neuroendocrinology, 98*(4), 254–266. https://doi.org/10.1159/000355632

Paarlberg, R. (2023). Is organic better? Not if you follow the evidence, researcher says. *The Harvard Gazette.* https://news.harvard.edu/gazette/story/2023/09/is-organic-better/

Patterson, R. E., & Sears, D. D. (2017). Metabolic effects of intermittent fasting, *Annual Review of Nutrition, 37,* 371–393, https://doi.org/10.1146/annurev-nutr-071816-064634

Pelz, M. (2022). *Fast like a girl: a woman's guide to using the healing power of fasting to burn fat, boost energy, and balance hormones* (1st ed.). Hay House.

Pelz, M. (n.d.). *A beginners guide to fasting: Everything you need to know about fasting.* DrMindyPelz.com. https://drmindypelz.com/a-beginners-guide-to-fasting/

Phinney, S. D., Volek, J. S., & Lexington, K. (2011). *The art and science of low carbohydrate living: An expert guide to making the life-saving benefits of carbohydrate restriction sustainable and enjoyable.* Beyond Obesity.

Price, C. J., & Hooven, C. (2018). Interoceptive awareness skills for emotion regulation: Theory and approach of mindful awareness in body-oriented therapy (MABT) [Conceptual analysis]. *Frontiers in Psychology, 9.* https://doi.org/10.3389/fpsyg.2018.00798

Reuter, P. R., Forster, B. L., & Brister, S. R. (2021). The influence of eating habits on the academic performance of university students. *Journal of American College Health, 69*(8), 921–927. https://doi.org/10.1080/07448481.2020.1715986

Richard, S. L., Renn, B. N., Kim, J., Tran, D.-M. T., & Feng, D. (2023). Mental health is related to metabolic syndrome: The Hispanic community health study/study of Latinos. *Psychoneuroendocrinology, 152,* 106085. https://doi.org/10.1016/j.psyneuen.2023.106085

Riebl, S. K., & Davy, B. M. (2013). The hydration equation: Update on water balance and cognitive performance. *ACSM's Health & Fitness Journal, 17*(6), 21–28. https://doi.org/10.1249/FIT.0b013e3182a9570f

Seidler, K., & Barrow, M. (2022). Intermittent fasting and cognitive performance – targeting BDNF as potential strategy to optimise brain health. *Frontiers in Neuroendocrinology, 65,* 100971, https://doi.org/10.1016/j.yfrne.2021.100971

Seufert, V., Ramankutty, N., & Mayerhofer, T. (2017). What is this thing called organic? – how organic farming is codified in regulations. *Food Policy, 68,* 10–20, https://doi.org/10.1016/j.foodpol.2016.12.009

Sharifi, S., Rostami, F., Babaei Khorzoughi, K., & Rahmati, M. (2024). Effect of time-restricted eating and intermittent fasting on cognitive function and mental health in older adults: A systematic review. *Preventive Medicine Reports, 42,* 102757, https://doi.org/10.1016/j.pmedr.2024.102757

Shirai, T., & Tsushita, K. (2024). Lifestyle medicine and Japan's longevity miracle. *American Journal of Lifestyle Medicine, 18*(4), 598–607. https://doi.org/10.1177/15598276241234012

Smith-Spangler, C., Brandeau, M. L., Hunter, G. E., Bavinger, J. C., Pearson, M., Eschbach, P. J., Sundaram, V., Liu, H., Schirmer, P., & Stave, C. (2012). Are organic foods safer or healthier than conventional alternatives? A systematic review. *Annals of Internal Medicine, 157*(5), 348–366.

Stallones, L., & Beseler, C. L. (2016). Assessing the connection between organophosphate pesticide poisoning and mental health: A comparison of neuropsychological symptoms from clinical observations, animal models and epidemiological studies, *Cortex, 74,* 405–416, https://doi.org/10.1016/j.cortex.2015.10.002

Tahmi, M., Palta, P., & Luchsinger, J. A. (2021). Metabolic syndrome and cognitive function. *Current Cardiology Reports, 23*(12), 180. https://doi.org/10.1007/s11886-021-01615-y

Tang, F., Wang, G., & Lian, Y. (2017). Association between anxiety and metabolic syndrome: A systematic review and meta-analysis of epidemiological studies. *Psychoneuroendocrinology, 77,* 112–121, https://doi.org/10.1016/j.psyneuen.2016.11.025

The Galen Foundation. (1999). *Fasting For Survival Lecture by Dr Pradip Jamnadas.* https://www.youtube.com/watch?v=RuOvn4UqznU&t=1318s

Therapist Aid. (2021). *Urge surfing: Distress tolerance skill.* https://www.therapistaid.com/therapy-worksheet/urge-surfing-handout.

Tribole, E., & Resch, E. (2020). *Intuitive eating: A revolutionary anti-diet approach.* St. Martin's Essentials.

Varady, K. A., Cienfuegos, S., Ezpeleta, M., & Gabel, K. (2022). Clinical application of intermittent fasting for weight loss: Progress and future directions. *Nature Reviews Endocrinology, 18*(5), 309–321. https://doi.org/10.1038/s41574-022-00638-x

Volek, J. S., Yancy, W. S., Gower, B. A., Phinney, S. D., Slavin, J., Koutnik, A. P., Hurn, M., Spinner, J., Cucuzzella, M., & Hecht, F. M. (2024). Expert consensus on nutrition and lower-carbohydrate diets: An evidence- and equity-based approach to dietary guidance [review]. *Frontiers in Nutrition, 11.* https://doi.org/10.3389/fnut.2024.1376098

Vujovic, N., Piron, M. J., Qian, J., Chellappa, S. L., Nedeltcheva, A., Barr, D., Heng, S. W., Kerlin, K., Srivastav, S., Wang, W., Shoji, B., Garaulet, M., Brady, M. J., & Scheer, F. A. J. L. (2022). Late isocaloric eating increases hunger, decreases energy expenditure, and modifies metabolic pathways in adults with overweight and obesity. *Cell Metabolism, 34*(10), 1486–1498.e1487. https://doi.org/10.1016/j.cmet.2022.09.007

Walsh, J. (n.d.). *Eating disorders and drinking water.* Change Creates Change. https://changecreateschange.com/eating-disorders-and-drinking-water/

Weaver, R. R., Vaughn, N. A., Hendricks, S. P., McPherson-Myers, P. E., Jia, Q., Willis, S. L., & Rescigno, K. P. (2020). University student food insecurity and academic performance. *Journal of American College Health, 68*(7), 727–733. https://doi.org/10.1080/07448481.2019.1600522

White, C. (2020). Why regenerative agriculture? *The American Journal of Economics and Sociology, 79*(3), 799–812. https://doi.org/10.1111/ajes.12334

WHO. (2022). *Pesticide residues in food.* World Health Organization. https://www.who.int/news-room/fact-sheets/detail/pesticide-residues-in-food

Wu, Y., Song, J., Zhang, Q., Yan, S., Sun, X., Yi, W., Pan, R., Cheng, J., Xu, Z., & Su, H. (2023). Association between organophosphorus pesticide exposure and depression risk in adults: A cross-sectional study with NHANES data. *Environmental Pollution, 316*, 120445, https://doi.org/10.1016/j.envpol.2022.120445

Zuin, M., Roncon, L., Passaro, A., Cervellati, C., & Zuliani, G. (2021). Metabolic syndrome and the risk of late onset Alzheimer's disease: An updated review and meta-analysis. *Nutrition, Metabolism and Cardiovascular Diseases, 31*(8), 2244–2252. https://doi.org/10.1016/j.numecd.2021.03.020

16 Self-Care

Positive mental health and a lifestyle that supports optimal living could include contributions like movement, time spent in nature, mindfulness, dental hygiene (yep you heard that right), and sleep. By building them into our daily habits we can strengthen our coping skills, expand our emotional bandwidth, and better manage stressors, giving us that "ounce of prevention" that helps us avoid a crisis that will then require the "pound of cure" to resolve the situation. As with so many things that impact mental health, lifestyle and nutrition habits are bi-directional. A healthy lifestyle supports good nutrition habits, and good nutrition habits give us the stamina and clarity to maintain a healthy lifestyle.

SELF-CARE PRESSURE

Self-care can feel a bit overrated. Promotional promises and life-changing hacks and checklists for what we "should" be doing are pushed at us with every turn. While many are meant to motivate us, if we're not yet ready to be motivated, guilt and shame can grow as we stare at the laundry list of things we are failing to accomplish. It does not help that as humans we have a natural tendency to compare ourselves to others. And, in the age of social media, others' lives seem so appealing. We can easily begin to feel like total failures. Feeling overwhelmed by not being able to stay on top of all of our self-care goals (because let's face it, we never will) and checking some self-care accomplishment boxes is, ironically, counterproductive for self-care.

Feeling inadequate for not having better self-care is not going to help our mood or mental state. Adding to your guilt is not what this chapter is about. This section of the book is meant to be a practical and supportive guide. Our focus here is to help you understand more deeply why self-care is important, the essential components that can bring real value, and how best to create a sustainable, relevant, and affordable plan. Your final self-care plan may not be social media worthy, but hopefully, it will help you feel a little better and will give you some ideas on how to keep adding in those lifestyle changes that make the biggest difference in supporting you to thrive.

Of Note . . . H.A.L.T. – A QUICK CHECK-IN WITH YOURSELF

Our lives are busy! Sometimes, it is hard to acknowledge how we feel before we find ourselves irritable and reacting to people and situations with anger and impatience. One tool to help you pause and check-in with yourself is to use the H.A.L.T. method. The H.A.L.T. acronym was originally created by David Streem, M.D., a psychiatrist and addiction specialist. The idea is simple. When you start noticing yourself feeling upset, ask yourself, "Am I feeling Hungry, Angry, Lonely, or Tired?" If you answer yes to any of these questions, address the root cause to decrease your discomfort. Each of these states has a solution. If you are feeling Hungry, eat something (ideally a healthy snack or meal). If you are feeling Angry, express yourself in a safe and effective way, such as journaling, movement, or talking with a friend. If you are feeling Lonely, reach out to someone. If you are feeling Tired, (you guessed it!) take a short nap or plan for a better night of sleep.

MOVEMENT AND MENTAL HEALTH

It is common knowledge that movement is good for our overall health, however, most of the focus has been on physical health. Movement is essential for good mental health as well. Research has demonstrated that physical activity can reduce symptoms of anxiety and depression at a rate similar

DOI: 10.1201/9781032647647-22

to other forms of treatment, including many medications (Carek et al., 2011; Rebar et al., 2015). Exercise, whether low-intensity or high-intensity, can lead to improvements in mood by triggering the release of endorphins and enhancing sleep quality (more on sleep later). Endorphin release decreases pain (both physical and mental) and increases feelings of pleasure, which decreases symptoms of depression and anxiety and provides positive reinforcement for exercising again in the future.

Exercise also improves *brain plasticity,* which is the brain's ability to mature through growth and reorganization as a positive and adaptive response to changes in the environment. Brain plasticity is a sign of brain health. Exercise encourages brain plasticity by stimulating neurogenesis (the process by which the brain grows new neurons) and new neural connections which improve brain function. One of the key regions of the brain that is supported by exercise is the hippocampus (involved with learning and memory), which improve our ability to solve problems more effectively and make meaningful lifestyle changes. Exercise also influences the function of the thyroid and adrenal glands, which are crucial for mood regulation and resilience, and increases oxygen production, which stimulates our ability to relax, plan, and execute (Basso & Suzuki, 2017).

Regardless of age, consistency is key, so integrating physical activity into daily routines is essential to prevent drifting into a sedentary lifestyle. A study by Raichlen et al. (2023) demonstrated that a sedentary lifestyle increases the risk of developing Alzheimer's disease among older adults. The researchers attributed the increased risk to reduced blood flow to the brain, impaired ability to maintain healthy glucose levels, and increased systemic inflammation. Exercise enhances our ability to pay attention, remember, process information, plan, and make thoughtful decisions (Chang et al., 2012). Movement can make you smarter!

Movement that challenges our brain as well as our body can be especially useful as we age. A study of older adults found that playing a video game that pushed them to learn new movements improved measures of physical health (e.g., blood pressure, balance) as well as the ability to pay attention and focus (Anguera et al., 2022). A low-tech option is to attend dance classes where they are challenged to learn new movements and steps. This combination of movement, coordination, and learning has been shown to improve cognitive function, while the socialization and music associated with dance improve mood (Predovan et al., 2019). These findings suggest that an integrated approach to movement combined with mental challenges looks promising for older adults seeking to maintain or improve their cognitive health.

You may be wondering if exercise can make a difference once you have already been diagnosed with a psychiatric disorder. A review assessed the evidence that supports the use of exercise to decrease symptoms of major depressive disorder (Noetel et al., 2024). They concluded that exercise is an effective treatment for depression, especially walking, jogging, yoga, strength training, and dancing, and was equally effective for people with different levels of depression and with or without comorbidities such as diabetes. Exercise was comparable to psychotherapy and medication for reducing depressive symptoms, with vigorous exercise being better for those who could tolerate it. The study's authors concluded that structured exercise programs should be included as a core treatment for depression alongside psychotherapy and antidepressants.

A note on exercise for those who may find going to the gym uninteresting. All types of movement, including dancing, hiking, and gardening, are beneficial if our heart rate increases. All you need is the ability to move at whatever level feels good and is available for your body. Try combining short intense bursts of movement that get your heart pumping with quiet gentle movement that helps you relax. A little every day can make a big difference to feeling calm, happy, and better able to problem-solve for the day ahead.

BENEFITS OF NATURE

When you exercise, consider doing it outside when the weather permits. Being outdoors in itself can have healing effects. Barton and Pretty (2010) found evidence supporting a dose-response relationship between exposure to nature and mental health benefits, showing that the more time you spend in

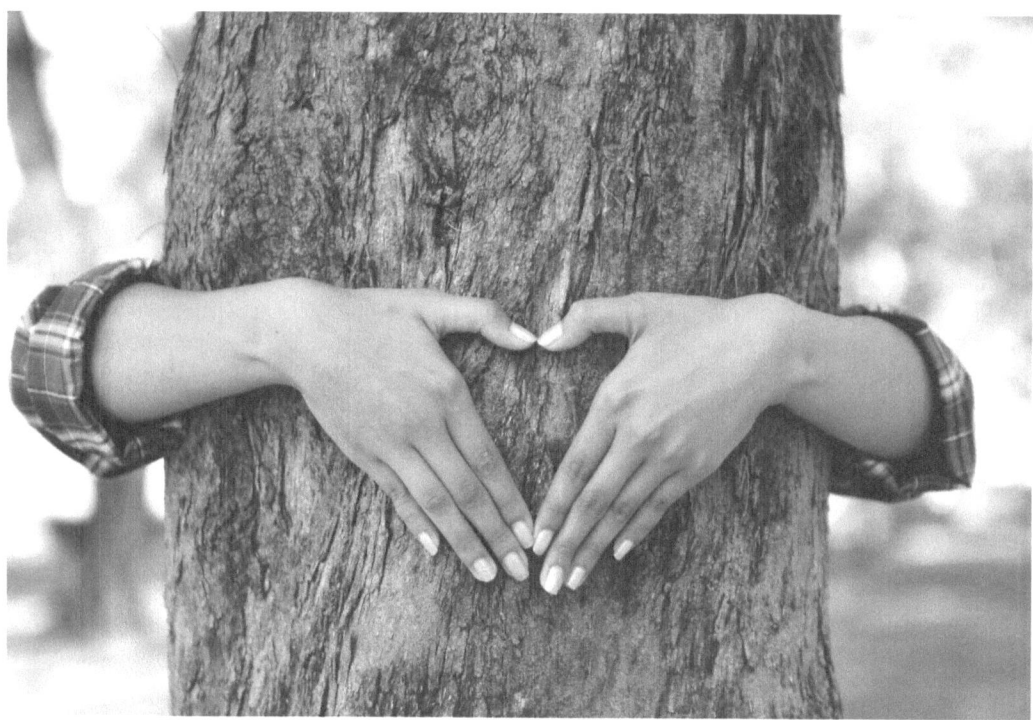

FIGURE 16.1   Time in nature provides mental health benefits. Credit Alohaflaminggo (Shutterstock).

nature, the greater the mental health benefits you are likely to attain. They identified that even short periods in nature can lead to improvements in mood, self-esteem, and overall mental wellbeing. Time in nature gives us needed recovery time from attention fatigue by giving your brain a break.

We tend to breathe more deeply when we are in natural settings. The air is cleaner and better oxygenated due to plant activity, which provides more oxygen to our brains. When we are stressed, we tend to hold our breath, restricting oxygen flow to our brain and body. This becomes a feedback loop. The more stressed we are, the less oxygen we inhale. The less oxygen our brain has available, the less we can plan and problem solve, leading to more stress. Time in nature cues us to slow down, breathe, and relax, which improves our cardiovascular health (such as blood pressure and heart rate), and moves us from our sympathetic to our parasympathetic nervous system so that we can heal (Haluza et al., 2014). When we are in rest and digest mode, our immune system is better able to fight infection and inflammation, including brain inflammation, which is essential to obtaining optimal mental health.

A fun fact is that spending time in nature exposes you to *phytoncides* (pronounced fy-ton-sides). Phytoncides are volatile organic compounds emitted by plants, particularly trees. These compounds are part of the plant's natural defense system against insects, fungi, and bacteria. Phytoncides have been found to have beneficial effects on human health, particularly when people are exposed to them in natural environments such as forests or green spaces. Research suggests that inhaling phytoncides can lower stress hormones like cortisol, reduce blood pressure, and enhance immune function. These effects contribute to the overall health benefits associated with spending time in natural settings, known as "forest bathing" or "shinrin-yoku" in Japanese culture (Li, 2022).

Another important element of being outdoors is the ability to experience awe, inspiration, and mindfulness. In their work on mindfulness and nature, Djernis et al. (2019) propose that practicing mindfulness in natural environments amplifies the benefits of both mindfulness and nature exposure, fostering a deeper connection with the environment and promoting relaxation and stress relief. Mindfulness in nature heightens attentional focus and present-moment awareness, which can relieve mental fatigue and enhance mood. Even looking at pictures of nature decreases activity in the amygdala (the almond-shaped emotional processing center of the brain) and has a calming effect (Yamashita et al., 2021).

MINDFULNESS AND MEDITATION FOR MENTAL HEALTH

All religious traditions have some form of meditation, whether it is called prayer, contemplation, or more structured meditation practice. One does not need to practice or follow a specific religious philosophy to benefit from this practice. A key element of meditation is mindfulness to help focus and calm the mind. As mentioned in Chapter 10, mindfulness practices originate in Buddhist traditions but have been adapted into secular contexts, such as Mindfulness-Based Stress Reduction (MBSR), Mindfulness-Based Cognitive Therapy (MBCT), and Acceptance and Commitment Therapy (ACT), which are widely used in psychology and healthcare settings to promote wellbeing, reduce stress, and enhance emotional resilience.

Mindfulness refers to a mental state characterized by focused attention on the present moment, without judgment or attachment to thoughts, emotions, or sensations that arise. In other words, it involves being here and now, aware of one's thoughts, feelings, bodily sensations, and the surrounding environment in a non-reactive manner. A mindfulness practice entails regularly setting aside time to develop and cultivate these skills. It has been shown to have numerous benefits for stress reduction and mental health when practiced regularly (Kabat-Zinn, 1994). One simple (but not easy) thing that promotes mindfulness is to limit multitasking.

Of Note . . . DOWNSIDES OF MULTITASKING

Multitasking is defined as engaging in more than one task at the same time. For example, being on the phone while writing this sentence. This general definition is a bit of a misnomer since our brain is not able to perform multiple tasks at once. A better description is *task switching*. Doing more than one thing at a time requires the mind to switch focus and attention from one task to another, creating a gap in how we receive and code information. Reducing multitasking (known as monotasking) gets easier (but not easy) when we practice mindfulness.

We understand the struggle! It is real! It is like our brain is a computer with too many tabs open: news, fashion, politics, and cuddly creatures. After a while, nothing new will load and we are staring at a spinning wheel. This metaphor for our multitasking brains serves as a practical reminder. When we are working on our computer, it is helpful to close some of the tabs to improve performance. The same is true for our brain browser. How many times have we been listening to music while working on a research paper, answering email, and chatting on Slack? We have all done it! Some of us may be doing some variation of multitasking right now. The point is to practice self-compassion, self-correct, and limit our distractions. That is the hack! Work to limit distractions in a conscious and intentional manner, attempting to clearly focus on one task at a time.

Cultivating monotasking feels more important now than ever, especially with the pull that technology has on our ability to focus on tasks. Daily we spend over 3 hours on our smartphones and check them about 60 times a day (Harmony Healthcare IT, 2024). With notifications being front and center in our lives, even those of us who use the embedded time management apps to limit our phone use (e.g., the Do Not Disturb function), it is hard to resist that intermittent reinforcement that we get from checking our phones constantly. Have you ever silenced your notifications only to find that you have the urge to check your phone more often just in case you missed something?

If you are a student, it is tempting to multitask during class, especially when lectures or teachers are not as engaging. Online classes and taking notes on a laptop can make it particularly hard to avoid distractions, which can be detrimental to your learning outcomes. A naturalistic study looking at multitasking in a classroom setting found that, not surprisingly, engaging in the use of a laptop during class led to multitasking such as shopping and reading emails, and negatively impacted outcomes on learning and test scores (Jamet et al., 2020).

So how can we combat these modern-day challenges of multitasking, especially when we always have an advanced computer (smart phone) in our hands ready to distract us? Here are some tips for cultivating monotasking habits. When you are performing a task, engage fully in the task, paying attention to each movement, sensation, and detail. You might want to start with simpler tasks like folding laundry or walking to class. As your mind wanders, gently bring it back to the task at hand without self-criticism. Just notice. Remember to keep breathing throughout the task. Resist the urge to rush or mentally jump ahead to the next task. Allow yourself to fully complete one task before moving on. Notice how it feels to be fully present in the moment and in the activity. Carry this mindfulness practice into your daily routines. Use mindfulness techniques to bring awareness to your tendencies to multitask and gently redirect your focus when needed.

RESEARCH EVIDENCE FOR THE BENEFITS OF MINDFULNESS AND MEDITATION

There is significant research that supports the benefits of mindfulness and meditation, with different theories about why it works and the underlying mechanisms for how it impacts mental health. In a review by Hölzel and colleagues (2011) of neuroscience and psychological research, several mechanisms of action were identified. Meditation promotes neuroplasticity, which improves cognitive functions such as attention, memory, and emotion regulation. The focused attention involved with mindfulness improves our ability to sustain attention and more effectively switch between tasks. Functional MRI studies show that experienced meditators have positive changes in brain regions associated with attention, so there appear to be structural brain differences from long-term meditation practices.

Mindfulness influences emotion regulation by promoting non-judgmental awareness of emotional experiences, which leads to decreased reactivity to negative emotions and increased resilience to stressors. We can be aware of uncomfortable emotions without feeling we must immediately act upon them to protect ourselves. Mindfulness cultivates awareness of bodily sensations which facilitates more sensitively responding to physical and emotional states. If we are aware of what our body needs and responds in a timely manner, we are better able to take care of ourselves before it accelerates into a crisis.

Mindfulness meditation improves cognitive abilities such as enhanced attention, increased working memory (where we temporarily hold a limited amount of information), and cognitive flexibility. These changes are recognized as participants being less distracted, more effective at holding and manipulating information, and better able to adapt and shift their approach when facing demanding situations which contribute to more effective problem-solving (Zeidan et al., 2010).

DENTAL HEALTH

We know that good dental hygiene makes for nice looking teeth that effectively chew our food. What is less known is the impact of healthy teeth and gums on mental health. In Chapter 5, we discussed the importance of good mastication (chewing) to break down food into small particles that can be easily digested in the intestines so that we can absorb the nutrients. Good mastication requires strong, healthy teeth, and a willingness to slow down and chew our food thoroughly. Here

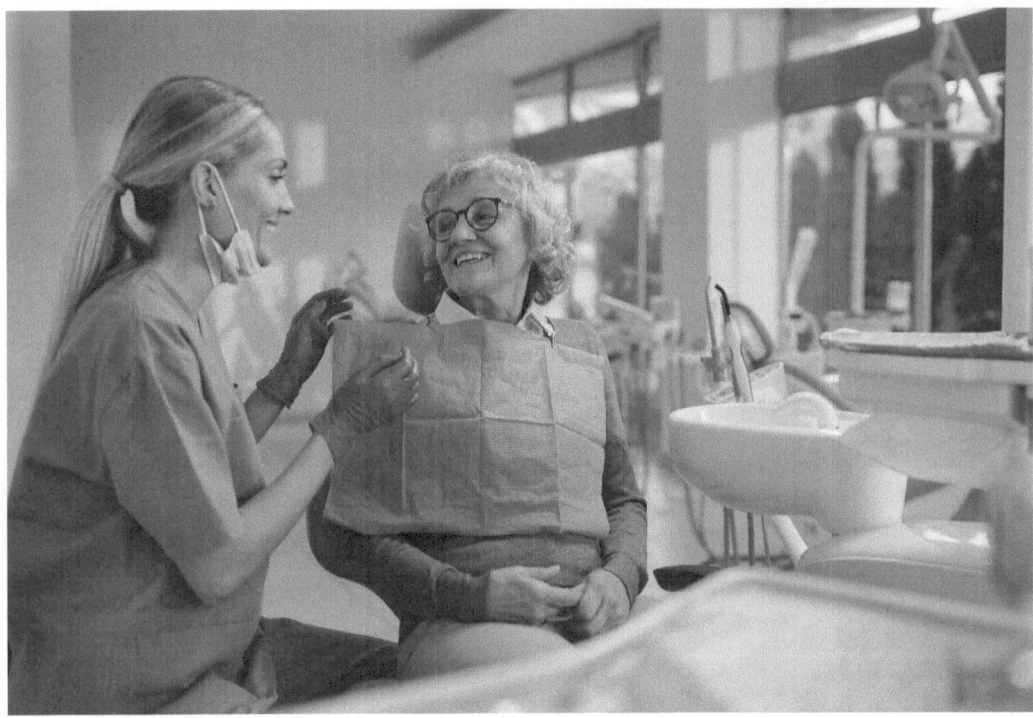

FIGURE 16.2   Regular visits to the dentist support good mental health. Credit: Drazen Zigic (Shutterstock).

again, mindfulness can be useful. Mindful mastication is the healthy habit of slowing down and carefully chewing our food until it is broken down in our mouth to a smooth paste. This can take some getting used to, since many of us eat very quickly and chew only enough to get the food down our throat. At first, the sensation of keeping the food in your mouth while you chew can be uncomfortable and feel strange, but eventually it becomes normal for most people.

In Chapter 7, we discussed the brain inflammation model of depression and the fact that systemic inflammation caused by an infection or injury in one part of the body can increase inflammation in the brain. Inflammation of our gums and mouth is a common contributor to systemic inflammation. It is all interconnected. There is also a bidirectional influence between dental hygiene and mental illness. For example, depression increases the risk of poor dental hygiene (i.e., it is hard to find the strength to brush and floss your teeth when you are feeling depressed). At the same time, poor dental hygiene can lead to inflammation in the gums and mouth, which can then lead to more depression. The good news is the connection can go the other way as well. Epidemiological studies have demonstrated a positive correlation between changes in mouth health (such as clearing up periodontitis with improved dental hygiene and care) and decreased symptoms for mood and trauma-related disorders, especially depression (Martínez et al., 2022). Building new habits to improve how we care for our teeth can be one more tool to improve mental health.

This one behavior change has the potential to impact many people. Gum disease such as periodontitis, which is a chronic oral bacterial infection, affects nearly 40% of adults in the U.S. and is the most prevalent inflammatory disease in adults. A 10-year longitudinal study of periodontitis as a risk factor for depression showed a higher incidence of subsequent depression among patients with periodontitis regardless of age and sex. While this study does not clearly demonstrate causality, it does suggest that periodontitis may be an independent risk factor for subsequent depression (Hsu et al., 2015).

Hashioka et al. (2019) examined the evidence for a causal link between periodontitis and psychiatric disorders, including Alzheimer's, major depression, Parkinson's disease, and schizophrenia.

They identified three possible mechanisms of action for the relationship between gum disease and psychiatric conditions: (1) inflammation that impacts neural connections and cellular activity; (2) periodontal bacteria molecules that travel up and directly invade the brain either through the bloodstream or via cranial nerves; and (3) the periodontal bacteria activate the brain immune cells (microglia) that act as the brain's first line of defense against damage and pathogens in the central nervous system. All of this to say that there is some evidence that periodontitis negatively affects the brain in ways that increase the risk of mental illness.

Bottom line, taking care of our teeth and gums is part of self-care. Not only brushing and flossing as recommended by dentists, but also getting regular check-ups. Dental hygiene is often one of the first things to do when we feel overwhelmed or fatigued, which can make seeing the dentist both physically uncomfortable and emotionally embarrassing. Professional dental care can be expensive, and insurance may or may not be accessible or offer relevant coverage, which makes good daily dental hygiene even more important. It is important to find a dentist who is kind and compassionate, where you can ask questions and not feel guilty for imperfect dental hygiene. Take the time to interview a dentist and understand their philosophy and style of practicing dentistry to establish a relationship before you find yourself sitting with their fingers in your mouth. Luckily, many college and university campuses recognize the importance of a healthy mouth and offer low-cost dental care on campus for their students.

SLEEP

Our love–hate relationship with sleep is fascinating, to say the least. On the one hand, we depend on sleep for survival. On the other hand, we often struggle to let go, relax, and turn our brains off enough to rest. Our sympathetic nervous system remains overactive, and we are unable to relax. Technology, chronic stress, lack of exercise, caffeine, alcohol, inflammatory foods, medication, and untreated medical conditions all impact our sleep.

THE IMPORTANCE OF SLEEP

Sleep serves essential functions that we often take for granted. We have evolved to need sleep to help us with memory consolidation, synaptic plasticity (i.e., high functioning brain neurons), brain development, and energy conservation (Diekelmann et al., 2009). When we are rested, we are generally in better spirits and our ability to problem solve improves. When we are tired, we feel it in our bones, in our body and mind. We are easily distracted, make silly mistakes, feel on edge, and often feel grumpy.

Evolutionarily, when we were fighting the infamous sabretooth tiger, those with poor sleep had slower reflexes and did not think as clearly, putting them at higher risk of being eaten. In today's world, while we are not battling sabretooth tigers, we are battling many other things, like amorphous remote work hours, complex relationships, enticing technology, social isolation, a sedentary lifestyle, multitasking, and poor eating habits. So, sleeping well is as important for our survival now as it was millions of years ago, but for different reasons. Today the sabretooth tiger is not the most salient predator; our lifestyle is.

SLEEP AND HEALTH

For someone struggling with sleep, the first step is to rule out medical issues such as sleep apnea. *Sleep apnea* (also known as obstructive sleep apnea) is a sleep-related breathing disorder with repetitive pauses in breathing and periods of shallow breathing that cause decreased oxygen levels and poor sleep quality. Approximately 39 million U.S. adults have sleep apnea (Ling, 2024). Obesity is one of the main components contributing to sleep apnea. In obese people, fat deposits in the upper respiratory tract (e.g., the soft palate of the mouth) narrow the airway and decrease muscle activity, creating periods during sleep when the airway is partially closed or obstructed (Jehan et al., 2017).

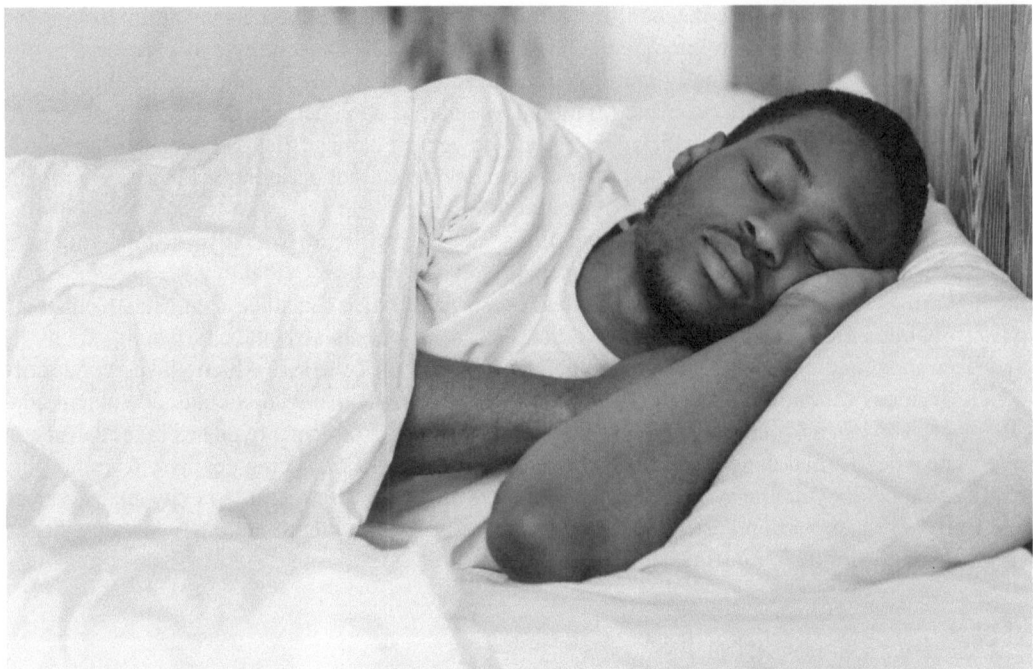

FIGURE 16.3   Consistent quality sleep is essential for health. Credit: Hero Images on Offset (Shutterstock).

Current treatment focuses on using a C-PAP machine that pumps oxygen and has a mask that covers the nose and mouth to deliver continuous oxygen to your lungs and brain while you sleep. While a C-PAP machine can provide some immediate relief, it does not address the root cause of weight gain that must be addressed for long-term improvements in sleep. Here we see another mechanism that links nutrition to mental health through its impact on the quality of our sleep.

As mentioned in Chapter 9, sleep deprivation is a risk factor for problems with mood, cognition, gut health, obesity, and chronic disease. There is a large body of evidence that connects sleep deprivation and mental illness. Disturbances in sleep patterns contribute to the onset and maintenance of mood disorders such as depression and bipolar disorder, with evidence of mechanisms such as disruptions in neurobiological processes and hormone regulation (Harvey, 2011).

SLEEP HYGIENE

Our ability and willingness to prioritize sleep is essential. Sleep hygiene is the set of skills and tools we use to maximize our sleeping potential. Predictable routines during the day that indicate to our body when it is time to wake, eat, move, work, play, and rest set the tone for having consistent high-quality sleep at night (de Biase et al., 2014). Given the high rates of sleep deprivation, most individuals can benefit from making the following improvements to their sleep hygiene:

Consistent Sleep Schedule: Go to bed and wake up at the same time every day, even on weekends. This helps regulate your body's internal clock. If you are well rested, a late night on the weekend is not a problem. However, if you have been struggling with feeling fatigued or sad, then protecting your sleep schedule becomes of primary importance.

Relaxing Bedtime Routine: Establish a calming routine before bed, such as reading a book, taking a warm bath, or practicing relaxation exercises. Avoid stimulating activities like using electronic devices or arguing with someone before bedtime.

Optimized Sleep Environment: Make sure your bedroom is conducive to sleep by keeping it cool, dark, and quiet. Use blackout curtains, earplugs, or a white noise machine if necessary. If you typically sleep with your pets, find another location for them to sleep. Their restlessness and movement can wake you from deep sleep, even if they are quiet.

Limited Exposure to Screens: Avoid screens (phones, tablets, computers, TVs) at least 30 minutes before bedtime. The blue light emitted by screens can interfere with your sleep–wake cycle. Unless you live in a studio apartment or dorm room, a good place to start is to remove all screens from your bedroom, including your cell phone. It can charge in another room while you sleep. If you are using your phone as your alarm clock, but a physical alarm clock, preferably one that doesn't tick loudly.

Eat and Drink Mindfully: Avoid large meals, caffeine, sugar, and alcohol close to bedtime. These can disrupt sleep or make it harder to fall asleep. For chronic insomnia, it may be important to avoid caffeine for three weeks to see if it is affecting your sleep in any way. Some people are surprised to find they start sleeping better when they remove all caffeine from their diet.

Regular Exercise: Engage in daily physical activity but avoid vigorous exercise close to bedtime. Exercise during the day promotes better sleep at night.

Stress Reduction: Practice relaxation techniques such as deep breathing, meditation, or yoga to help reduce stress during the day and promote relaxation before bed. Writing in a journal at bedtime can help release worries and fears so that your brain can settle down and let you sleep.

Limit Naps: If you need to nap, keep it short (20–30 minutes) and earlier in the day to avoid interfering with nighttime sleep.

Manage Early Awakenings: If you wake up in the middle of the night and it is not time to get up, do NOT toss and turn. Get up and walk around, ideally in a pattern (e.g., around the coffee table) for 10 to 15 minutes until your body feels tired. Then go back to bed. It is tempting to lie there and wait to go back to sleep. That rarely works because it can make you feel frustrated and agitated. Try this instead. It feels counterintuitive, but it works.

Seek Help if Needed: If you consistently have trouble sleeping despite practicing good sleep hygiene, consult with a healthcare professional. They can help identify underlying issues and recommend appropriate treatment.

FOOD FOR THOUGHT: BUILDING HEALTHY HABITS

We hear about good habits and bad habits all the time, but we often feel helpless to make any lasting changes to our lifestyle. In this section, we explore some ideas about how to develop and maintain healthy habits. We hope this inspires you to learn more about this topic.

Habits are behaviors that are so ingrained in our mind and body that they happen automatically. We do not have to make a conscious effort to engage in them. This can include simple things like how we get dressed. Do you put on the right sock first and then the left one? Do you put on both socks first then the shoes, or one sock and shoe at a time? Chances are that up until now, you have never thought about this because it is a habit, an automatic behavior. It is also relatively low stakes. How you wear your socks probably does not matter much in your day-to-day life. Whether you store them in the dedicated drawer or leave them on the floor is probably a lot more relevant, especially if you live with others.

When we look at how one develops a habit, a good place to start is Pavlov. Most students are familiar with Pavlov's dog conditioning experiments that form the early basis of classical conditioning theory. Pavlov paired the promise of food with a bell so that at some point when the bell rang the dogs salivated anticipating food even in the absence of any visible signs of food. In a way, the foundation of new habit formation, whether conscious or not, is tied to conditioning if we pair a reward with a desired outcome. For example, increasing consumption of fruits and vegetables can be tied to the reward of improved energy and mood.

When we engage in behaviors that are reinforced by pleasing us, we have activated our reward pathways which include the release of dopamine. Evolutionarily, our mind and body opt for the path of least resistance which will provide the most reward with the least amount of effort. When we try to make changes, we often start by using our willpower to overcome the natural draw toward pleasurable activities, but as discussed in Chapter 15, willpower is a very limited source of energy and is generally not sufficient to make long-term changes. Therefore, it can be helpful to understand how habits are formed and how long they take to develop.

Landmark research by Lally et al. (2010) suggested that it can take from 1 to 8 months to create a new habit. On average, it takes about two months of consistent repetition to build a new habit. The key components are consistency, repetition, and automacy (the ability to do something without thinking about it).

One essential ingredient to make habits stick is to make the tasks less aversive. Typically, new habits are challenging to create and healthy habits even more so because at first, they do not activate our dopamine reward system. Pairing a new habit with an established habit can ease transition and make the new habit more pleasurable more quickly. For example, if your goal is to practice meditation, you could add a ten-minute meditation when you first arrive home from work so that it becomes part of your winddown behavior, which already feels good.

Setting clear goals is an important part of changing habits. Willpower or self-control in the absence of a clear motivating goal will not yield the desired results (Van der Weiden et al., 2020). Elements that increase our ability to form good habits are frequently and consistently performing some aspect of the desired behavior, increasing the inherently rewarding nature of the behavior, and practicing the new behavior in a comfortable environment. We need to feel safe to experiment and maintain a fun and celebratory attitude about any behaviors that move us in the right direction. Be cautious about using food as a reward, as it can sometimes overshadow the natural reward of completing the task, so we end up just pushing through and getting it over with in our eagerness to get to the food, especially if it is fun food (Avena, 2023).

SMART goals are a systematic style of goal setting that has been found to lead to more consistent outcomes. Coined by George Doran in 1981, SMART is an acronym that stands for Specific, Measurable, Attainable/Achievable, Realistic, and Timed/Time bound (Doran, 1981). The use of SMART goals in clinical settings can be helpful when the client can check in with their therapist or nutritionist to explore different options and try things out (Bailey, 2019). While SMART goals are very popular in the coaching and fitness communities, there is limited research on the use and effectiveness of this framework (Swann et al., 2023). However, anecdotally, many people have found this style of goal attainment to be beneficial.

It is important to start with small, easily attainable goals and then build on them. This can be a challenge if our goals are lofty, poorly defined, or dare we say, not very SMART. Creating SMART goals necessitates breaking down complex goals into small steps. For example, if your goal is to limit multitasking, you want to start small. Perhaps begin by identifying one task that you want to engage in mindfully. Or you may determine that the main focus of your multitasking is your phone. In that case, consider limiting how many times you can check your phone. You read that correctly! Notice how reading that last sentence makes you feel right here and now. Are you feeling anxious? Are you reaching for your phone? Did you just decide to ignore this habit change as a possibility in your life? Bear with us.

A SMART goal may be to check the phone less than 60 times a day. That may feel more attainable and less stressful than a more difficult goal like only checking your phone five times a day. Ask yourself: how many times is a realistic (and truly necessary) number of times for me to check my phone? Consider if your phone use is situational, meaning there are times when you need to check your phone more frequently and other situations when you can put it away. Notice if your phone is a way to avoid something in your life (e.g., social interactions, procrastinating working on an important task), in which case part of the plan needs to include how you will manage the worry that is causing your avoidance behavior. Perhaps there are times when it would be helpful to set your phone in the other room to help you focus on the task at hand (e.g., working on homework, when on a date, or going to sleep).

Make a plan by writing down the first steps you want to try using the SMART goal template. Add dates and specific details about what you hope to accomplish. For example, your SMART goal may be to limit the number of times you check your phone to 50 times per day (Specific), using an app to track your behavior (Measurable), which is only a little lower than your average use (Attainable). You will maintain this restricted phone checking behavior for three days to see how it feels, and then decide if you want to maintain or discontinue this behavior change (Realistic and Time Bound). As you accomplish the first set of goals, you will need to create additional SMART goals by asking yourself similar poignant questions for how to add the next steps.

Writing down SMART goals provides valuable structure and brings a greater sense of accountability. It is an important element to increase the likelihood of goal attainment (Locke & Latham, 2019). If you have not taken the time to think about it and document your goals, they may not have become important enough to you to warrant change. Writing down goals and tracking your behavior help keep you accountable so you can push through the discomfort of new behaviors to build new habits and lasting change.

REFERENCES

Anguera, J. A., Volponi, J. J., Simon, A. J., Gallen, C. L., Rolle, C. E., Anguera-Singla, R., Pitsch, E. A., Thompson, C. J., & Gazzaley, A. (2022). Integrated cognitive and physical fitness training enhances attention abilities in older adults. *NPJ Aging, 8*(1), 12.

Avena, N. M. (2023). *Sugarless: A 7-step plan to uncover hidden sugars, curb your cravings, and conquer your addiction.* Union Square & Co.

Bailey, R. R. (2019). Goal setting and action planning for health behavior change. *American Journal of Lifestyle Medicine, 13*(6), 615–618.

Barton, J., & Pretty, J. (2010). What is the best dose of nature and green exercise for improving mental health? A multi-study analysis. *Environmental Science & Technology, 44*(10), 3947–3955.

Basso, J. C., & Suzuki, W. A. (2017). The effects of acute exercise on mood, cognition, neurophysiology, and neurochemical pathways: A review. *Brain Plasticity, 2*(2), 127–152.

Carek, P. J., Laibstain, S. E., & Carek, S. M. (2011). Exercise for the treatment of depression and anxiety. *The International Journal of Psychiatry in Medicine, 41*(1), 15–28. https://doi.org/10.2190/PM.41.1.c

Chang, Y. K., Labban, J. D., Gapin, J. I., & Etnier, J. L. (2012). The effects of acute exercise on cognitive performance: A meta-analysis. *Brain Research, 1453,* 87–101.

de Biase, S., Milioli, G., Grassi, A., Lorenzut, S., Parrino, L., & Gigli, G. L. (2014). Sleep hygiene. In S. Garbarino, L. Nobili, & G. Costa (Eds.), *Sleepiness and human impact assessment* (pp. 289–295). Springer Milan. https://doi.org/10.1007/978-88-470-5388-5_27

Diekelmann, S., Wilhelm, I., & Born, J. (2009). The whats and whens of sleep-dependent memory consolidation. *Sleep Medicine Reviews, 13*(5), 309–321. https://doi.org/10.1016/j.smrv.2008.08.002

Djernis, D., Lerstrup, I., Poulsen, D., Stigsdotter, U., Dahlgaard, J., & O'Toole, M. (2019). A systematic review and meta-analysis of nature-based mindfulness: Effects of moving mindfulness training into an outdoor natural setting. *International Journal of Environmental Research and Public Health, 16*(17), 3202. https://www.mdpi.com/1660-4601/16/17/3202

Doran, G. T. (1981). There's a SMART way to write managements' goals and objectives. *Management Review, 70*(11).

Haluza, D., Schönbauer, R., & Cervinka, R. (2014). Green perspectives for public health: A narrative review on the physiological effects of experiencing outdoor nature. *International Journal of Environmental Research and Public Health, 11*(5), 5445–5461.

Harmony Healthcare IT. (2024). *Black Mirror or Black Hole? American Phone Screen Time Statistics.* https://www.harmonyhit.com/phone-screen-time-statistics/?clreqid=a5b99b78-5919-4ddd-a2d7-5cb3c4e66e6d&kbid=58587

Harvey, A. G. (2011). Sleep and circadian functioning: Critical mechanisms in the mood disorders? *Annual Review of Clinical Psychology*, 7(1), 297–319.

Hashioka, S., Inoue, K., Miyaoka, T., Hayashida, M., Wake, R., Oh-Nishi, A., & Inagaki, M. (2019). The possible causal link of periodontitis to neuropsychiatric disorders: More than psychosocial mechanisms. *International Journal of Molecular Sciences*, 20(15), 3723.

Hölzel, B. K., Lazar, S. W., Gard, T., Schuman-Olivier, Z., Vago, D. R., & Ott, U. (2011). How does mindfulness meditation work? Proposing mechanisms of action from a conceptual and neural perspective. *Perspectives on Psychological Science*, 6(6), 537–559.

Hsu, C.-C., Hsu, Y.-C., Chen, H.-J., Lin, C.-C., Chang, K.-H., Lee, C.-Y., Chong, L.-W., & Kao, C.-H. (2015). Association of periodontitis and subsequent depression: A nationwide population-based study. *Medicine*, 94(51), e2347.

Jamet, E., Gonthier, C., Cojean, S., Colliot, T., & Erhel, S. (2020). Does multitasking in the classroom affect learning outcomes? A naturalistic study. *Computers in Human Behavior*, 106, 106264.

Jehan, S., Zizi, F., Pandi-Perumal, S. R., Wall, S., Auguste, E.,000 Myers, A. K., Jean-Louis, G., & McFarlane, S. I. (2017). Obstructive sleep apnea and obesity: Implications for public health. *Sleep Medicine and Disorders*, 1(4).

Kabat-Zinn, J. (1994). *Mindfulness meditation for everyday life*. New York: Hyperion.

Lally, P., Van Jaarsveld, C. H., Potts, H. W., & Wardle, J. (2010). How are habits formed: Modelling habit formation in the real world. *European Journal of Social Psychology*, 40(6), 998–1009.

Li, Q. (2022). Effects of forest environment (Shinrin-yoku/Forest bathing) on health promotion and disease prevention -the establishment of "Forest medicine." *Environmental Health and Preventive Medicine*, 27, 43. https://doi.org/10.1265/ehpm.22-00160

Ling, V. (2024). *Sleep apnea statistics and facts you should know*. National Council on Aging (NCOA). https://www.ncoa.org/adviser/sleep/sleep-apnea-statistics/

Locke, E. A., & Latham, G. P. (2019). The development of goal setting theory: A half century retrospective. *Motivation Science*, 5(2), 93.

Martínez, M., Postolache, T. T., García-Bueno, B., Leza, J. C., Figuero, E., Lowry, C. A., & Malan-Müller, S. (2022). The role of the oral microbiota related to periodontal diseases in anxiety, mood and trauma-and stress-related disorders. *Frontiers in Psychiatry*, 12, 814177.

Noetel, M., Sanders, T., Gallardo-Gómez, D., Taylor, P., del Pozo Cruz, B., van den Hoek, D., Smith, J. J., Mahoney, J., Spathis, J., Moresi, M., Pagano, R., Pagano, L., Vasconcellos, R., Arnott, H., Varley, B., Parker, P., Biddle, S., & Lonsdale, C. (2024). Effect of exercise for depression: Systematic review and network meta-analysis of randomised controlled trials. *BMJ*, 384, e075847. https://doi.org/10.1136/bmj-2023-075847

Predovan, D., Julien, A., Esmail, A., & Bherer, L. (2019). Effects of dancing on cognition in healthy older adults: A systematic review. *Journal of Cognitive Enhancement*, 3, 161–167.

Raichlen, D. A., Aslan, D. H., Sayre, M. K., Bharadwaj, P. K., Ally, M., Maltagliati, S., Lai, M. H., Wilcox, R. R., Klimentidis, Y. C., & Alexander, G. E. (2023). Sedentary behavior and incident dementia among older adults. *JAMA*, 330(10), 934–940.

Rebar, A. L., Stanton, R., Geard, D., Short, C., Duncan, M. J., & Vandelanotte, C. (2015). A meta-meta-analysis of the effect of physical activity on depression and anxiety in non-clinical adult populations. *Health Psychology Review*, 9(3), 366–378.

Swann, C., Jackman, P. C., Lawrence, A., Hawkins, R. M., Goddard, S. G., Williamson, O., Schweickle, M. J., Vella, S. A., Rosenbaum, S., & Ekkekakis, P. (2023). The (over) use of SMART goals for physical activity promotion: A narrative review and critique. *Health Psychology Review*, 17(2), 211–226. https://doi.org/10.1080/17437199.2021.2023608

Van der Weiden, A., Benjamins, J., Gillebaart, M., Ybema, J. F., & De Ridder, D. (2020). How to form good habits? A longitudinal field study on the role of self-control in habit formation. *Frontiers in Psychology*, 11, 494700.

Yamashita, R., Chen, C., Matsubara, T., Hagiwara, K., Inamura, M., Aga, K., Hirotsu, M., Seki, T., Takao, A., & Nakagawa, E. (2021). The mood-improving effect of viewing images of nature and its neural substrate. *International Journal of Environmental Research and Public Health*, 18(10), 5500.

Zeidan, F., Johnson, S. K., Diamond, B. J., David, Z., & Goolkasian, P. (2010). Mindfulness meditation improves cognition: Evidence of brief mental training. *Consciousness and Cognition*, 19(2), 597–605.

Index

Note: Locators in *italics* represent figures and **bold** indicate tables in the text.